# THROUGH THE LOOKING GLASSES

## THE SPECTACULAR LIFE OF SPECTACLES

# TRAVIS ELBOROUGH

Little, Brown

LITTLE, BROWN

First published in Great Britain in 2021 by Little, Brown

1 3 5 7 9 10 8 6 4 2

A CIP catalogue record for this book
is available from the British Library.

Hardback ISBN 978-1-4087-1284-9

Typeset in by M Rules
Printed and bound in Great Britain by
Clays Ltd, Elcograf S.p.A.

Papers used by Little, Brown are from well-managed forests
and other responsible sources.

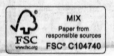

Little, Brown
An imprint of
Little, Brown Book Group
Carmelite House
50 Victoria Embankment
London EC4Y 0DZ

An Hachette UK Company
www.hachette.co.uk

www.littlebrown.co.uk

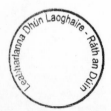

*To my parents,*
*who I didn't see much of in 2020*

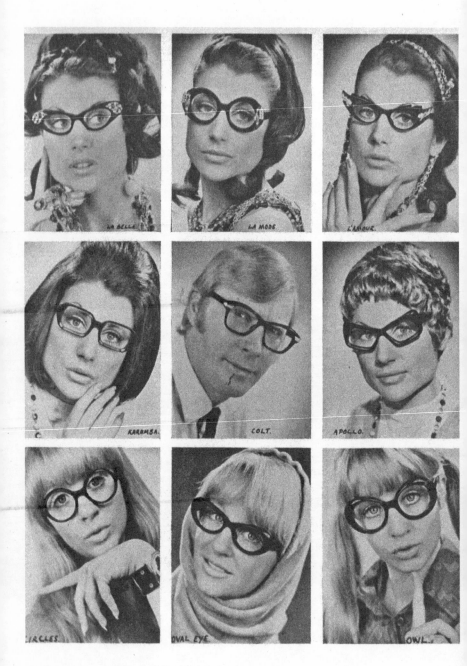

Welby Fine Frames Ltd of Tunbridge Wells, trade advertisement 1970.

# Contents

Everything was made for a purpose; everything is necessary for the fulfilment of that purpose. Observe that noses have been made for spectacles; *therefore* we have spectacles . . .

Dr Pangloss in *Candide*
by VOLTAIRE

# INTRODUCTION

## Making a Spectacle of Myself

It surprises me how little I remember about my first pair of glasses. Their arrival, arguably, changed the entire course of the rest of my life. I've been encumbered with spectacles of one kind or another ever since. Yet I am hard pressed to recall a specific moment when my eyes failed so disastrously that glasses were suddenly deemed necessary. It should, surely, be among the most shattering moments of childhood. Something up there with the death of a much-loved pet, with its intimations of human mortality. Or the flunking of an exam or a rejection by the school football team in terms of being publicly branded mentally or physically deficient.

To a child back then, glasses appeared so much more objects of the grown-up world; certain teachers, parents, neighbours and newsreaders wore spectacles, just as they also drove cars, smoked and drank. Among the kids at school there were perhaps only one or two others in my year who had to wear them. And while adolescents often yearn to obtain the accoutrements of adulthood early (fags, booze and motors here we come), glasses, as pieces of medical kit akin to optical prosthetic limbs – Zimmer frames for unsteady eyes, if you will – represented an alarming leap towards premature senility rather than any easing into maturity.

At home I think there was a general erring on the side of sitting nearer the television screen (rather than crouching behind the sofa) for Doctor Who on Saturday evenings, lest I miss any of

Tom Baker's antics outsmarting malevolent aliens in the disused quarries and ventilation shafts he was fated to frequent each week. In the back garden and at the local park, cricket and tennis balls, never especially subservient to my will at the best of times, evaded attempts to catch or trap them. Objects of historic or natural interest, pointed out by my pedagogically inclined parents on summer holidays in the West Country, often looked rather misty from wherever I was standing – regardless of the weather. There were the predictable issues with road signs and bus route numbers. And so it went on until, finally and miraculously, I was presented with a pair of spectacles.

This first pair – bog-standard, square-framed NHS numbers in sturdy brown plastic issued with a snap-shut cloth-covered tin case – arrived, if I remember correctly (and I am not sure I do), in the aftermath of some school medical check-up.*

If the arrival of glasses on my own nose is a matter of rather hazy personal history, the story of their invention in the first place, as we shall see, is even more opaque, and the name of their inventor a mystery that is still to be solved.

Life without them, however, would be almost unimaginable for me, as is probably the case for the 4 billion adults in the world whom the Vision Council of America calculated in April 2020 wear glasses today. An oculist dealing in patched-up second-hand glasses is, noticeably, one of the traders to endure amid the wreckage of society in Doris Lessing's apocalyptic novel *The Memoirs of a Survivor*. In similar territory, I am haunted, in particular, by 'Time Enough at Last', an episode of *The Twilight Zone* based on a Lynn Venable story in which Burgess Meredith (the future Penguin to Adam West's Batman) plays Henry Bemis, a myopic, hen-pecked bank clerk who wants nothing more than the time to read. He is granted his wish when an H-bomb explosion leaves him as the last man on Earth,

---

* Peter Capaldi, upon signing up to become the twelfth incarnation of the Time Lord, put the character in the same socio-historical bracket as these glasses, saying, 'I don't remember *Doctor Who* not being part of my life, and it became a part of growing up, along with the Beatles, National Health spectacles and fog. And it runs deep. It's in my DNA.'

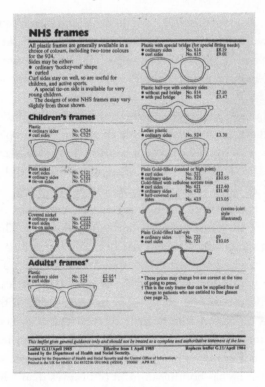

NHS glasses range, NHS leaflet April 1985.

only for Bemis's pebble-lensed glasses to fall off his face and smash on the steps of the public library. Tears roll down his face as he sits peering at a blurry page and surrounded by piles of books he will now never be able to read.

Pedants have maintained that the lenses in the glasses Meredith wears look suspiciously more like those for treating long-sightedness than short-sightedness. Also, even a severe myope could probably just about be able to make out text close-up; their greater difficulty would be with anything slightly further afield. Such cavils, however, do nothing to reduce the chill the tale induces by reminding all spectacle wearers of their dependency. Like the blinded Samson in Gaza, without our specs many of us would be close to eyeless. And as with Bemis in that episode, a good deal of our time is spent simply groping around for glasses, briefly set down and then misplaced. My and my wife's bedroom nightstand, on which we carefully place our two pairs of black horn-rimmed frames before switching out the light, looks overnight like the opening title sequence to *The Two Ronnies*.

School career advisers pointed out that the police did not accept those without 20/20 vision. A rule that seemed to imply that the enforcement of the law could not be trusted to anyone lacking perfect eyesight. That glasses are somehow unnatural, dishonest and a form of cheating, allowing their wearers to see what otherwise might be hidden from them, has been, as it happens, a constant theme since they first emerged in the Middle Ages. The medical profession's antipathy to them has been almost as long-standing. Georg Bartisch, described as the 'founder of modern ophthalmology' and who published *Ophthalmodouleia*, a formative study of the eye and eye disease, in Dresden in 1583, is one of the earliest physicians on record who heartily disapproved of spectacles. 'It is much better,' Bartisch wrote, 'and more useful that one leaves spectacles alone. For naturally a person sees and recognises something better when he has nothing in front of his eyes than when he has something there. It is much better that one should preserve his two eyes than he should have four.' Two hundred and fifty years later, his compatriot Johann Wolfgang von Goethe would rail against bespectacled interlocutors, writing: 'For what do I gain from a man into whose eyes I cannot look when he is speaking, and the mirror whose soul is veiled to me by a pair of glasses which dazzle me.'

That glasses alter a person's appearance, giving their wearers a different look, in all senses of the word, has often been another black mark against them. Glasses were denounced as 'disagreeable adjuncts' by the essayist L. Higgins in 1885 and said to be 'very disfiguring to women and girls' by the optometrist Dr Norburne B. Jenkins in 1900. As recently as 2010, a survey of 3000 women in Britain by the Sight Care Group of independent opticians claimed that half of those who wore specs felt uglier with them on, two-thirds left them off on nights out and 50 per cent wouldn't wear them on a date.

Italo Calvino's story *The Adventure of a Near-Sighted Man* relates the experiences of a myope whose whole world has been opened up by his spectacles, but who returns after some years' absence to the provincial city of his birth and finds that while he can finally see former classmates and old billiard-playing companions, no one recognises him. The glasses, he accepts, 'were a kind of mask' – and this concept of spectacles as a disguise is most famously one of the distinctions between the truth- and justice-seeking visiting alien from Krypton Kal-El, aka Superman, and his milquetoast human alter ego the newspaper reporter Clark Kent.

Superman was dreamt up in Cleveland, Ohio in the 1930s by the American writer Jerry Siegel and the Canadian-born illustrator Joe Shuster. Both men, who met at high school, were children of Eastern European Jewish immigrants and bespectacled. Yet for most glasses wearers, the character of Kent has been more of a thorny issue. He may allow Superman to live covertly among humankind and is obviously a nice guy, but he is also clumsy and short-sighted, incapable of flight, and not the one doing the duffing up of wrong-doers and the general superhero stuff. In short, he is all too human, rather than an ubermensch, and Kal-El is always more super without his glasses on.

Kent was presented as brainy, good with words – a reporter on the *Daily Planet* no less (a clever move by Shuster and Siegel, since newspaper syndication was vital to the strip's success, and what editor could resist a superhero who daylights as a journalist?). That spectacles are the preserve of the learned and clerkly stretches right back to their earliest invention and their adoption by monastic scholars with manuscripts to illuminate and biblical commentaries to copy out. One of the oldest figurative representations of a person in spectacles in Britain is a sculpture of a nun (or possibly a lay brother: the carving rather skimps on gender indicators) on a corbel in the eaves of the church of St Martin in Salisbury, Wiltshire, dating from the 1430s, though it may be up to a century older than that.

As will become clear too, in the centuries since then optical aids of various shapes and sizes have enjoyed their moments of fashionability. In more recent decades, and conveniently coinciding with the onset of my own adolescence, there were cerebral-seeming pop stars such as David Sylvian, Lloyd Cole and Morrissey who wore their glasses with pride. And so we couldn't in any way confuse them with Nik Kershaw or Kenny Loggins. The journey of the former Smiths front man from the gladioli-scattering and hearing-aid-sporting warbler of 'This Charming Man' to the Stephen Yaxley-Lennon-supporting wearer of Britain First pin badges has been one of the most depressing to witness. The devotion Morrissey once received from the bookish, the awkward and the ostracised – some of the very people most likely to be bullied by racist thugs – seems almost impossible to comprehend now. In hindsight, the signs were there. But in the 1980s, fealty to the singer and his group was expressed by both the adoption of vegetarianism and certain sartorial signifiers – fifties quiffs, loose-fitting jeans, cardigans and spectacles.

Morrissey had been 'forced', in his words, to wear glasses at thirteen, though, as he once confessed, he really needed them 'much sooner'. Glasses, in his opinion, 'had this awful thing attached to them that if you wore them you were a horrible green monster and you'd be shot in the street'. His decision to appear on stage in spectacles, he would claim, was merely perfunctory, and he did also use contact lenses. Nevertheless they became, like the hearing aid, the wilted blooms and the meat-free diet, part and parcel of his pop persona, and were much imitated by admirers. As he told Gary Leboff of *Melody Maker* in 1987, 'I wore NHS glasses, which I still do, so it wasn't a mantle or a badge. And suddenly I saw all these people who didn't need to wear spectacles doing so in imitation of the Smiths and bumping into an awful lot of walls. Other bands have tours sponsored by Levi's – maybe we should find a large firm of opticians.'

For those of us who needed spectacles not to bump into walls, the upside was that our glasses were rendered far more socially acceptable, almost trendy. Especially when worn in conjunction with the youth culture *uniforme du jour* of my peer group: a long Crombie coat, Doc Martens boots, black jeans and a suitably faded T-shirt of a suitably obscure group lingering in the lower regions of the indie 'alternative' charts.

Since that time glasses have been an essential part of my identity. Again, as much about how I look as how I see (bizarrely, I was once propositioned by a male drunk at a bus stop on Charing Cross Road on the grounds that I looked the spit of Sue Perkins). At the age of forty-seven, and after putting it off for nearly two years, I finally bit the not inconsiderable financial bullet and accepted the fact that I needed varifocal glasses. If the pain of purchasing these particular spectacles was borne mainly in the wallet, my ego was nevertheless correspondingly left bruised. Time has been reasonably kind to me. I still have a full head of mostly brown hair and all my own teeth. But here were my eyes showing their age and, as the optician tactfully explained, mine too. As windows to my soul, they'd always been somewhat faulty. Now, however, they were letting me down, not so much by being weak, but by shattering a much cherished illusion that I was still a youngish man.

In the famous 'Seven Ages of Man' speech in William Shakespeare's *As You Like It*, glasses are synonymous with becoming an old codger, Jaques describing the 'sixth age' as shifting 'Into the lean and slippered pantaloon, / With spectacles on nose and pouch on side'. For me, of course, there has pretty much been a pair of spectacles for each of my ages up to this point. In their infancy, however, spectacles were only lensed to correct the eye conditions of the aged. A couple of hundred years would pass before oculists and spectacle makers finally got round to the idea of catering for youthful myopes. As will also become plain, what may seem like the simplest things, such as side pieces over our ears to keep our glasses firmly in place, were equally tardy arrivals in a story that takes us from the Dark Ages to the Enlightenment, through to industrialisation and beyond to the digital-augmented reality of Google Glass.

Spectacles offer us a frame in which to consider massive shifts in human experience. As aids to the spread of knowledge, they helped underpin the Renaissance and ushered in scientific rationalism.

Their first creators might have been jobbing craft folk, but glasses have graced the eyes of the pious and the heretical, the royal and the revolutionary, dissenters and dictators, artists, authors, inventors, architects, engineers and artisans, and accordingly have transformed both our perceptions of the world around us and its physical form. They are truly devices that have changed the course of human history, for close to a millennia allowing us to see better for longer, and granting the gift of sight to those who otherwise might have languished without it. Without glasses, whole libraries would have been left empty for the absence of books written by their wearers. The computer I am typing this on could possibly never have been designed, the science underpinning its most basic functions never realised. Whole swathes of daily life would be unimaginable without the contributions of those whose eyes have needed optical aids. Even those who have never worn glasses themselves are the beneficiaries of societies forged by the bespectacled since the Middle Ages.

This book attempts to scoop up some of that history while relating how spectacles themselves have developed over the centuries. Among its inspirations was the possibility, detected during a routine sight test, that I might have glaucoma and ultimately be beyond glasses. At the time of writing, and following several examinations at the Homerton and Moorfields, I appear to be in the clear – though they are, as a doctor at the latter hospital drily observed, 'still keeping an eye on me'.

Between its initiation and completion, Covid-19 intervened, a pandemic that if you were to believe the wilder corners of the internet originated in the consumption of a Chinese remedy derived from bats to cure eye problems. That the most famous breaker of lockdown rules in the UK was the former government adviser Dominic Cummings, choosing to test his eyesight by driving, child in tow, to Barnard Castle in County Durham rather than booking an appointment at, say, Specsavers, is another of life's little ironies. Especially as vision loss has become one acknowledged symptom of post-Covid patients.

What follows, though, is an account of the life and times of spectacles, one driven by my own myopic foibles and preoccupations. It is a wearer's guide, if you will, and subject to the whims of my own shortened perspective. Its field of vision is perhaps blurry on occasion and even out of focus, but one that hopefully allows spectacles to be seen as the truly eye-opening devices they are.

# PART ONE

# 1

# Burning Glasses and Saintly Vision

In the whole scheme of human history, glasses could be said to be a comparatively recent invention. The British optometrists Ida Mann and Antoinette Pirie once went so far as to maintain that spectacles were 'not an essential part of civilisation' since, as they argued, rather impishly, 'neither Plato, nor Aristotle, Confucius nor Mohammed, Charlemagne nor William the Conqueror ever wore spectacles, and yet the world went on in much the same way, philosophies, religions and wars included, as it does now'. Their 'now' was 1946, and the phrase 'much the same way' is dubious to say the least, but we can see their point. There were many thousands of years when we got by perfectly well without them. But the thing, quite obviously, is that some bright spark did invent them, and as with the arrival of the wheel or dry cleaning, the course of our existence was irreparably altered as a result. It might, in some respects, seem surprising that it took quite so long for someone to alight on what today appears such a comparatively simple idea. Our ancient forebears, after all, were not incurious about eyes or optics, nor entirely unskilled in the art of glass making. Its manufacture in and around Mesopotamia can be dated to four millennia ago, if not before, the terrain between the Tigris and Euphrates rivers, by happy chance, bequeathing the local artisans ample supplies of the basic necessary ingredients: sand, lime and soda.

It was in this region too that in 1853 the British archaeologist

Austen Henry Layard uncovered a disc of rock crystal dating from around 750 BC that might conceivably be the oldest known lens yet discovered. The so-called Nimrud (or Layard) Lens was found during Layard's excavations of the ruins of a palace at Nineveh, briefly the largest city in the ancient world and the capital of the Neo-Assyrian Empire, which lies just outside Mosul in modern-day Iraq in what was formerly Upper Mesopotamia. Oval-shaped and with one slightly convex and one plane face, the crystal, which is in the British Museum's collection, had evidently been ground and polished, and looks and acts a little like a simple magnifying glass. Its obvious, if crude, optical qualities led to it immediately being hailed as a lens. In the century and three-quarters since then it has been subject to a proliferation of claims regarding its original purpose. Among the most outlandish is the suggestion that it could have been deployed in a primitive telescope with which the Assyrians surveyed the moons of Jupiter and the rings of Saturn. This notion has been dismissed entirely by most scholars who note that the crystal's convex plane is too unevenly ground ever to have served such ends. Indeed the general consensus, backed up by more recent archaeological research, is that the crystal is probably not a lens at all and was ground for some other purpose entirely. Another possibility is that it was made as an inlay for a piece of furniture. The Assyrians, for all their undoubted qualities, left nothing further to convince experts that they ever got a handle on using crystals, or glass, for magnification, or fire making.

There is plenty of evidence, on the other hand, that the Ancient Greeks were well versed in the art of using crystals and glass for incendiary means. The Peripatetic philosopher Theophrastus was a pupil of Aristotle, and succeeded him to become head of the Lyceum school in Athens in around 322 BC. In his name-on-the-tin treatise *On Fire*, he records that a fire could be kindled by directing the sun's rays through a so-called 'burning glass' – an idea that some two millennia later was second nature to the feral boys of William Golding's *Lord of the Flies*, who used the lenses of Piggy's spectacles (which we will return to later) to raise a bonfire in the hope of attracting a rescuer to free them from their island isolation.

In his *Natural History* of AD 77, the Roman historian Pliny the Elder, however, wrote about stones or glass coming to the aid of weak or ailing eyes. He mentions the supposed soothing qualities of smaragdi, translucent precious stones such as green beryl or emerald. In a much discussed and infuriatingly vague passage, he states that Nero, whom he also records was short-sighted, watched the gladiatorial games with a stone of this ilk at his side. There are readings of this passage that tantalisingly seem to suggest the myopic emperor may have been using a kind of lens to see more clearly. But there is little else to back this thesis up, and others have argued that Pliny might equally plausibly be referring to a kind of mirror which might perhaps have allowed the emperor a more shaded view of the action. Alternatively, an emerald might have been wielded, rather like the eyeshades donned by newspaper editors of old, to help deflect the glare of the sunlight in the amphitheatre from his poor eyes.

That Nero, one of Rome's most infamous tyrants and notorious for his murderous rages and insane jealousy, was green-eyed on occasions of bloody contests in itself seems almost unduly fitting. But the belief that emeralds and green beryls possessed special health-giving qualities for the eyes appears to have been widely held in antiquity. Centuries earlier Theophrastus too had commended them, maintaining that their green colour was good for the eyes. He noted a trend for emerald and green stone rings, where the gems were permanently at hand to offer a kind of visual relief, to be gazed at when required. While the anonymous compilers of the near contemporary Greek philosophical work of scientific enquiry known as the *Aristotelian Problemata*, some of which dates from the third century BC, argued that constantly viewing solid objects exhausted the eyes. They reasoned that emeralds, as transparent green substances that contained 'a considerable amount of moisture', were less harmful to look at as they were less restrictive to vision. In all of this, however, there is no real concrete suggestion of enhancing what was seen through the stone, in the manner of a lens.

For that we have to turn to Seneca, the Roman statesman,

historian, Stoic and one-time tutor to Nero who was eventually compelled to commit suicide in AD 65 after he was accused of plotting against the increasingly paranoid emperor. In his *Natural Questions*, Seneca describes the effect of looking at stuff through water, where he notes 'that everything is much larger'. He goes on to mention that 'writing, however tiny and difficult' becomes 'larger and clearer' if he observes it through a 'glass sphere, or globe, full of water'. Here, then, is the earliest known written account of a magnifying glass in action. It seems unlikely that this was an isolated experiment. And we can easily imagine Seneca having recourse to such a device on numerous other occasions during the final years of his life. He devoted this period to study and writing, having been effectively banished from public life and Rome.

Yet there are reasons for us to be cautious about believing that magnifying glasses or anything like them could ever have enjoyed much widespread use in this epoch, even among the most optically challenged of the Empire's thinkers, or movers and shakers. In a culture where recitation and dictation were the norm, Rome's elite had armies of young secretaries, stenographers and literate slaves to call upon. The likes of Julius Caesar, Cicero, Horace, Pliny the Elder and his nephew, 'the bleary-eyed' Pliny the Younger, scarcely needed to pick up a pen nor read a parchment themselves.

Pliny the Elder's own copious literary production was, for example, only achieved by the ingenious deployment of readers and notaries. Among his last acts was to regale a scribe with descriptions of the eruption of Vesuvius before embarking on a fateful, and for him fatal, rescue mission to the smoking shores of Herculaneum.

All of this was, in a sense, and from our point of view, a hindrance to the invention of spectacles. For the Romans had a practical and highly efficient system in place that no water-filled globe or roughly ground rock crystal could really improve upon. If anything, the system mitigated against anyone bothering to finesse better lenses for those blighted by bad eyesight, as nobody could see a need for them. And to an extent that situation would not really change until the Middle Ages.

Another spoke in the wheel, as far as the ancients and the evolution of eyewear goes, was the various competing accounts of the relationship between the eye and the objects it perceived. The main issue was that since the time of the Ancient Greeks there had been two conflicting schools of thought about how the eye itself worked, both of which had arguments in their favour, and noble and eloquent advocates on their side. On the one hand there were the extramissionists like Plato and Euclid who believed that the eye was active, and that sight was the result of a stream of light, or fire, emanating from the eye like the beam from a torch that then apprehended the objects in front of it. Against them were intromissionists such as the pre-Socratic Democritus, and the likes of Aristotle, Epicurus and the Roman Lucretius, who saw the eye as the recipient of something from the object itself. The latter three all put forward ingenious theories where miniature particles from objects – in effect, their simulacra – were carried through the air to our awaiting eyes.

Aristotle, in particular, questioned the theory of vision that Plato had outlined in the *Timaeus*. If, he wondered, our eyes really did emit light, as Plato had maintained, why could we not see in the dark? He would go on to conclude that it was 'unreasonable to suppose that seeing occurs by something issuing from the eye' and maintained that the eye must receive rays rather than the other way round.

The whole idea of our eyes apprehending the world via beams of fiery light might sound like something from a science fiction B-movie now. But extramissionist theories of vision of one sort or another, with their rather appealing blend of ego and empiricism, were, in the end, to predominate thinking about optics until well into the Renaissance.

This was in no small part because one of the founding figures of medical science, a man whose influence would endure for 1500 years after his death, espoused a version of extramissionist vision. Claudius Galenus, or Galen, was the Greco-Roman physician and philosopher born in AD 129 who attended to emperor Marcus Aurelius; he proved that urine was formed in the kidneys (rather than the bladder as previously thought) and discovered that arteries carried blood.

When it comes to the eye, he is justly credited by the modern optical historian A. Mark Smith with providing the world with the first 'truly systematic anatomical and physiological account of vision' and is acclaimed as a medical theoretician and anatomist who 'insisted on testing theory with anatomic fact'. Galen's descriptions of the fundamental features of the eye would not in fact be superseded until the seventeenth century. Working mostly with the eyes of oxen for dissecting specimens, Galen itemised the retina, the cornea, the iris, the uvea and tear ducts. He also wrestled with the problem of binocular vision, i.e. why we see a single image when we have two eyes set apart from one another. Turning to the question of whether 'a body that is seen ... either sends something from itself to us and thereby gives us an indication of its peculiar character or if it does not itself send something, it waits for some sensory power to come to it from us', he came down in favour of the latter after looking at a mountain and pondering the issue of perceiving distance and scale. He reasoned that since an image of a mountain would have to shrink drastically to enter the pupil then it made more sense for a person's sensory powers to go to the mountain and grasp its enormity than the other way round.

But underlying his whole physiology was an idea formulated by the Ancient Greeks and adapted by the Stoics, that all living things were animated by a vitalising force of air and fire called *pneuma* (essentially 'breath, or wind, of life' or 'spirit'). In his iteration of this concept, sight accordingly was the result of 'visual pneuma' moving from the brain and out into the eyes, though not beyond them, through the hollow optic nerves.

Having observed that cataracts – a condition depicted in statuary from Ancient Egypt dating from the Fifth Dynasty, circa 2465-2323 BC – caused blindness by creating a barrier between the cornea and the crystalline lens, Galen concluded, logically enough, that the lens was 'the principal instrument of vision'. This was another idea that would hold, the odd knock aside, until Johannes Kepler came along in the 1600s at the height of the Renaissance and finally demonstrated the function of the retina. By then, spectacles were common enough. But the principles underpinning how and why visually corrective lenses worked continued to be a matter of theoretical conjecture until the publication of Kepler's *Astronomiae Pars Optica* in 1604.

## Monkish speculations

The arrival of spectacles nearly four centuries earlier in the late medieval period seems down more to the practical skills of glass makers than physicians and philosophers. Though that is to downplay the potential role of the learned in the push to their initial creation and proliferation – a subject considered in Umberto Eco's 1980 novel *The Name of the Rose*.

Set in a Benedictine Abbey somewhere in northern Italy in 1327, during a period when the papacy had moved from Rome to Avignon in France and was in dispute with various mendicant orders over matters material and theological, the book is a famously highbrow whodunit whose plot revolves around the agreeably grisly murders of half a dozen monks. The man charged with solving this mystery is a visiting Franciscan friar, William of Baskerville, who, as his name partially suggests, is a detective in the mould of Sherlock Holmes.* And Baskerville comes equipped not with a magnifying glass but with a pair of newfangled spectacles.

The incidents in the novel are purportedly related years after the event by Baskerville's own Watson, Adso of Melk. In the period of the murders Adso was a youthful Benedictine novice serving the friar as a disciple and scribe. Now an aged monk, he confesses to being able to finally set down his reminiscences of those distant

---

* In the period between the publication of the first Holmes adventures and their eventual embrace by the reading public, Arthur Conan Doyle, who'd previously qualified as a physician in Edinburgh and practised in Southsea, studied ophthalmology in Vienna. On returning to London in 1891, he took premises in Upper Wimpole Street and tried to establish himself, without success, as an eye doctor. The failure of this venture was soon softened by the sudden demand for more Holmes stories, and Doyle abandoned medicine for good to concentrate on writing full time.

days only with the aid of a pair of spectacles his former master forced upon him when they parted years ago. Adso ruefully notes that Baskerville obviously perceived a time in the future when glasses would come in useful for him. A time to which, in his youthful ignorance, he remained wilfully blind. Seeing much more clearly than anyone else is Baskerville's special power, in a novel which is as much about looking for signs as a workaday hunt for a murderer. Though watching is what detectives do.

Spectacles in Eco's fictional schema, then, are the devices which help frame a killer and enable the deeds of the guilty (and the good) to be recorded. Their presence also speaks of the arrival of previously unimaginable ways of looking at the world. In the novel, Baskerville's specs make a notable appearance in the work-shop of the abbey's head glazier, Nicholas Morimondo. The friar and Adso significantly find Morimondo at his bench and in the process of applying stones and pieces of coloured glass to a silver-framed reliquary – one of those cabinets for storing a splinter of the true cross, or the thumb bone of some pious saint who met an excruciating end at the hands of the impure and unbelieving. And after being shown Baskerville's spectacles for the first time Morimondo excitedly recounts hearing about glasses from a cer-tain Brother Jordan from Pisa, over twenty years earlier.

Here Eco is tipping his hat to one of the earliest known references to spectacles and spectacle-making we have. And that document is the text of a sermon delivered, tellingly, in a Dominican monastery by one Friar Giordano da Pisa (also known as da Rivalto) in 1306.

A theologian, philologist, lecturer and founder of the Confraternity of the Holy Redeemer at Pisa, Giordano was born in that city (or in a nearby castle in Rivalto, hence his other name) in around 1260. Educated at the local monastery of St Catherine of Alexandria and then at the universities of Bologna and Paris, he was to become one of the most popular and innovative preachers of his age. He caught the ear of the general public by sallying forth into the world on foot and giving sermons in a vernacular Italian peppered with dialect from his native Tuscany.

Having taught and preached in Siena, Viterbo and Perugia, in 1303 he was appointed principal lector and general preacher at the monastery of Santa Maria Novella in Florence. In that city he appears to have become an almost manic street preacher, venturing forth daily to address rapt crowds whenever the spirit gripped him. It was said that God was often so moved by his oratory on these occasions that he would make a flaming red cross appear on Giordano's forehead as a sign of his approval. This holy version of Washington presidential hopefuls' I Approve This Message appears in the subsequent iconography of Giordano. The preacher is almost universally depicted in paintings from the late Middle Ages to the present day with a great scarlet X-marks-the-spot hovering over his head. Just such a portrait hangs in the church of St Catalina in Pisa, where he was buried following his death in Piacenza en route to Paris and a new teaching post at the Sorbonne in 1311. In this picture Giordano, his bald pate embellished with a red blotch, looks alarmingly like the last leader of the Soviet Union, Mikhail Gorbachev (or at least how he was envisioned by the puppeteers of the satirical TV show *Spitting Image*). Still, venerated for carrying the word of God to the masses and reputed to have performed the odd miracle, he acquired a devoted cultish following and was eventually beatified by Pope Gregory XVI in 1838. In the close to two centuries since then, Giordano has enjoyed the added accolade of being universally acclaimed for helping open the world's eyes to glasses.

Of the many, many lessons Giordano gave, most have inevitably been lost. But the sermon in which he mentions spectacles is one of a number of addresses dating from between 1303 and 1306 of which we have thorough records. Known as the Florentine Lenten, these are the sermons that the preacher gave each year at Lent. This period of Christian penance in the month leading up to Easter is traditionally observed by almsgiving, fasting (or at least more abstemious eating) and mortification of the flesh. It was especially dear to the Dominicans, who as committed ascetics weren't averse to bouts of self-flagellation in imitation of the sufferings of Christ.

But Giordano, in this particular passage, speaks in praise of a material object, one that he evidently deems an unabashed benefit and an aid to learning (something the scholarly Dominicans were all in favour of) rather than an unnecessary luxury – a position that, as we shall see, was not shared universally in his epoch, or far beyond it.

Here, then, is what some loyal scribe recorded of his speech: 'It is not yet twenty years since the art of making spectacles, which have made for good vision, one of the most useful arts on earth was discovered ... I, myself, have seen and conversed with the man who made them first.'

If we take Giordano at his word, and scholars see no reason to doubt his sincerity, this means that the first spectacles can be dated to around 1286. It is also most likely, following the sermoniser's own movements at that time, that they were created by a crafts-man in or around Pisa.\* The Pisan cause receives further support from another historical document. This dates from just seven years after the sermon and concerns a contemporary of Giordano at the Dominican monastery of St Catherine of Alexandria in Pisa, the Friar Alessandro della Spina, who it is clear not only encountered 'the man who made them first' but also studied his methods and replicated his art.

In 1313, the first chronicle of St Catherine of Alexandria was drawn up by Friar Bartolomeo da San Concordio. Della Spina, then only recently deceased, was among the former brothers esteemed to have led a worthy enough life to be granted a brief character sketch in this volume.

San Concordio described della Spina as 'a modest good man'

---

\* The esteemed late Italian historian of optics Vincent Ilardi (1925-2009), who devoted decades to researching the origins of spectacles and telescopes, main-tained that Giordano entered the monastery of St Catherine of Alexandria in Pisa as a novice in 1280, was studying in Paris and Bologna between 1284 and 1286, but was most probably back in Pisa before beginning his teaching career in Siena in 1287. He argued that Giordano's failure to mention either Bologna or Paris in the sermon is another factor in Pisa's favour. Ilardi reasoned that if he had first encountered glasses in those great citadels of commerce and learning, he would surely have said so. That he didn't implies that they were not known in those university cities yet.

who 'knew how to sing, write' and 'illuminate' manuscripts. He could undertake 'everything which mechanically skilled hands' could do, and having seen something that 'had been made, [then] knew how to make it'. Eyeglasses, the chronicle continues, 'had first been made by someone else', someone 'who was unwilling to share them'. So della Spina 'made them and shared them with everyone with a cheerful and willing heart'.

Quite what the unnamed spectacle inventor made of this largesse – in today's terms della Spina's actions look like a potential infringement of intellectual property rights at the very least – has been lost to history. The reluctance of this person to 'share' their invention has been attributed by various writers to a not unreasonable desire to maintain a monopoly on the trade.

As a member of an order who took its vows of poverty pretty seriously, della Spina could hardly have been looking for a slice of the financial action here. Nor can it seem likely that he wished to make the inventor poorer per se. Unless, of course, the inventor was a particularly miserly character, a medieval Scrooge of the spectacles who abused his staff and used his monopoly to charge customers exorbitant rates. In which case the friar might have been justified in bringing him down a peg to teach him the errors of his ways. Still, it's worth recalling that Giordano chose to refer to spectacles in a sermon. Amid the word of God, glasses were part of the good news he brought to the people of Florence that day. The Dominicans were, from their establishment in 1216, an avowedly evangelical and semi-peripatetic order. St Dominic took as a founding principle Christ's instruction to his disciples from St Mark's Gospel to 'go into the whole world and preach the gospel to every creature'. Dominic, it has been claimed, also 'saw the need to use all the resources of human learning in the service of Christ', and this is precisely what della Spina was doing.* He must have observed the benefits glasses might bring to Bible study, for instance, or the art of illuminating manuscripts. In consequence

---

* Symbolising St Dominic's outward-looking nature, a dog with a torch in its mouth is among his emblems.

he could foresee that more of the Lord's works would be done, and his gospel further disseminated. Accordingly, sharing the knowledge of how to make glasses became an issue of Christian duty for the friar.

It is unlikely, in any case, that the secret of glasses making could have remained a secret for very long. The first pairs of glasses, even if taking thousands of years to arrive on the scene, were simply two single lenses set in a handled frame of bone, wood or metal that were riveted together. These could then be perched on the nose, though only ever precariously so. While skill might be needed to prepare and grind the lenses (and we will return to that shortly), once seen, the basic concept of a pair of glasses is one that, as the optical historian Vincent Ilardi pointed out, almost 'any artisan' of the period or 'a talented friar-artisan like Della Spina' could have replicated without too much trouble.

This idea is even incorporated into the plot of *The Name of the Rose*. At one point in the novel, Baskerville's glasses are snatched in an attempt to prevent him deciphering an ancient parchment that could hold the key to the mystery. The detective is forced to enlist the glazier Morimondo to help him make a replacement pair.

Baskerville states earlier in the novel that his glasses were 'given to him by a great master, Salvinus of the Armati'. This again is a nod to those in the know by Eco, for in the long and blurry history of eyeglasses, Armati was once popularly held to be the inventor. His name was only relegated to an interesting anecdote in the annals of eyewear in the 1950s, when the historian Edward Rosen proved beyond almost any doubt that the story was a fiction, one first perpetrated and promoted in the seventeenth century by Ferdinando Leopoldo del Migliore – in Rosen's words an 'ardent Florentine patriot' whose dedication to that city state extended to maintaining, against all contrary evidence, that della Spina was also 'a Florentine, and not Pisan'.* Migliore was to make these

---

* Rosen noted that Spina is a district in Pisa, which most likely supplied the monk's family with their surname, and there is also the Ponte della Spina bridge in the city.

claims in a historical survey of Florence he published in 1684 in a section describing the church of Santa Maria Maggiore. One of the oldest (if not *the* oldest) in Florence, the church, which dates from the ninth century, if not before, has undergone many restorations, and had been substantially rebuilt shortly before Migliore's time. Reflecting on the loss of particular monuments during that work, he wrote:

> There was another memorial which went to ruin in the restoration of that church. It was ... very precious because by means of it we came to know the first inventor of eyeglasses. He was a gentleman of this country [Florence], which is so highly renowned for genius in every subject requiring keenness of mind. He was Messer Salvino del' Armati son of Armato, of a noble family ... The statue of this man in ordinary dress was to be seen reclining on a large slab with letters around it, which said the following:
>
> Here lies Salvino degli Armati, son of Armato, of Florence, inventor of eyeglasses. May God forgive his sins. A.D. 1317.

As it happens, it was the supposed inclusion of the word 'inventor' in the inscription on Salvino's memorial that set scholarly alarm bells ringing. Philologists argued that the term was virtually unknown in the fourteenth century, and didn't come into common use until the sixteenth century. The inscription could perhaps have been added at a later date. But if so it seems odder still that no one had ever mentioned the name of Salvino in relation to the earliest spectacles before Migliore.

If it is now finally possible to tick this Florentine son off the list of potential eyeglass pioneers, others continue to question whether Pisa could be the true birthplace of spectacles. Here the issue concerns the quality of the lenses and the pre-eminence of Venetian artisans in this area. Venice to this day produces some of the finest glassware in the world. In the Middle Ages, and especially after the so-called Fourth Crusade of 1202-4, its craft folk were blessed with several geopolitical and technical advantages over their Italian peers. Everything, in a sense, turns on that epoch's obsession with holy relics.

This will take some unpicking, but it is vital to the broader story of spectacles. If we return again to *The Name of the Rose*, it is worth recalling that when Baskerville and Adso first meet the glazier Morimondo he is tinkering with a reliquary.

## Boning up

To contemporary eyes, of course, the faith placed in the miraculous powers of dubiously sourced body parts, wood chippings and garments only underlines the reason this era in Europe is sometimes referred to as the Dark Ages. Here is premature death (usually grisly and involving sustained torture), superstition, gullibility and unsavoury hygiene all rolled into one. That such relics might be touched, or genuflected before, to ward off plague (*the* plague from 1346 on) only adds to the notion of the hideous backwardness and barbarity of these times. How could they not *see* there were enough splinters of the true cross knocking around to timber a bridge from Rome to Jerusalem?

But the cult of saints and their relics, as the medievalist James Robinson has observed, is 'one of the identifying characteristics of the Middle Ages'. Its origins go back to the earliest days of the Catholic Church, and the martyrdom of Christ's apostles and the first Christians at the hands of the Roman imperial state. It was Nero, according to Tacitus, who officially initiated the persecution of Christians, scapegoating them for the Great Fire of Rome in AD 64 to deflect blame for the blaze away from himself. What he started, perhaps with an emerald stone cooling his firestorm-strained eyes, was continued in earnest by most of his successors until Constantine granted free worship with his Edict of Milan in AD 313. Where the graves and remains of their fallen fellow religionists had, by necessity, been venerated covertly, now pilgrimages could be made to the places of their glorious deaths or internments. Carefully stowed relics, holding some promise of a direct line to the divine, were able to become objects of public worship. And under Constantine, the first Christian Roman emperor, the decidedly pagan practice of erecting temples (aka churches) around the graves (or death sites) of the revered (and then dedicated to their memory) was established. St Peter's Basilica in Rome, perhaps most famously, was founded by Constantine upon the tomb of Jesus's chief apostle, Peter's sacred bones sanctifying this lavish endeavour as those of a lesser if no less spiritually nourishing rank would do elsewhere in the centuries to come.

In Venice's case, the lack of an indigenous martyr was not to prevent this island republic from establishing what is among its most famous religious monuments on the basis of relics conveyed from elsewhere. The basilica of St Mark's was initially formed around the remains of the same named gospel writer and, by tradition, secretary to St Paul. St Mark's decayed body was, by most accounts, pilfered from its resting place in Muslim-controlled Alexandria and carried back to Venice by a couple of dutiful Christian sailors. These religiously inclined mariners are said to have outwitted the local customs officers by disguising the corpse, conveyed in a barrel, under a layer of pork fat, just to add further insult to Islamic sensibilities.

But the whole business of relics had by then already received a boost from Constantine's mother, Helena. In AD 326, and acting as the First Lady of the Empire, she undertook a pilgrimage to the Holy Land, where through dogged research all the key locations of Christ's life and ministry, death and resurrection – along, miraculously, with such priceless artefacts as the bulk of the True Cross and nails from the crucifixion – were discovered. And no doubt to the enormous satisfaction of all concerned, Helena was to send a decent-sized piece of this cross and a nail or two to her son, who was at this point on the brink of consolidating his empire by moving the imperial capital east to the Greek city of Byzantium.

Unlike Rome, where on occasion the Tiber had practically foamed with the blood of dead Christians, Byzantium, or Constantinople as it was to be renamed, suffered from a severe deficit of martyrs. Almost in overcompensation, and to shore up its future under the eyes of God, Constantine and his heirs were to make it one of the greatest repositories of relics ever assembled.

The bulk of these treasures were in due course to find their way to Venice after the sacking of Constantinople by Venetian-led Crusaders in 1204. The skull of John the Baptist and the arm of St George were among the items from Constantinople that were swiftly rehoused in the church of St Mark's. Joining them, importantly, were what historian W. Patrick McCray in his 1999 study of glass making in Venice describes as 'several wonderful examples of worked crystal'. These works would spur Venice's own artisans on to greater heights. The republic was to benefit in other ways that would directly affect the production of glass on the archipelago. Crucially, the Crusaders' ventures allowed the Venetians to establish a series of trading bases on the eastern Mediterranean and the west of the Aegean which gave it easy access to the Levant and beyond, eventually to China. Marco Polo was, after all, a Venetian.

It has often been maintained that spectacles were already known in China, their invention there perhaps pre-dating Europe by as much as a century, and that it was Polo who brought the first descriptions of them back to Venice towards the end of the thirteenth century.

Until recently accused of making it no further than the Bosphorus and held, in any case, to be an inveterate liar on the basis of some of the more outlandish descriptions of places, people and animals contained in *Travels of Marco Polo*, the trader and explorer is less readily dismissed as a medieval fantasist these days. For all that, extensive combing of every extant edition of the *Travels* and in its various translations by scholars for whom such pedantry is close to a calling has failed to turn up a single reference to spectacles. Nevertheless, Venice in this period was extremely open to fresh ideas from the east as the more general output of its glass workers attests. We'll return to the question of glasses and China later, but for the moment it's the influence of the near rather than far east on the republic's artisans that is of interest.

Through its newly developed trading relations with Cyprus, Syria and Alexandria, Venetians encountered the innovative techniques practised around the Levant to produce glass with far fewer impurities in it.

The key ingredient in traditional glass is silica, of which the most basic source is sand. But sand varies in quality and can contain traces of iron, calcium and aluminium oxides that affect the colour and shape of the finished glass. Therefore the purer the silica the better. Pliny records that the sands of the Belus River on the Syrian coast were, for this very reason, prized by Roman glass makers in his day. Ancient glass makers would also resort to crushed quartz or ground rock crystal as other, purer, sources of silica. However, pure silica has a melting point of around 1700°C, a temperature far in excess of anything furnaces in those times could muster. To reduce the melting point of the silica ingredients, an alkali fluxing agent had to be added to the mix. The naturally occurring mineral mixture natron, which had been mined since Roman times from the Wadi-el-Natrun desert region of Egypt between Cairo and Alexandria, was one alkali the Venetians had previously availed themselves of. But as McCray argues, their glass making was only to progress to its inventive heights after they began sourcing quantities of raw glass and an alternative purer alkali, the soda-rich plant ash, from the Levant. The procurement of which, he states, was 'entirely dependent' on the trading relations Venice was to enjoy with that region in the wake of the Fourth Crusade.

The technical know-how learnt from their counterparts in the near east was to infuse Venetian glass with the artistic influence of Islam. The Venetians' subsequent mastery of glass-blowing, in particular, is widely attributed to their updating of traditions established in Syria and Egypt. In return, Venetian merchant galleys subsequently journeyed eastward with glass wares they traded for olive oil from Crete, cotton from Cyprus and Turkey, and spices from the East Indies. Another of their innovations was sheet glass for window panes. This idea was initially developed by medieval German glaziers, who relied on plant ash from the beechwood that abounded in the local forests as a flux in their glass. But improved upon by Venetian artisans it was being fitted into the windows of royal palaces, the houses of wealthier merchants, cathedrals and the more well endowed of churches by the middle of the thirteenth century.

The latter institutions were to urge glass makers on, demanding they make bigger and better panes. These were for almost fish-tank-style reliquaries, typically placed beneath altars, where the whole skeleton of a saint, or a bundle of their bones, would be displayed behind a sheet of protective glass. The sacred remains could be seen and gazed at with suitable reverence, but not manhandled by overenthusiastic pilgrims seeking cures for their physical and/or spiritual ills. The origins of these somewhat macabre tableaux stem from a rather literal reading of a verse from the Book of Revelation, that most cryptic of biblical texts, that runs, 'I saw under the altars the souls of them that were slain for the word of God and the testimony which they held.'

Of course most relics were considerably smaller than a whole skeleton. And in the aftermath of the plunder of Constantinople, thousands of tiny fragments of blessed hair, skin, bone, clothing, lumber and iron were to come on to the market. Almost every church in the western world, no matter how modest its budget, could obtain a relic within its price range. Size, of course, isn't everything, and the scale of the object of devotion, then as now, was no indicator of its value. In the Top Trumps of medieval Christianity one drop of Christ's blood obviously scored higher than the complete remains of some second division martyr. But where a glass pane might be used on a large altar reliquary, so more diminutive items came increasingly to be placed inside reliquaries finished with plates or discs of polished rock crystal that not only allowed the item to be viewed but also had a slight magnifying effect. One of the finest examples of this type of reliquary can be found in the treasure room of Halberstadt Cathedral in Germany. Made between 1220 and 1225, it contains twenty-one miniature relics, among them a splinter from the Holy Cross and a thorn from the Crown of Thorns, each shielded by an individual plate of clear rock crystal in a kind of cabinet of curiosities. And it was while crafting these cabinets that monk glaziers became more fully acquainted with the concept of magnification and began to use polished crystals as visual aids elsewhere, with ageing scribes and illuminators quick to see the benefits.

## The optics of the situation

Indeed, it was the English philosopher, theologian and Franciscan friar Roger Bacon who first wrote about lenses in this respect. In his *Opus Majus*, completed around 1267 – potentially nearly a full twenty years before spectacles were first conceived – he outlines the basic principle of corrective lenses, stating that 'if anyone examines letters or other minute objects through the medium of crystal or glass or other transparent substance, if it be shaped like the lesser segment of a sphere, with the convex side toward the eye, he will see the letters far better and they will seem larger to him . . . For this reason such an instrument is useful to old persons and to those with weak eyes, for they can see any letter, however small, if magnified.'

Bacon is one of the models (along with the scholastic thinker and fellow English Franciscan William of Ockham) for Eco's Baskerville. But unlike his fictional counterpart, it seems doubtful that the friar ever got beyond theorising about optics. His writing here, most historians contend, owes more to philosophical speculation than hands-on practical experimentation, as there is no clear evidence either way to support the idea that he used such lenses himself. He was also partially responding to an earlier work by the tenth-century Islamic polymath Abu Ali al-Hassan ibn al-Haytham (commonly Latinised to Al-Hazen), and one that Baskerville also commends to young Adso in *The Name of the Rose*, telling him that he 'must read some treatise on optics' and that 'the best ones are by the Arabs'.

Born in Basra in what is now southern Iraq in AD 965, Ibn al-Haytham began to formulate his own theories on vision and optics while languishing for a decade in prison, having failed the Fatimid caliph Al-Hakim bi'amr Allah over an ambitious, if all but unachievable, scheme he'd proposed to dam the Nile. This was magnanimous for the caliph, who legend claims once ordered all the dogs in Cairo to be slaughtered because their incessant barking got on his nerves. In any case, Ibn al-Haytham used his time behind bars wisely, reading all the classical works on the subject, which if largely lost to the west for a time, survived during the bleakest years of the so-called Dark Ages thanks to the efforts of the Islamic scholars of the House of Wisdom in Baghdad. Here Islamic scribes ensured their preservation by translating many of the original texts in Greek by Plato, Galen, Aristotle and others into Arabic. (Just such a 'lost book' by Aristotle provides another plot point in *The Name of the Rose*.)

Ibn al-Haytham duly emerged from gaol to conduct the series of experiments that would see him retrospectively hailed as 'the first true proponent of the modern scientific method' and complete his mammoth seven-volume treatise the *Kitab al-Manathir*, or *De Aspectibus*, or *Book of Optics*. It was a book whose influence would reverberate across the fields of science, mathematics and art throughout the Renaissance and far beyond; an asteroid would be named in his honour in 1999. In Florence, and following its translation into Italian in the fourteenth century, his discussions on perspective were taken up by the likes of the architect and writer Leon Battista Alberti, the sculptor Lorenzo Ghiberti and the artist Piero della Francesca. Consequently they stimulated the production of artworks that strove to imbue scenes on flat canvases and friezes with a greater illusion of three-dimensional depth.

Ibn al-Haytham's anatomical descriptions of the human eye, particularly in his account of how the cornea worked, were not to be bettered until the time of Kepler. He was the first person to posit the idea that the optic nerve might transmit visual sensations to the brain. He overturned entirely the emission theories of Plato and Galen, that vision was the result of rays radiating out from our eyes. Ibn al-Haytham found it impossible to understand how rays might reach distant stars from the very instant our eyes were opened. Similarly he also couldn't see, if such a system prevailed, how or why it should be painful to look at the sun after stepping out of the dark. He therefore concluded that logically light must travel to the eye and not the other way round. Having established this, he formulated a theory of light that grappled, most accurately to that date and long after, with the underlying physics of refraction and reflection. Key among his insights was to surmise that all objects, and not just mirrors, could reflect light from a primary source like the sun or fire. What was seen by us, he reasoned, was then dependent on conditions in the atmosphere. Also included in the work was a discussion of the properties of convex lenses.

The *Kitab al-Manathir* was translated into Latin in the twelfth century and widely circulated in monasteries and university libraries of the period, hence both the real-life Bacon and the fictional Baskerville's familiarity with the text. Amusingly, the one element of Ibn al-Haytham's writings that Bacon seemed unable or unwilling to accept was his trouncing of ray-gun-style vision. In *Opus Majus*, the Franciscan presented yet another version of the classic Platonic model despite all the arguments marshalled against such theories by the Arab thinker. However, the convex lenses Ibn al-Haytham described appear to have had a thickness greater than their radius, rendering them unsuitable for reading. Here, then, Bacon improved upon Ibn al-Haytham's idea and hinted at a breakthrough that in the end was to be realised by efficient artisans rather than monkish theoreticians – though the latter would, as scribes and readers and writers of arcane texts, of course benefit enormously from the invention.

The utility of lenses as an aid for reading, quite specifically, over, say, sewing, needlepoint or metalwork, for which they could, arguably, be equally useful, is a crucial detail in one of the oldest legal documents concerning glasses ever to come to light. The reference to 'vitreos ab oculus ad legendum' or 'glasses for the eyes for reading' appears among the state trade regulations for the guild of crystal-glass workers in Venice in 1301. This statute, building on earlier rules first set down in 1284, expressly forbids glass makers from passing off high-quality glass as crystal and vice versa. The implication here is that Venetian glass was both good enough to fool the unsuspecting and was being used for reading spectacles by this date. The combination of this information with the verifiable antiquity of its source was another feather in the cap for Venice, and for those who have sought to promote it over Pisa as the birthplace of glasses making.

Venice, as the Spanish novelist Javier Marias once observed, is a city that 'has to be seen'. But Pisa, if anything, seems an even more fitting place for the earliest spectacles to hail from topographically. A long-standing rival to the island republic for Levantine trade and a commercial port city with an established glass industry of its own, Pisa was founded on the shores of the Tyrrhenian Sea, on a marshy headland between the rivers Arno and Auser (now known as Serchio). Originally a coastal settlement, the city would find itself further and further inland as the alluvial deposits of those two rivers encroached upon the ocean. By the first century AD Pisa was two and a half miles from the coast; by the tenth it was four; today it's a solid six miles inland. Its perpetually shifting shoreline and the region's generally unstable alluvial ground are the reasons its most notorious landmark, the campanile to the cathedral, leans as it does. Commenced in 1173 and not finished until nearly two centuries later, the tower's lilt was already so pronounced by 1298 that the first investigation into straightening the structure was commissioned in that year. But to live in a place where the horizon is in retreat and buildings commonly shift about is perhaps to be afforded a view of the world that's more open to change in matters of perspective. Is it really surprising, for example, that one of its most famous sons is Galileo Galilei? A man reputed to have conducted experiments into gravity from the bell tower, and who would go on to perfect the telescope and by pointing it at the stars turn our universe on its head by proving that the sun, not the Earth, is at the centre of the solar system, before sadly losing his own sight amid charges of heresy. The first spectacles, as has been stated, were made with convex lenses and could correct presbyopia, the condition of long-sightedness that makes focusing on close-up objects difficult, along with hypermetropia or long-sightedness itself. The former condition is caused by a loss of flexibility in the eye's natural lens, which becomes less elastic and less translucent as we age. A sixty-year-old typically receives around a third of the amount of light to their retinas compared with a ten-year-old. Most people over forty suffer from it, regardless of any prior eye conditions such as myopia (short-sightedness). The most basic common remedy for its symptoms is to hold books, newspapers, tickets, washing instructions, really anything you want to see clearly, at arm's length. The act of pushing these objects into the middle distance helping the eye to accommodate it. For Pisans, the idea of stuff moving away from you visually was second nature, and perhaps the urge to correct it optically hailed from a deep-seated desire to return the city to its marine roots.

## God-given vision

Wherever they first emerged, in Italy it appears both Pisa and Venice were eventually to be outclassed by Florence in any case, which would become acclaimed for the quality of its eyeglasses. W. Patrick McCray cites as an example the fourteenth- and fifteenth-century inventory books of the Gonzaga family. This elite house, which ruled over parts of Lombardy, Piedmont, and Nevers in France until the seventeenth century, purchased numerous pieces of fine luxury glassware from the workshops of Murano in Venice, but notably ordered their eyeglasses from Florentine artisans. McCray argues that Venetian guilds once so innovative ended up being stifled by their own traditions, leaving both Florentine and later Bohemian manufacturers to develop clearer glass better suited for optical lenses, and to dominate the market. Documents from the 1450s and 1460s unearthed by Vincent Ilardi confirm the preference for spectacles from Florence among the Dukes of Milan too, who, as he writes, in this period 'were ordering prestigious Florentine eyeglasses by the hundreds to give away as gifts to their courtiers'.

The sense here of glasses as 'giftable' objects of prestige rather than potentially embarrassing medical implements (can we, for instance, imagine the Dukes of Milan presenting their courtiers with Florentine-crafted ear trumpets or wooden legs?) is also present in some of the earliest representations of them in art. The first picture of a person wearing spectacles we have comes from 1352. The wearer in question is Hugh of St Cher, the French Dominican cardinal described by one chronicler as the 'great churchman, legislator, reformer, religious superior, theologian, exegete, preacher, writer, statesman, confidant of popes', and hailed as 'Blessed Hugh, Commentator' by Fra Angelico, who snuck him into one of his crucifixion scenes. The depiction of Hugh with glasses is no less anachronistic. The Dominican died in 1263, over two decades before the earliest estimated date of their invention. This portrait is one of a series of frescoes of forty Dominican worthies painted by Tomaso Barisini da Modena on the Chapter House of that order's San Niccolò monastery in Treviso, in the Veneto region of Italy, some 20 miles from Venice. As an artist of this period, Tomaso is held up as a pioneer of a more realistic style of painting, one that anticipated the work of Flemish masters in the following century. In this cycle especially he represents Dominican scholars, theologians and saints going about their godly business in scholarly study cells, with all the appropriate paraphernalia (books, ink wells, quill pens, and even primitive pairs of scissors) within reach. Hugh is not alone in being painted with an optical aid either. The Italian preacher Pietro Isnardo da Chiampo of Vicenza and Nicholas Caignet de Freauville, the French Cardinal of Rouen, appear with a reading mirror and magnifying glass, respectively. Tomaso could have exercised greater realism by depicting the latter (who died in 1325) with spectacles rather than Hugh. And in giving him glasses the Venetian-born painter arguably set a worrying precedent that would see all manner of historical and semi-mythical figures pictured with spectacles they could never have worn in their own lifetimes.

Hugh, nevertheless, was a scholar, holding the post of master of theology at the University of Paris and lecturing in canon law and philosophy before serving as an adviser and envoy to Pope Gregory IX and being raised to the cardinalate by Innocent IV. Said to have laboured with 'untiring industry as a compiler of explanations of the Sacred Text', Hugh's biblical commentaries were numerous enough for an eight-volume edition of his exegetical works eventually to be published, in 1754. In the annals of scriptural studies, his reputation rests on three significant projects. These are an index of the Bible, the first concordance of the Bible, and a correction of the so-called Latin Vulgate of St Jerome.

Interestingly, Tomaso did not depict St Jerome himself with glasses in a fresco he subsequently provided for the neighbouring church at the San Niccolò monastery, though this would become a common enough trope for artists throughout the later Middle Ages and on into the Renaissance.

As with many a saint, Jerome's life, works and legends offered painters plenty of scope for visual representation. Like an Action Man doll, Jerome in paint comes in an array of outfits and complementary accessories, depending on which element of his story is being highlighted. There is ascetic, celibacy-seeking Jerome, usually shown beating his bare chest with rocks or occasionally being whipped by angels. There is Jerome the devoted secretary to Pope Damasus I, elevated to the rank of cardinal and dressed in a mitre and/or wearing plush red robes. There is Jerome the lion tamer, with a big cat either forever supplicant at his feet or shown, as the myth has it, having a thorn plucked from its paw by the saint himself. But inevitably as the man who strove, with failing eyesight and thanks to the aid of a team of devoted amanuenses, to put the whole of the Bible into Latin, his most common pictorial set-ups are bookish and ecclesiastical. As with Tomaso's image of Hugh, the art of scriptural translation is seemingly incapable of being accomplished in the painterly mindset outside of a monkish cell kitted out with a desk laden with books, papers and quill pens, and a candle nearing its end. The Jerome of these pictures is unfailingly wizened, and a human skull also regularly features as a table piece, emphasising, along with those nearly spent candles, the transience of worldly existence and the saint's proximity to God and salvation.

And again, although he died in Bethlehem in AD 420, spectacles are another of his accoutrements in painterly studies from the fourteenth century on. He appears wearing them in works by the Dutch painter Lucas van Leyden, the Italian Lionello Spada and the French painter Georges de la Tour, among others. But perhaps more commonly they appear at rest on his desk or even hanging, quite daintily, on their own special hook, as per a fresco of St Jerome executed by Domenico Ghirlandaio for the nave of the church of the Ognissanti, Florence, in 1480.

St Jerome, in simpler times even erroneously credited with the invention of glasses (perhaps because he was pictured so often with them), was to be adopted as the patron saint of spectacle makers. He was far from the only saint to be retrospectively granted eyeglasses by artists. In these golden days of symbol-heavy religious painting the recipients of spectacles ranged from the Old Testament prophet Moses to St Peter, the apostle to whom the risen Christ first appeared. All were people, shall we say, of vision. For the enlightened recipients of God's wisdom, the addition of glasses is a tribute to their extra spiritual perspective, studiousness and diligence in spreading the gospel. Yet spectacles remained in certain Christian circles objects of suspicion. Here were devices that altered reality, putting the previously unseen in sight. If such defects were God-given, all part of the natural pre-ordained cycle of life, were men or women entitled to correct them? And in a largely agrarian world, time was indeed cyclical, moving through recurring seasons.

The early Christian Church inherited from Platonic thought a touch of scepticism about the visual sense anyway. While the 'hearing ear and the seeing eye' were blessed, as the Lord had 'made them both', the former was often the preferred medium for Christ's spiritual message. Hearing is actually stated as a source of Christian faith in a verse of the book of Romans (10:17): 'So faith comes from hearing, and hearing through the word of Christ.'

In a reverse of that hoary adage about small children, the decidedly more wrathful Hebrew God was mostly *heard* rather than *seen*. In the Old Testament it's nearly all about the *voice*. His presence is only very occasionally instanced by the appearance of a flaming bush, or his will indicated by the issuing of commandments on stone tablets that will then have to be read. In the gospels of the New Testament, Jesus is often reluctant to perform miracles, refusing on several occasions to *show* the supernatural power of God when he'd rather *tell*, persuading the unconverted by preaching to them instead. And following Jesus's own miraculous return from the dead, the apostle Thomas is initially incredulous, refusing to believe his eyes, insisting on physically touching the wounds on Christ's hands and side before he'll accept the resurrection. Those who followed him, though, would, in effect, be left with hearsay. In the King James version of St John's Gospel where the story of Thomas is related, Jesus tells the doubting disciple that while 'thou hast seen me ... blessed [are] they that have not seen and yet have believed'. This statement implicitly puts the act of faith beyond the merely observable. For the majority of Christians in the Middle Ages, illiteracy ensured that the bulk of their religious instruction was to be received aurally from their priests, and a good chunk of it recited in a Latin they neither spoke nor read.

Before the arrival of the printing press and the expansion of literacy, it was for the same reason that those who needed glasses in the thirteenth and fourteenth centuries remained a comparatively small group. And one, as we have already seen, heavily composed in life and art of the clerkly, the living usually managing to put aside any theological doubts they might have held about these devices upon encountering their practical benefits. The medieval medical profession, on the other hand, continued to discourage their use, urging their patients to ingest fennel seeds or anoint their eyes with such horrific-sounding lotions, potions and salves as the one promoted by the fourteenth-century London surgeon John of Arderne rather than wear glasses. Arderne recommended a nightly unguent composed of twice-cooled and melted butter combined with vapours from 'the sour urine of a man ... mixed with a little fat of a capon liquified by the sun's heat or a fire'. It was a concoction that Arderne claimed to have used himself, maintaining in the manuscript of his treatise on the subject, *De Cura Oculorum*, that it had allowed him to keep reading, writing and studying into his seventieth year.

Even Guy de Chauliac, considered the first medical writer to mention spectacles and professor of medicine at the University of Montpellier, presented them as a very last resort. Residing in Avignon for the last twenty-five years of his life, where he served as surgeon to the papal court, de Chauliac composed his book *Chirurgia Magna* in 1363, the fourth chapter of which was to become the standard medical textbook for the next two centuries. In it he advises the use of various balms for ageing eyes, including

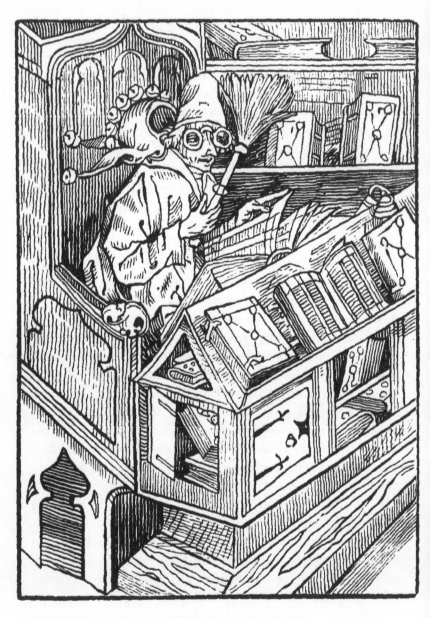

Woodcut illustration from Sebastian Brant's *Das Narrenschiff*
(The Ship of Fools), 1494.

bathing them in fennel water. But he writes somewhat despairingly that 'if these things do not avail, recourse must be had to spectacles of glass or beryl'.

In France, perhaps because of the lengthy presence of the papacy in Avignon with its attendant ranks of scribes, bureaucrats and theologians (and despite de Chauliac's later medical advice), spectacle making seems to have begun fairly early in the fourteenth century. By 1465 a spectacle makers' guild was well enough established to be presented alongside the haberdashers and upholsterers in a review of Parisian craft workers conducted by Louis XI.

The general preference for higher-quality polished beryl rock crystal for lenses alluded to by de Chauliac resulted in spectacles initially being christened *bericles* there. The German term *brille* has the same root. But *bericles* would gradually be replaced in French by 'lunettes', the name still in use today, a reference to the moon-like round shapes of the lenses – just as the word 'lenses' itself derives from an abbreviation of *lenticchia*, the Italian for 'lentils', after their similarity to the bulging beady pulses cultivated in Italy since farming began.*

There is no record of spectacle making in Britain in the fourteenth century. But a pair of glasses (valued at two English shillings) were listed in an inventory at Exeter Palace of the personal effects of Bishop Walter de Stapledon, the Lord High Treasurer of England, who died in 1326. The bishop had previously undertaken diplomatic missions on the continent and acted as a chaplain to Pope Clement V in France and could conceivably have obtained his spectacles on the European mainland, though the possibility that English monks and artisans could just as easily as their continental cousins have mastered the techniques of manufacturing spectacles by then should not be ruled out. At that price, however, it's likely that de Stapledon's spectacles were at the luxury end of the market and most likely fashioned with crystal lenses and frames of a precious or gilt metal. Pairs framed with

---

* In his memoir *The Factory of Facts*, the Belgian-American writer Luc Sante records that one of the culinary specialities of the Walloon city of Verviers is a type of spectacle-shaped biscuit called *lunettes* that were traditionally served on saint's days.

brass, iron or wood were selling comparatively cheaply, going by the exchange rates of the day, at a mere six Bolognese *soldi* (shillings) in Italy during this same period. It is not until over a century later that the first spectacle makers are documented in London, though customs records show that spectacles and spectacles cases were being imported in some quantities from Holland from the end of the fourteenth century. The two resident craftsmen, Matthew and Paul van (de) Bessen, strikingly, were Dutch and listed as living and working in Southwark in the 1440s and 1450s when this south-of-the-river suburb was home to numerous Dutch, German and Flemish artisans. It is also a Flemish pedlar at Westminster Hall who implores the brassic narrator of the fifteenth-century satirical poem *London Lyckpenny* to buy 'fyne felt hatts, or spectacles for to reade'.*

Archaeological finds, such as the pairs of rivet frames discovered with a thousand other medieval artefacts in compacted centuries-thick dust under the oaken floorboards of a nunnery choir in a monastery at Weinhausen in Germany in 1953, confirm that spectacles were well enough known in Germany, Austria and the Low Countries long before their manufacturing was officially documented in places like Frankfurt (in 1450), Strasbourg (in 1466) and Nuremberg (in 1478). The latter city would become by far the most significant mass producer of glasses in Europe and was by the 1470s also, as it happened, at the forefront of the German print trade. One of the most technically advanced illustrated books of the fifteenth century, the *Liber Chronicarum*, a kind of proto-potted history of the world, is also known as *The Nuremberg Chronicle* as it was produced in the same Nuremberg workshop where Albrecht Dürer served his apprenticeship.

---

* In 1974 the remains of a pair of rivet spectacles were recovered from a medieval rubbish dump discovered during excavations at Trig Lane, near Blackfriars. Dating from 1440, they are the oldest spectacles ever found in England. Though lensless and today looking in their partially broken state more like the claw from an amusement arcade grabbing game, they were clearly originally comprised of two identical circular frames. Each was most likely shaped from a bone plate cut with a metal tool like a pair of dividers from the metacarpal of a bull, and then pinned together.

## Books: a revelation

Curiously, the story of the evolution of printed books, and in particular the innovations of Johannes Gensfleisch zur Laden (more familiarly known as Gutenberg after his patrician family's pile in their native Mainz), is itself inextricably intertwined with getting a better look at reliquaries. For the starting point of what would prove to be a convoluted path to Gutenberg's press with malleable metal type – one littered with false starts, failed prototypes, aggrieved former business associates, legal writs and large financial outlays – began in Strasbourg with a scheme to manufacture thousands of mirrored badges for pilgrims expected to descend en masse on Aachen in 1439.

Bordering Belgium and the Netherlands, Aachen, the most westerly city in modern Germany, was anointed by Charlemagne, Charles the Great, who made it the capital of his empire in AD 790.

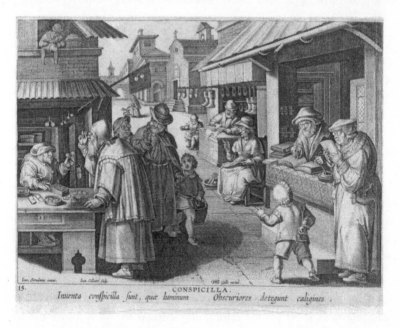

Conspicilla Inuenta conspicilla sunt, quæ luminum, obscuriores detegunt caligines, engraving, Phis Galle, circa 1600.

The cathedral that would come to house his earthly remains after his death in 814 was built on the ruins of a sulphurous Roman thermal spa, and became one of the holiest sites of medieval pilgrimage after Charles's canonisation by Emperor Frederick I in 1165. Adding to its appeal for those seeking to even the scores on their chance of salvation, the cathedral held numerous other relics aside from Charlemagne's own, which were stored in a casket of pure gold. The robe Mary wore the night Jesus was born and the loincloth Jesus sported on the cross were, and remain, among the cathedral's most cherished possessions. Such was the demand to visit Aachen that in 1349 the cathedral was forced to formalise access to its relics, and from that date onwards only put them on show for a limited two-week period every seven years, a ritual that continues to this day. Of course in the Middle Ages, when faith in these items was much more fervid, this did little to slake the desire to come to Aachen; if anything, it only fed it. During this fortnight in 1432, over 10,000 people a day were traipsing through the cathedral close, all desperate to get a glimpse of the relics, and at one point a nearby building collapsed and seventeen people were killed and a hundred more injured.

Pilgrims had long bought and worn metal badges decorated with the appropriate saint as a commemorative token cum relic-infused talisman of their odyssey. But at Aachen in 1432, and faced with the sheer difficulty of getting anywhere near the objects of veneration, the more enterprising also obtained little portable metal convex mirrors whose wide-angled views not only aided the visitor to see a distant relic amid the scrum but were also understood to help direct some of the healing rays that supposedly emanated from these holy items towards the true believer. And suddenly the idea of combining the two was born. Why not have a pilgrim's badge with a small polished mirror inset in a frame decorated with a figure or two of reverence? The only snag was that all the goldsmiths and metal workers of Aachen could not produce enough, so their guilds reluctantly agreed to allow outsiders to make and sell pilgrim's badges for the duration of the relic season, and for them to do the same again in seven years' time.

It was to this date that Gutenberg and his associates looked, and all their energies were directed to mass-producing some 32,000 mirrored badges for the 1439 Aachen pilgrimage. That no one up until then had mass-manufactured anything like this number of mirrors did not deter them. Gutenberg, whose father was closely associated with the archiepiscopal mint at Mainz, and from where it is assumed he acquired his subsequent knowledge of the gold-smith's arts, was the technical wizard behind the operation. What he was actually working on and quite how or why he moved from mirrored badges to a press with moveable type is yet another mystery, though many of the first printers were gold or silversmiths, including Procopius Waldfogel, a man whose own similar press in Avignon is thought by some to have been in operation as early as 1444, pre-dating Gutenberg's by nearly four years. England's first printer, William Caxton, is a bit of an anomaly having previously spent his working life in the wool trade.

Perhaps the most crucial event in the tale, on which the eventual mass dissemination of knowledge via the printed word possibly hangs, was that the 1439 Aachen pilgrimage was postponed for a year due to further outbreaks of the plague. This delay may have robbed Gutenberg and his backers of their chance to make a quick buck from sucker pilgrims – had he perfected the mirror-making in time, obviously. But it appears, aside from accelerating a rift with his business partners, to have nudged him more firmly in the direction of type. The mass-produced mirrored badges were never to materialise, while his highly practical means of printing would emerge from Gutenberg's workshop back in Mainz a decade later.

It was evidently an idea, like spectacles themselves, whose time had come, hence the various competing claims to the invention. But we have the extraordinary coincidence that without relics and reliquaries, spectacles may never have been invented; and also that without relics and reliquaries Gutenberg would not have created his press – a device that would ultimately result in millions more people needing spectacles to read the texts that could now be printed cheaply and at scale.

# 2

# Of Myopia and Men

It says as much about similar types of majoritarian bias such as
that suffered by the left-handed that it was nearly 200 years after
spectacles for presbyopia (and hypermetropia) were first invented
that seemingly anyone got round to making glasses to cure short-
sightedness. Such an oversight looks to be ... well, short-sighted.
And here again the language is telling.

To have good distance sight is not only to be granted the ability to see faraway objects more clearly, it is, in common parlance,
also connected to such noble qualities as foresight and the ability
to make shrewd judgements about future events. Even the gift of
prophecy. There is obviously a certain logic to this. In the days
before spyglasses, the ability to see the approach of a better-armed
adversary on foot, horse or by ship allowed evasive action, for
instance, to be taken, and in good time. Battles were fought and
lost and empires, continents, nations and cities vanquished on such
minor advantages as being forewarned and therefore forearmed.

By contrast, short-sightedness is lumbered with almost entirely
pejorative associations. A glance at the entry in the current *Oxford
English Dictionary* reveals glosses such as 'characterized by or
proceeding from want of foresight or limited mental vision' and
'[l]acking in foresight or in extent of intellectual outlook'. Even its
supposedly studiously literal definition gives us 'having the focus
of the eyes at less than the *normal* distance; unable to distinguish

objects clearly at a distance; myopic'. The italics are mine, but that 'normal' comes with more than a few assumptions.

Since it is something of a rarity in the real world, it is perhaps better to speak of 'perfect' rather than 'normal' vision. But the basic measurement, enshrined in duels with pistols and, perhaps more pertinently, the Snellen eye test, is the ability to see distant objects clearly at 20 feet (6 metres). It is to the Snellen test – named after Herman Snellen, the Dutch ophthalmologist who developed a type of chart with phalanx-like ranks of letters of descending scale – that we owe the famed double whammy of 20/20 vision (6/6 in metric measurements). Or visual acuity, to be more accurate, as this is what the Snellen test calculates. 20/20 vision derives from the distance of the chart from the patient (our classic pistols-at-dawn twenty paces), plus that subject's ability to read characters on a specific lower line (commonly the eighth that runs D E F P O T E C). Each line above that represents a graded deterioration in visual acuity at that distance. If the patient can't quite make out the letters on the 20/20 line but can see the ones above that they'll have a visual acuity of 20/25, and then 20/30, and so on as the letters get larger and larger. The last and lowest score possible is 20/200. Here only the single big 'E' at the top of the chart will have been declared legible and the patient would normally now be classified as legally blind.

If it is not uncommon to have worse than 20/20 visual acuity, it is equally possible to have better than 20/20 visual acuity. Anyone sharp-eyed enough to read the very bottom, smallest letters on the chart will score a visual acuity of 20/10, twice that of the often presumed gold standard.

Much of what can or cannot be seen at distance is determined by the size and shape of the eyes. This is what distorts how light from faraway objects reaches our retinas, and then the kinds of images that are conveyed to our brains via the optic nerve to decode. To put it very crudely, short-sightedness, perversely is caused by eyes that are too long and long-sightedness, generally, the reverse.

A good-sized eye, in terms of hitting the 20/20 benchmark, has been calculated as one where the space between the front of the cornea and the macula (the centre of the retina at the back of the eye) is 0.945 inches (2.4 centimetres). With such an eye, the rays of light from, say, a tree 20 feet away will be refracted in such a way as to form a clear tree-shaped picture on the retina. If, however, the eye is slightly longer in length, the rays of light from the tree will be bent too much before reaching their intended target. The picture will form somewhere in the vitreous jelly in front of the retina rather than on the retina itself.

What reaches the retina then is a sort of vapour trail of the tree's after-image. The faraway piece of forestry will be rendered as a greeny-brown blur to the brain of the larger-eyed viewer. The only ways of rectifying this, without recourse to glasses with con-cave lenses, are by reducing the pupil to a pinhole (i.e. squinting) to create an artificial depth of field or moving closer to the tree. The latter will bend the light rays reflected from the tree on to the retina, and eventually bring its image fully into focus – though the extremely short-sighted may only ever be able to see a section of its bark or branches up close, and never be able to get far enough away to perceive the tree as a complete entity.

Those born mildly long-sighted or hypermetropic, on the other hand, especially when young and their crystalline lens is clear and spryly responsive to the ciliary muscle, may be able to overcome any problems with blurriness or difficulties in seeing near objects by the accommodation process, i.e. pulling it into focus. But with age, and over time as the lens grows tougher and more resistant to the ciliary muscle, that gradually becomes harder and harder. Though in many instances in ages gone by, relatively minor long-sightedness may not have been a huge handicap.

Back in 1286 or thereabouts when spectacles were originally developed, the number of those who could read or write, or ever needed to, was tiny. If life wasn't quite as nasty, brutish and short as is often supposed, providing you survived childhood, it was still the case that famine, disease and violence could reduce life expec-tations, killing off plenty before they got round to suffering from presbyopia, leaving only a limited pool of people in the Middle

Ages who might require the earliest glasses which were primarily to aid ageing readers. Though if, as epidemiologists Maria Patrizia Carreri and Diego Serraino maintain, 'landholders, monks and members of the Vatican were likely to be better fed, clothed, sheltered and had access to better medical care and survived longer' than their less fortunate contemporaries, there appears to be a strong correlation between those who lived longer and those who might have needed to continue to consult written documents and books after the wearying of their crystalline lenses.

Of course in a pre-industrial age when physical characteristics determined professions far more profoundly, the short-sighted might also have been expected to be heavily represented among monks, at least. For the ability to see close-up, if not far away, biologically equipped the medieval short-sighted for such priestly professions as calligrapher, scribe, copyist and book-keeper – jobs where intense concentration on the fine detail was required. The myopic also therefore made good tailors, engravers, weavers, goldsmiths, cobblers, notaries and merchants, but perhaps obviously enough rather poor hunters, soldiers, sailors, shepherds and herdsmen. These professions inevitably entailed the scanning of distant horizons, battlefields, oceans and fields, for prey, rival forces, shorelines and errant livestock. A consequence of this division of labour – always a slightly unequal one, since the short-sighted were only ever in the minority – was, of course, to put the myopic in the realm of less heroically active employment. Their professional tasks, after all, were undertaken for the most part indoors and at workbenches and desks rather than out in the open with animals and/or arms. Of course as the Middle Ages progressed and western societies evolved more sophisticated bureaucracies, trading arrangements, farming techniques and printing methods, myopes would come to enjoy greater positions of privilege and political power as Churchmen, lawyers, accountants and administrators. However, the acutely myopic, particularly those of humble origins, might also be confined to medieval hospices with the similarly economically inactive elderly, infirm and insane. The 'near blind', the historian Tomas Maldonado has noted, is a common category of inmate in the records of such institutions. These people, Maldonado suggests, were probably among the more fortunate with plenty of impoverished myopes 'seen as undesirables' and even 'forced to live outside the walls of the fortified settlements' among 'the motley rabble of outcasts'.

Perhaps a factor in their exclusion, and an issue for myopes of all classes, is that uncorrected short-sightedness makes social interactions much more difficult. In the highly stratified world of earlier times, lords and ladies of the manor expected due deference and doffed caps. Convivial relationships with local employers, fellow workers, neighbours and friends were (then and as now) greased with polite greetings and subtle acts of courtesy. The myopic in these circumstances could be held to be aloof, rude or insubordinate for their inability to respond to the expected cues. The near and not so near blind might struggle to recognise members of their own family on the other side of the street, let alone distant acquaintances. An error of vision might be perceived as a slight. The better-sighted, even if aware of the other's myopia, might still be left wondering if they had been purposely ignored rather than merely visually out of range. The suspicion is that the short-sighted person is only seeing what they want to see. Or that they are somehow using their myopia selectively to get out of things they don't want to do, only adding untrustworthiness to the many negative traits of these awkward, bookish shirkers of hard graft.

Nearly 500 years after the arrival of glasses with concave lenses to correct the condition, even otherwise respected medical professionals could still be found bemoaning the general appallingness of the short-sighted. In an article entitled 'Physical Defects in Character' and published in 1930, a certain Dr Rice explained in some detail why he believed the myopic child invariably grew into a rum old adult. The passage in question is worth quoting at length for its football coach-like take on childhood development:

A near-sighted child cannot do well on the playground because he cannot see. He will not like to hunt because he cannot see the game or the sights of his gun. He will not like to tramp because distant objects are poorly seen and, for that reason, not appreciated. He will not like races or aviation or travel or sports of any sort. As a rule these persons do not like the theatre, or the motion picture, and are likely to have the idea that the latter, especially, is entertainment for children only, or they might say for morons. It is because they cannot see the pictures clearly. But in school the situation is different. It is so easy to see and so wonderful to read as there are none of the diverting influences that draw the attention of the normal child, or the motor-minded boy, to the fields, the park and the woods. The child who knows that he cannot excel over his fellows in games gets a big satisfaction out of the conquest of the mind that he can command. After all, he reasons, this is what is really important. Ball games, hunting and fishing are a waste of time. What does it matter if one cannot do those things? He sees the fine details. When his classmates make mistakes the book-worm jumps to his feet with his hand in the air. He pleases his teacher but he loses his friends. He gets a reputation as a know it all and a grind and is popular only the days before the final examination. He does not count in athletics or parties, he is not one of the bunch. Such a child as we have described is not dependent on others for entertainment and is liable to grow rather contemptuous of the abilities of others. He does not adapt himself to the surroundings, and is not willing to make compromises. He is often severe in his righteousness and his rightness and may become a disagreeable personage.

Ida Mann and Antoinette Pirie, writing just a few years later on the dangers of not giving glasses to the short-sighted child, were to make some similar observations, implying that the myopic could be prone to Walter Mitty-like daydreaming too:

A child who develops short sight fairly early in school life and is allowed to grow up without glasses acquires usually a distinctive and slightly peculiar character, since it is cut off from and simply does not understand many of the things that help in the development of the normal child in a long-sighted world. First of all, it is intensely interested in books and in all fine detail and very bored with games. This is understandable, as if you cannot see a ball till it is within three yards of you, you have very little chance of catching or hitting it accurately, and if you are no good at games you cannot be expected to be interested in them. You can, of course, read for hours without effort and so tend to live in a world of books and fantasy, in which you wander dreamily about, getting a name for standoffishness, since you pass your friends in the street and never bother to pay much attention to the real world.

## The Holy See

Given such views, it might then seem somewhat ironic that one of the most famous myopes known to have availed themselves of early concave-lensed spectacles was Pope Leo X. His example contradicts the preceding handwringing predictions for the social prospects of myopic youth: he was both a worldly statesman, one with rather extravagant material tastes for a man of God, and an immensely enthusiastic huntsman. As even Vincent Ilardi notes, Leo (christened Giovanni di Lorenzo and born into the prominent Florentine Medici family in 1475) was 'a bon vivant' who 'enjoyed parties' and 'baser amusements' and 'does not fit the typical personality of myopes ... usually introverted, bookworms, "nerds", shunning sociability'. Yet myopia and hypermetropia are largely hereditary conditions, the size of eyes, like the shape of a nose or the colour of hair, passed on through the generations.* And it has been argued that the Medici clan's short-sightedness most

---

* However, contemporary studies also show that environmental factors, especially spending time indoors and looking at nearby objects, including screens and books, when young may affect eye growth and increase any propensity to short-sightedness. Alarm bells have already been raised about the possible long-term effects of home-schooling and digital learning during the Covid-19 epidemic on the eyesight of a whole generation of children. (See Chapter 13 for more on the rising instance of myopia in recent decades.)

likely contributed to their initial success in the fields of finance, wool and politicking. Leo's forebears, precluded for the most part by persistent weak eyesight and inconstant physical health from successful soldiering, found their outlet in banking and commerce. Having amassed their fortune, they were able to wield serious political power by often exceedingly unsavoury means and bank-roll endeavours artistic and scientific in their Florentine fiefdom. Their well-attested patronage of the visual and literary arts was itself most probably another symptom of short-sightedness – a condition that, as Mann and Pirie put it, sometimes leads to an intense interest in 'books and in all fine detail'.

Leo aside, much of the evidence of the Medicis' myopia is slightly circumstantial. Nevertheless, convincing enough references to their 'bad sight' and 'poor eyes' abound in the contemporary records. And in descriptions of the individual Medicis' appearances there are numerous references to their 'beautiful large eyes' – possibly a sign of myopia, since the myopic eyeball is usually larger and often with bigger pupils. Alternatively, it might indicate thyroid disease in the family rather than optical issues. Lorenzo the Magnificent, saluted by Niccolò Machiavelli as 'the greatest protector of art and literature', was elsewhere reported to have had prominent if weak eyes. Artists tasked with immortalising members of the dynasty often, it seems, took care to emphasise the family's distinctive if defective eyes in their pictures. Lorenzo's brother, the 'brilliant'-eyed Giuliano, assassinated at twenty-five, was, for instance, drawn with his eyelids half shut in portraits by both Bronzino and Botticelli. While Lorenzo's son Piero (known to history as Piero the Unfortunate for surrendering Florence to King Charles VIII of France in 1494), said to possess 'remarkably beautiful eyes', was subjected to what might be described as two eye-catching studies by Botticelli and Gherardo di Giovanni del Fora. To the modern viewer Piero looks more bug-eyed than beautiful in these pictures. His watery-green eyes appear as bulbous as golf balls and half curtained with lids that look as heavy as shopfront shutters. It has been suggested that myasthenia gravis could be the cause of such drooping lids.

But despite this ocularly odd lineage, only Leo is definitively known to have worn glasses to correct his short sight. Though never pictured with his spectacles, which he is said to have dispensed with in public after his elevation to the papal throne in 1513, Leo was shown holding a single concave lens in a gold-handled frame in a portrait of him with two cardinals, Giulio de Medici and Luigi de Rossi. Painted by Raphael in the fifth year of Leo's reign, he is dressed in a crimson cap and robes, and seated at a desk or table draped in a scarlet cloth on which an illuminated Bible rests. He holds the lens in his left hand and is flanked on either side by the cardinals in their red robes and caps. They stand behind his chair, a sturdy-looking near-throne upholstered with a thick cushion in crimson velvet with red braid trimmings.* The scene is slightly ambiguous. What might be a small silver and gold bell also sits on the table by the Bible, suggesting that possibly the Pope has used it to summon these minions. But the aggrieved expression on his corpulent face implies that the Pope has been interrupted by them unexpectedly while contentedly studying the scriptures with his myopia-adjusting lens. Frowning a bit, he certainly seems to be eyeing Giulio to his right with what looks like open hostility. While Luigi behind him to his left grips the chair with both hands and glances shamefacedly out at the viewer, as if embarrassed by whatever events are going on.

In either scenario it's possible that Leo's face, however grumpily, is merely registering their presence – which since he is not wearing his glasses, nor looking through his lens, may not have occurred until they were almost on top of him. Leo's myopia was severe enough to mean he struggled to see clearly anything further than four inches away from him. Not that this seems to have prevented him from hunting, a sport he and a good many of his cardinals undertook each autumn in the countryside outside Rome, despite

---

* Much of the painting is, in fact, red, a colour associated with Christ's blood and Christian martyrdom and worn accordingly by His emissaries on Earth in the upper echelons of the Roman Catholic Church. And therefore leaving Raphael with a somewhat limited colour palette to play with here.

the Pope's twin handicap of being grotesquely overweight. But just as his lack of physical mobility was compensated for by a horse with enough stamina to bear his bulk, so it is recorded that an optical device, usually billed as a 'crystal concave lens', was used to overcome the limitations of his sight when pursuing beasts of the chase. In a letter to the Marchioness Isabella of Mantua in May 1518, Antonio de Beatis provided a first-hand account of Leo using a very similar lens to the one in the Raphael painting to finish off a deer at close quarters during a recent hunt. The animal had seemingly become trapped in a cloth barrier that served as the paling to keep the beasts within range. The Pope, spotting the unfortunate animal as it struggled to escape, headed after it. Reaching the prone stag, he dismounted and waddled the final feet towards it with a lance in one hand and the lens held up to his eye with the other. Fixing the prey firmly in sight, he then set about delivering the mortal blow. Under the rules of the hunt this counted as a fair kill. But it doesn't seem especially sporting nor likely to have enhanced the dignity of his office much. Something he was obviously concerned enough about to avoid wearing spectacles when performing his normal duties – lest he seem less infallible, perhaps.

Papal accounts, however, confirm that Leo continued to use glasses in private. Within the first three months of his coronation he spent fifty-six ducats on spectacles and twenty-five ducats on a single monocle. Some of these glasses would have been purchased as gifts, to demonstrate the new Pope's magnanimity. But this is still a fortune at a time when the most luxurious pairs of spectacles, framed in precious metals and with the finest crystal lenses, cost around a ducat and Leo was paying the keeper of his hunting dogs a salary of four ducats a month.

Even if the Pope had wanted to wear his glasses when going about his daily business – delivering liturgies, commissioning sacristies by Michelangelo, excommunicating Martin Luther for drawing up his ninety-five theses condemning the practices of the Catholic Church – he may have encountered a few practical problems anyway. Practical problems that much like a pair of scissors for the left-handed stem from the very fact that glasses were first designed to help ageing presbyopic eyes to continue to do close work, not to aid a short-sighted minority to see further every day. And as already stated several times now, they stayed that way for nearly two centuries.

The earliest evidence we have of glasses for short-sightedness is found in Italian ducal documents from the middle of the fifteenth century and only finally collated and verified in the 1970s. What might be the oldest reference to glasses with lenses for distance appears intriguingly, considering the Medicis' reputation for myopia, in a letter sent to Leo's grandfather, Piero di Cosimo de Medici (also known as Piero the Gouty after the ailment that frequently confined him to bed), from Ardouino da Baesse on 24 August 1451. Ardouino, in Ferrara, writes to acknowledge the receipt of four pairs of glasses from Florence. He complains, though, that one of the pairs has arrived with broken lenses and asks if a near-sighted replacement could be arranged, since all the other three pairs are for 'distant vision'.

More substantial proof of glasses for short-sightedness in Florence in this period comes in an exchange of letters between the Duke Francesco Sforza of Milan and Nicodemo Tranchedini da Pontremoli, his ambassador to the Tuscan city. In a missive dated 21 October 1462, the duke asks Tranchedini to acquire three dozen pairs of eyeglasses 'placed in cases so that they will not break' for him from Florence, since, as he comments, 'it is reputed that they are made more perfectly [there] than in any other place in Italy'. He specifies that a dozen of these eyeglasses should be 'those apt and suitable for distant vision, that is for the young; another [dozen] that are suitable for near vision, that is for the elderly', and finally a third dozen for what he calls 'normal vision'. Tranchedini fulfilled the duke's request and dispatched the spectacles with a letter addressed to his secretary on 4 November. Which means that the order must have been completed in less than a fortnight. This level of efficiency in processing a bulk order indicates that spectacle making in Florence had become a highly sophisticated mass-manufacturing operation by then. More importantly, this letter confirms it was also by now regularly churning out spectacles for 'young' (i.e. myopic) eyes as well as those for the 'elderly' – and at quite reasonable rates too. The final price for the duke's thirty-six eyeglasses, which Tranchedini stresses are of the highest quality, was just three ducats, which works out at around seven *soldi* a pair. Subsequent correspondence between the duke and Tranchedini reveals that the ambassador was myopic and used Florentine eyeglasses himself.

It is, of course, conceivable that concave spectacles for shortsightedness were produced long before the 1450s, and that since such lenses are a mere inversion of the convex type that spectacle makers all over Europe were familiar with, there is no reason to suppose that craftsmen in other cities could not have figured out how to make them by this time. If, that is, they'd put their minds to it. Yet nothing has come to light so far to suggest they did. Again, with all their energies directed to supplying glasses for the 'normal'-sighted majority who in an increasingly literate world dominated by new accountancy systems and international trade needed to hang on to their close sight as they aged, the myopes were less of a priority.

In Florence, however, glass workers and spectacle makers in this era were living in an intensely creative intellectual and artistic crucible, a city where the system of linear perspective that opened the door to far more representative Renaissance art was formally set down by Filippo Brunelleschi, the architect who gave Florence's Cathedral of Santa Maria del Fiore its domed roof in 1436. Matters of distance – how it might more convincingly be depicted in a two-dimensional painting, how buildings and streets could be laid out to produce the most aesthetically pleasing of views – were topics that interested Florentine thinkers, artists and artisans. And with a de facto ruling house of myopes there would potentially be a greater incentive for those engaged in optics to consider the problem of distance vision. The person who perfected spectacles to assist short-sightedness could expect to enjoy the patronage of some of the wealthiest and most powerful members of Florentine society. Their necessities here, conceivably, proving the mother to this invention. There is, it should be stressed, no direct causal link between the Medicis and concave-lensed spectacles, only a coincidence of time and place. Still, it seems more than serendipitous that of all the spectacle-making cities in the world, Florence under the Medicis was the first to cater for the short-sighted.

One difficulty for these first short-sighted spectacle wearers, however, was that while lenses had finally arrived to suit their needs, the shape of the frames themselves initially remained much the same. If now more likely featuring a bridge to connect the two circular lenses rather than a basic rivet, these frames, tooled in metal or bone, were nevertheless still designed to perch on the nose. This was perfectly fine for sitting down and studying something close-up, but far less cop if you wanted to roam out into the world and gaze at things in the distance that previously were beyond view, or chase after boar on a horse, say, as they wouldn't stay put for long. Hence perhaps Leo's own choice of a hand-held single concave lens for hunting rather than the spectacles he is generally believed to have eschewed. The issue would continue to vex spectacle wearers and makers alike for centuries to come. An elaborate but largely unsatisfactory and uncomfortable solution advanced in Leo's own day was to fix the glasses on to a forehead frame. This was usually a band of metal which was worn on the head in the manner of the diagnostic mirrors sported invariably by doctors in Leo Cullum's classic *New Yorker* cartoons, if perhaps far less often in the medical profession at large.

## Catch the king's eye

As many historians of the Protestant Reformation have wryly commented, Pope Leo X was short-sighted in one other vital respect too. He failed to see that the discontent fomented in Germany by the theologian Martin Luther, who protested against the abuse of the indulgences sold to finance grand papal schemes such as the construction of the basilica of St Peter in Rome, would end up splitting the western Church in two. Who knows, perhaps Leo's foresight would have been better if he'd worn his glasses in office. Little could he have suspected that Henry VIII, upon whom in 1521 he conferred the title Defender of the Faith for penning his anti-Lutheran tract *Assertio Septem Sacramentorum Adversus Martinum Lutherum* (Declaration of the Seven Sacraments Against Martin Luther), would ever break with Rome. But then perhaps Henry eyed things differently because, unlike Leo, the monarch owned a suit of armour with a pair of rivet-style spectacles bolted on to the visor of its helmet.

This suit was a specially commissioned gift to the young English king from the Holy Roman Emperor Maximilian I. Fashioned in the Innsbruck workshop of Konrad Seusenhofer, goldsmith and armourer to the emperor, it was presented to Henry in around 1514. All that remains of the suit today is its extraordinary helmet, which is held at the Royal Armouries in Leeds. And its very extraordinariness is probably the only reason it survived and wasn't melted down for scrap soon after the Civil War – the most likely fate of the rest of the suit, along with several other items from the wife-dispatching king's armoury. The helmet boasts a grotesquely anthropomorphic visor, essentially a full metal mask of a human face with a nose piece, eye-shaped slits for viewing and a teeth-filled grille for the mouth. Further facial features, such as curled lips, skiable cheekbones and a chin indented as if to appear grazed with a day or so of stubble, add to its macabre life-like quality. Crowning the helmet are two great curly metal horns, beastly enough for Baphomet.

However, the addition of a pair of oversized round-rimmed copper rivet spectacles (probably originally finished with gilt), fixed on over the eye holes, means the overall effect is rather more madcap than sinister. The whole thing is perhaps more reminiscent of the Blue Meanies from the Beatles' *Yellow Submarine* cartoon than Dennis Wheatley and *The Devil Rides Out*. Which could also explain why the armour was long believed to have been bequeathed to Henry's court jester, Will Somers – a fool canny enough to go on to entertain the Protestant Edward VI and the Catholic Queen 'Bloody' Mary I.

As the king's waistline burgeoned, especially in the wake of a jousting accident in 1536 – an event that nearly killed him and pre-cipitated a marked decline in his physical and mental health – the suit's regal lifespan must have been fairly brief. Having come close to being blinded in an earlier jousting bout back in 1524, when an opponent's lance struck him just above the right eye and after which the king suffered from migraines for the rest of his days, Henry was plagued with ocular complaints in the latter years of life. His vision seems to have shrunk practically in direct contrast to the gains he made in weight and girth. With suppurating sores claiming his once athletic legs, the often immobile king was by 1544 ordering pairs of glasses from Germany in batches of ten. Royal accounts for that year record the purchase of 'ten pairs of spectacles at 4d the pair, 3s 4d'. Other repeat orders, the Tudor historian Robert Hutchinson has suggested, might imply that the king had a distinct proclivity for losing (and/or breaking) his spectacles.*

Eventually in the final two years of his life, and to save him the bother of having to clamp those spectacles on to his nose and the acute pain of reading and then signing the countless papers that came into the Privy Chamber, three of his most trusted function-aries – Sir Anthony Denny, John Gates and William Clerk – were sanctioned to sign off official documents on his behalf using a special 'dry stamp'. Including, as it turned out, his last will and testament.

After Henry's death in 1547 an inventory of his possessions was ordered. That tally took a full eighteen months to complete. Alongside the 9150 guns, cannons or other pieces of artillery, over 2000 pieces of tapestry, 2028 pieces of plate, seven rackets for tennis and 'a staff of unicorn's horns garnished with silver gilt and 9 stones in the top', the late king was calculated to own

---

* There is a portrait of Thomas More attributed to the Flemish school that depicts Henry's former Lord Chancellor, executed in 1535 for refusing to accept the king's divorce and the split from Rome, absorbed in his reading. A small book is clutched in both hands and a pair of spectacles lodged far down his nose, the flesh of his nostrils helping to keep them in place. What's particularly notice-able is that there is a crack in the left lens of these glasses. Whether the artist chose to include this detail as a metaphorical comment on his patron's inability to see the religio-political situation clearly or out of artistic veracity we cannot know. But it does show that even wealthy men were prepared to make do with slightly dodgy glasses if they allowed them to keep at their books.

forty-one spectacles and assorted reading aids, ranging from 'a brode glass to loke yppon a boke' (a broad glass to look upon a book), 'a grene stone ... to reade with', 'glasse to reede with' and multiple spectacles (spellings also as various) in gilt, horn or silver. The pair on his helmet appear unaccounted for but could potentially have been lumped in with the armaments. Or they might by that time have long passed into the possession of jester Will, and accordingly were quite possibly deployed to amuse Henry's heir whenever the pre-teen king was not earnestly furthering the Protestantisation of the English Church and state.

The one area of theology in which Henry VIII was ultimately in agreement with Martin Luther was that scripture should take precedent over any papal authority. And of all the changes to be unleashed by the Reformation begun in his reign – the dissolution of monastic houses, the ending of the adoration of saints and relics and the stripping of altars and rood screens of their elaborate decorations – his order in 1538 that a Bible in English rather than Latin should be placed in every parish church in the land would do most to encourage literacy in the population and so, by default, widen spectacle use in the long term.

If Henry, as a king, had a helmet augmented with spectacles, lowlier souls in this period appear more regularly to have looked to their hats as somewhere to affix their glasses. This was an option memorably exercised by the self-absorbed Panurge in *Gargantua and Pantagruel*, François Rabelais' exuberantly scatological early sixteenth-century comic masterwork. Beyond the pages of bawdy French satire it was commonly resorted to in order simply to ease the sheer discomfort spectacles might cause to the nose.

In *On the Use of Glasses*, published in 1628 and one of the earliest books on the topic, the Spanish pioneer of optical sciences Benito Daza de Valdés used a mock dialogue between a doctor and his student to consider just this matter. He suggested that to prevent 'too much swelling of the nose' spectacles might usefully be 'attached to a wing or a paddle'. This could then be 'inserted between the hat and the head' allowing spectacles to be used without touching the nose. The student retorts that this would be fine for a nobleman or a king but not practical for lesser mortals like himself who have continually to doff their caps. Valdés' doctor concedes the point but still goes on to berate those, like Thomas More, 'who put their glasses so heavily on the end of their nose that they can neither speak freely nor let the humour flow from there'. He is, however, seemingly heartened by the sight of 'others' whom he believes are 'better advised' and who have taken to attaching their spectacles 'to the ears by a cord in order to free the hands'.

This method of wearing glasses was immortalised in a famed portrait by El Greco of Fernando Niño de Guevara from around 1600. The Crete-born first master of the Spanish school of painting depicts the cardinal and Grand Inquisitor of Spain (a man credited with burning at least 240 heretics during the fleeting two or three years he held the latter post) seated on a heavy padded chair similar to that earlier enjoyed by Leo X, and just as luxuriously clad in the crimson religious robes of his office. De Guevara has a pointed salt and pepper beard and wears a pair of black roundish glasses, with a tiny bridge over the nose. These appear securely fixed to his head by two cords that run from the corner of each side of the frame in a horizontal V-shape above and below the ears and are then fastened at the back of the head. It's rather like he has donned a highly ineffectual mask (though glasses do obscure part of the face and therefore act, as always, as a kind of disguise). But in comparison with the detail El Greco has lavished on capturing the folds in de Guevara's stiff silk garments, the glasses in this painting have a crude, slightly tacked-on feel about them. Almost as if they have been scrawled on as a joke after the fact in the manner of those old Athena posters where the Mona Lisa might be graffitied with a cartoon beard and specs, or cheekily embellished with sunglasses and a joint.

In another portrait painted around the same time, Hieronymus Capivaccius (also known as Girolamo Capivaccio), the Paduan professor of philosophy and medicine who published a practical manual for would-be practitioners of the healing arts in 1597, was also shown sporting a pair of strung-on spectacles. This image subsequently circulated through the various engravings that

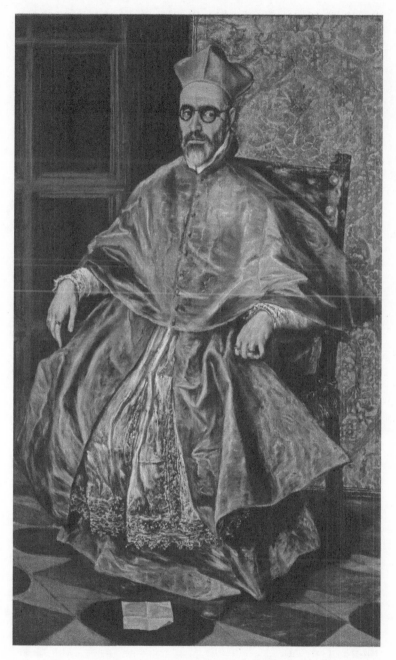

Portrait of Fernando Niño de Guevara, El Greco, 1600.

accompanied his printed works. But if obviously found in Italy and other parts of the continent, this style of spectacle seems to have remained largely confined to Spain – where, incidentally, wearing glasses, and the larger the better, became in the sixteenth and early seventeenth centuries briefly highly fashionable among the aristocracy and even for women in the higher ranks of society (more on this later, too). One foreign visitor to the country observed that 'The greater a person's fortune, the larger his spectacle glasses, to the extent that certain great men of Spain wear glasses as large as the hand.'

The bulk of the rest of Europe, meanwhile, failed to fall for glasses to anything like the same degree. And having judged the cords a foppish Iberian affectation, just as fiddly, irritating and uncomfortable as having glasses that slipped down the nose, this Spanish innovation was rejected by and large. Though with the further development of leather framed spectacles in Germany in this era, spectacle makers in Nuremberg in and around 1600 did produce some designs for glasses in horn and leather with straps that tied at the back of the head. In the drawings of them they look rather like goggles. Primitive forerunners, no less, to the type early motorists and World War One flying aces snapped on with a certain raffish air – an insouciant action that not so subtly broadcast the thrills and the deadly hazards of newfound speeds and man-made flight.

But no doubt more expensive to make, prone to wear, and perhaps tricky to keep tied in place, these early leather-strapped glasses failed to supplant simpler and cheaper nose spectacles. The near simultaneous arrival of metal wire, copper in particular, at this juncture allowed Nuremberg *Metallarbeiterinnen* to fashion both rims and a bridge for a basic pair of nose spectacles with just a few twists and turns of a single length of wire. And at a fraction of the cost of bone or even leather frames. Such wire nose spectacles, it must be reiterated, would continue to meet the needs of the majority of older presbyopia-afflicted wearers for the foreseeable future in any case.

# The Chinese way

Fascinatingly, the only other part of the world outside of Spain where spectacles with cords were a definite hit was east Asia, particularly in China and Japan, and it was long believed that spectacles of this sort were quite possibly invented in China. Some historians in years gone by even went so far as to posit the idea that the first spectacles were exported to Italy from China by Venetian traders such as Marco Polo. Aside from being a feasible-sounding story of cross-continental fertilisation, and one whose plausibility has been enhanced by verifiable accounts of how such Chinese innovations as paper, porcelain and gunpowder reached us, there is alas no proof either way for this. If anything, there is more to suggest that the traffic, at least in terms of Venice and glass (if not also glasses), probably went the other way. Certainly during a period in the 1330s when relations between the last Yuan dynasty emperor Toghon Temür (Shundi) and Pope Benedict XII in Avignon were at their most cordial, the Pope is known to have sent a retinue to China bearing an array of rich gifts that included examples of the finest Murano glass and crystal wares. But the subsequent Ming dynasty all but closed China to westerners in 1368. This policy of exclusion was to hold until 1514, when the sea passage opened by the Portuguese to India was extended to the Chinese coast and contact between China and Europe was tentatively restored.

Among those subsequently to beat a path to the east were Counter-Reformation missionaries from Franciscan, Dominican and Augustinian orders. And most significantly of all, members of the Society of Jesus, or Jesuits, founded in Spain in 1534 with the objective of 'converting the pagans'. By 1582, the Italian Matteo Ricci had founded a permanent Jesuit mission in China at Macao. Ricci was to become the first westerner to enter the Forbidden City and later translated Confucius into Latin. He also presented the Ming emperor Wanli (Zhu Yijun) with gifts such as European clocks and maps.* It has often been claimed that either he or one of the brothers of his order was also responsible for introducing spectacles to China at this time.

Yet there is much to suggest that the Chinese had a form of glasses long before that date. However, these spectacles were seemingly not fitted with lenses to aid presbyopia, hypermetropia or myopia. Instead their frames held discs of varying shades and transparencies of natural rock crystals and minerals, known as tea stones, that were believed to possess healing qualities. These were intended to shade the eyes from the glare of the sun or soothe inflamed eyes rather than enhance vision as such and were worn in a state of repose, much more like sunglasses or eyeshades than spectacles. Sadly it's impossible to say with any accuracy if these pre-dated the first European spectacles. Or whether they developed as a kind of distinctively Chinese interpretation of those brought over by the Venetians in the Mongol era. A type of non-spectacle spectacle, if you will, that evolved in line with China's own deep-seated spiritual and medical traditions during the country's long years of isolation, unaware of the miracle of concave lenses for myopia beyond its borders.

In *Glass Exchange between Europe and China: 1550–1800*, Emily Byrne Curtis notes that the opening line of a verse by the Chinese poet Li Fu refers to his reading glasses affectionately as a 'strange object' that has come 'from foreign lands'. Fu was writing in the 1740s, and yet nearly 200 years after the Jesuits' arrival in China still apparently regarded spectacles with optical lenses (in contrast, quite possibly, to the traditional Chinese frames with types of translucent quartz known as tea stones) as otherly and western.

Some fifty years later, Hugh Gillan, the physician to Lord

---

* Chinese cartography up to that point, and reflecting its years in near complete isolation from the world at large, was decidedly self-centred. Ricci would recall that 'The Chinese had printed maps of the world with titles such as "Description of the World" in which China was all, occupying the field with its fifteen provinces, and round the edge they depicted a little sea where a few islets were dotted about, on which they wrote the names of all the kingdoms of which they had ever heard; and these all put together would not have equalled in one size one of the provinces of China.'

Macartney, the English ambassador to China during the reign of Emperor Ch'ien-lung, saw craftsmen in Guangdong making spectacles who, as he recorded in 1793, still 'did not seem to understand any optical principles for forming them in different manners so as to accommodate them to various imperfect vision'.

Chinese importation documents record that Catholic missionaries continued to give European spectacles with corrective lenses as gifts well into the eighteenth century.

Yet a persistent element in almost all accounts of glasses in China in these centuries are references to the cords or strings used to keep them in place; Gillan certainly noted them in his journal. Contemporary pen and ink drawings of Chinese spectacle wearers and thousands of extant antique examples reveal that quite elaborate combinations of ropes and pulleys were often deployed, with additional weights, for example, attached to the ends of the strings like pendulums, to ensure they stayed put – a tradition that continued in some quarters of the nation until surprisingly recently.

Byrne Curtis argues that the historic use of heavier crystal and mineral lenses might go some way to explaining this cultural predilection for tying the glasses to the head. Even if so, it remains another intriguing coincidence that it was a predilection also shared by the Spanish nation – the land, after all, from which the Jesuits originally sprang. Similarly it is amusing to note that Fernando Niño de Guevara, the bestringed spectacle wearer in El Greco's portrait who embraced this Spanish fashion, was demoted by the Pope from Grand Inquisitor of Spain to Bishop of Seville for his fervent opposition to the Jesuits.

But in the next stage in the story of spectacles, merchants rather than clergy will lead the way, though those fleeing religious persecution will take a significant role in their advancement.

# 3

# An Enlightened Company

In the middle of the City of London, at 111 Cannon Street, just opposite a branch of Boots the Chemists and Cannon Street Station, a somewhat unprepossessing slab of limestone sits on display behind a pane of glass in the front wall of an undistinguished office block. Yet this rock, an object of utter indifference to most of the city workers in its vicinity, is *the* London Stone. A boulder that tradition maintains Brutus, Britain's mythic first king, brought from Troy and that the Kentish rebel Jack Cade struck his staff on and declared himself 'Lord of London' upon entering the capital in 1450 – an incident dramatised and embellished by Shakespeare in *Henry VI Part 2* where Cade also uses the stone as a makeshift throne. It has variously been claimed to have served as a monolithic Roman marker, a druidic altar (where in William Blake's poetic reimaginings gruesome human sacrifices were performed) and a sacred rock of destiny on which ancient British kings swore their oaths of ascension. Perhaps most preposterously, it has even been peddled as the rock from which King Arthur extracted his sword Excalibur.

Whatever other and possibly far murkier shenanigans went on at this spot in earlier times, late seventeenth-century documents from the Worshipful Company of Spectacle Makers provide one of the few credible records of the London Stone actually being put to a practical end. As the livery company granted a monopoly on the sale and manufacture of spectacles in London, it used the stone to smash to pieces items sold in contravention of its charter.

In this game of sedimentary rock versus spectacles, the glasses were the obvious losers. Though as noted in the account of the judgment against Mrs Elizabeth Bagnall, a widow whose haberdasher's shop was raided on 3 August 1671 and found to contain 'two and twenty dozen of English spectacles ... all very badd in the glasse and frames not fitt to be on sale', while the offending items were destroyed on the 'remayning parte of London Stone', a hammer was needed to finish off the job.

Having formerly starred in a Shakespearean play and been cherished as a remove-at-your-peril, ravens-in-the-tower piece of London's sacred geography, such a role seems beneath the stone's dignity. But the symbolism of using such a fixture to demonstrate the might of the City authorities would not have been lost on those who witnessed these showy trials.

At this point in the twenty-first century, the devil is in the data. Almost anyone can sell you anything, and self-avowed disrupters look to evade the most cursory of regulations operating outside of cyberspace. These days, the system of guilds that prevailed until mass industrialisation looks astonishingly, almost enchantingly, repressive. This was surveillance capitalism mark one, in the sense that every single craft was rigidly policed. In order to practise any particular trade, membership of an approved guild was required. In the case of spectacle making, a profession that didn't exist before the fourteenth century, its first practitioners had to operate in existing guilds until their numbers and expertise grew significant enough to be granted their own body. This process seems to have happened far faster on the continent. In Paris, for example, spectacle makers, if initially lumped in with mirror and later also toy makers, were already a recognised entity by 1465. By contrast, their counterparts in the City of London were so marginal that they were not even listed in an official survey of its trades published in the same period. Even after becoming a known quantity London's spectacle makers would have to be content with joining the Guild of Brewers until 1629 – effectively making all glasses in the capital beer goggles up to that point.*

No doubt there were practical reasons for these trades to converge in London. Some shared areas of expertise and mastery of the same basic materials, say. Horn, for instance, which could be turned into drinking vessels or spectacle frames alike. Or copper, which was traditionally the material for brewing vats, and might, in wire form at least, also be bent into shape as frames. Glassware might, of course, seem the most obvious linking point. And brewers were certainly experimenting with storing beer in glass bottles by the latter half of the sixteenth century. But all the research suggests that the commercial manufacture and sale of bottled ale would not really get under way until nearly a century later. By which point the spectacle makers had gone their own way.

The official history of the brewers company omits any reference to spectacle making. While the official history of the Worshipful Company of Spectacle Makers merely states that Robert Alt, the man who rallied support among 'friends and colleagues' for a petition to Charles I for a royal charter for the profession in 1628, was 'a Citizen and brewer' who 'practiced the craft of spectacle making in a shop on London Bridge'.

Alt's address on the bridge, if within the bounds of the City of London, nevertheless puts him in close proximity to the South Bank and Southwark. It is here where those two gentlemen of Flemish origins the van Bessens, the first documented spectacle makers in Britain, were living and working in the 1450s.

---

* In the pecking order of the City of London guilds set down in 1516, the brewers were ranked at number 14 in this commercial caste system. Two places, incidentally, below the esteemed Great Twelve Companies topped by the mercers, who were deemed the wealthiest and most prestigious of them all. The brewers' comparatively lowly ranking reflected their slightly disreputable reputation. Not so much for selling intoxicating liquids, but for watering their ale down and vending it in false measures – both common swindles back then. That spectacle makers, who proffered a product that altered the appearance of the wearer and made distant things appear nearer and near things further away, were relegated to a guild widely thought to be deceitful again hints at that persistent suspicion of glasses themselves.

Southwark was also an epicentre of brewing. Borough High Street was then lined with taverns catering to those journeying to and from London and earlier still on pilgrimages to Canterbury. Geoffrey Chaucer's own family had been vintners, trading with the Low Countries in particular. But it was Flemish and Dutch immigrants who settled in that area and brought with them continental notions of what beer should taste like. Crucially their recipes demanded that bitter hops be added to the more typical brew of fermented malted barley to improve the flavour.

I mention all this because it's another correlation between brewing and spectacle making – that headway was largely made in Britain by migrants from the Low Countries. When it came to optics in the late sixteenth and early seventeenth centuries, the period when London's spectacle makers chose to make their bid for autonomy, much of the running was being made in the land of dykes and pumping stations across the North Sea. Here, after all, was an emerging economic and cultural powerhouse. What would eventually become a whole new Protestant, if pluralistic, republic, one as dependent on international trade and fearful of rising tides as Venice before it. And just then entering an age that would be every bit as gilded in terms of wealth, economic ingenuity and intellectual and artistic creativity as any enjoyed by its Renaissance forerunner. A place set to become the first bourgeois market capitalist society. A nation that owed its increasing wealth to the spoils of shrewd stock-market speculation, slavery and colonial exploitation – an embarrassment of riches, to borrow the title of Simon Schama's classic study of the Dutch in this era.

Of all the innovations to emerge, though, from this confederation of Calvinist provinces in the alluvial delta of the Netherlands, there are two that can truthfully be said to have altered our entire perceptions of the world. And both quite conceivably emerged from the workshop of a single lens grinder and spectacle maker in Middelburg – the capital of the southwestern-most maritime region of Zeeland and a city whose circumstances, like those of Amsterdam, were to rise considerably after the fall of Antwerp to Catholic Spanish forces in 1585.

Hans Lippershey was an optical manufacturer born in Wesel on the Rhine in western Germany – though then yet another contested entrepôt fought over by the Dutch and the Spanish throughout the Eighty Years War – who seemingly found the stolidly Protestant if humanistically tinged Middelburg a more conducive place to ply his trade. Here in the late 1590s and early 1600s, alongside peddling spectacles, he conducted experiments with differing combinations of lenses that perhaps resulted in the creation of both the first compound microscope and the first refracting telescope, although other rival contenders for such claims exist, naturally enough. As it is, Lippershey usually has to share the credit for the microscope with Zacharias and Hans Janssen, a father-and-son team of fellow Middelburg spectacle makers; while Lippershey's designs for the telescope (including a binocular version), which he publicly demonstrated in 1608 and for which he applied for a patent, were almost immediately improved upon by Galileo. As if to rub salt into the wound, the Pisan-born astronomer would substantially refine the Lippershey-Janssens' Middelburg style of compound microscope for good measure too. Nevertheless, these Dutch-born devices can be said to have opened the door to the Enlightenment. They provided the necessary tools to embark on the course of modern scientific enquiry that was to follow, and one almost inconceivable without them. As the Norwegian writer Karl Ove Knausgaard has pointed out, they put 'the eye' at the centre of rational thinking, and in doing so helped supplant the idea of the mythic in which deeper meaning historically resided in what could not be observed.

And in England, as in Holland, these instruments were to be manufactured and sold by spectacle makers. Richard Reeve, from whom Samuel Pepys would buy a microscope in 1664 after marvelling at the device's ability to render 'a louse or mite ... most perfectly and largely', was a member of the Worshipful Company of Spectacle Makers. He was also appointed as the first official scientific instrument maker to the Royal Society, and supplied Robert Hooke, the author of the *Micrographia*, the ground-breaking 1665 study of microscopy, with one of his models too. Such developments seem a long way from beer, though Hooke did write about needing to dose an ant with brandy to get it to stay still enough for him to examine it properly.

But in distancing themselves from the brewers as such inventions were coming on stream, the Worshipful Company of Spectacle Makers were, consciously or not, to begin the task of assuming the mantle of sober men (and the odd woman) of science and business. The premises of the likes of Reeve offered the very instruments of enlightenment progress (if equally, in terms of the telescope, imperial expansionism) sought by people of quality such as Pepys. The company's founding charter sought, in particular, to suppress the sale of spectacles on the streets of the city itself by banning 'Hawkers and them that jett about'. It also strove to prevent any secondary market in spectacle parts by forbidding its members from selling either spectacle frames without lenses, or spectacle lenses without frames. Only the full package, as it were, was available from Worshipful makers themselves.

Still, their own shops largely remained workshops: places where spectacles and lenses were physically manufactured, or at least assembled. The stirrings of show rooms or primitive kinds of high-street retail spaces such as we might recognise today only just became discernible in this period. It was in 1625 that Charles I, for example, first granted London businesses the right to hang signs above their premises – 'FOR', as the deed put it, 'THE BETTER FINDING OF THEIR RESPECTIVE DWELLINGS'. Prior to that signs appear almost exclusively reserved for inns and taverns. Their appearance at this juncture speaks of an increasingly populous metropolis and an expansion of new specialist trades whose establishments might also need to be more prominent to visiting would-be clients.

Two years after spectacle makers acquired their charter, for instance, clockwork makers freed themselves from the blacksmiths to establish their own guild. (The tobacco-pipe makers were another guild to emerge in this era, with imports of 'brown gold' now regularly being shipped from Jamestown, Virginia.) Typically, the right to grind the glass faces for watches, a trade the spectacle makers claimed was justly theirs alone, would later become something of a bone of contention between the two guilds. To say nothing of the disputes that were to follow over the manufacturing of mathematical maritime instruments.

But the range of products spectacle makers made and sold was sometimes reflected in the signs adopted for their shops. The Worshipful Company's archives reveal members operating out of premises with such signs as 'The Great Golden Spectacles and Quadrant' and 'The Refracting Microscope'. Meanwhile others were to be discovered at the Pythagorean 'Three Spectacles', or such iconic signs as the 'Friar Bacon' and 'Sir Isaac Newton'. With the 'Archimedes and 3 Pair of Golden Spectacles' neatly combining the two. This latter emblem belonged to John Yarwell, who was evidently so taken with the sign that he kept it when he moved his premises from St Paul's Church Yard to Ludgate Street in 1697.

His trade card for the Ludgate Street address, headed 'Yarwell's True Spectacles' and featuring an image of the sign, provides a compelling snapshot of the type of glasses and plethora of other goods this particular spectacle maker offered for sale in this period. Yarwell seems to have been able to turn his hand to all manner of instruments, not all of them optical either. Alongside 'Telescopes of all Lengths for Day and Night', 'a new double microscope', 'Magnifying, Multiplying and Weather Glasses' and 'Reading glasses of all sizes', 'Speaking Trumpets' are offered as another Yarwell house speciality.

Other spectacle makers in this period were perhaps not quite so indiscriminate, but a number were. Beer, however, is noticeably absent from either Yarwell's or any of his contemporaries' trade cards.

Boasting of 'True Spectacles exactly ground on brass tools, after a new manner, approved by the Royal Society', Yarwell claimed his spectacles preserved 'the Eyes, either of young or old, so much that any person of Sixty years of Age, may see to Read the Smallest print as well as one of sixteen'. His customers had the choice too of 'Leather, Horn, Silver, Tortoise-shell and Steel-frames'.

## Shelling out and getting leathered by Continentals

Tortoiseshell was quite the new kid on the block at this point. The shells of what were actually Atlantic hawksbill sea turtles had then only recently started to arrive in Europe from the Caribbean. The frames, by rights, should really have been called 'turtleshell'. By the nineteenth century enormous stocks of these shells, most of them from the Bahamas, were being auctioned off at St Katharine's Dock on a quarterly basis. These auctions continued right up to 1939.

Not all of these shells were used for spectacles. A natural plastic, tortoiseshell was, and is, an extremely versatile and durable material that, until it was finally superseded by early synthetic substitutes like bakelite in the twentieth century, was used to make combs, knife-handles and jewellery and to surface and inlay cabinets and other pieces of furniture. Indeed it has been suggested that the fashion for women in Spain in the sixteenth century to wear large decorative tortoiseshell combs in their hair was possibly what led to it subsequently becoming such a popular material for spectacle frames in the first place.

Nevertheless, the process of separating the unfortunate turtle from its shell and then turning the shell into a spectacle frame was far from pretty, both unpleasant and arduous, involving a good deal of boiling all round. To prevent any damage to the plates of the shell, the animals were apparently routinely killed by turning them over on the sand and leaving them to die on their backs. Once they'd expired it was essential to boil the turtle's shell as soon as possible to ensure its colours didn't fade. Predictably, impatience often got the better of some of those involved in this business and many turtles were simply boiled to death. After the shells were removed, the plates were separated and sorted into different shades and thicknesses. Shipped raw, the shell plates would then be processed by their purchasers, who could transform them into pliable sheets with further rounds of boiling, steaming and pressing. A single slab of shell-sheet, about 6 inches long and 1½ inches wide, was all a spectacle maker needed for a complete frame. Easier to keep clean and gentler on the skin than most metals, tortoiseshell didn't warp or crack in extreme weather conditions and could be easily repaired by welding another piece into any break or gap in the frame.

Marine turtles have been a protected species since 1973 and trade in real tortoiseshell has been outlawed ever since. In John Yarwell's day it was in its infancy. As, incidentally, was whaling, another transatlantic trade that resulted in the near extinction of several species, but one that also furnished spectacle makers with baleen or whale bone, another material for frames. More controversial, however, was leather, which Yarwell, who ascended to the Worshipful Company's highest rank of master, was censured for using by its officials in 1692.

The company's firm line on leather spectacles stemmed, its official historian Frank Law believes, from their fear that their adoption would 'lead to a deterioration of workmanship employed in producing the more usual metal frames'. That spectacle makers in Nuremberg were also churning out leather frames in their dozens might also have influenced their decision. The ban seems to have been lifted, perhaps unsurprisingly, soon after Yarwell's final tenure as master of the company. For in 1694 John Marshall, another spectacle maker operating on Ludgate Street, was proudly, and seemingly without attracting the ire of the company, able to advertise 'neat Leather Frames for Spectacles, which are not subject to break as Horn or Tortois Shell', which he also described as 'the most serviceable of any other yet made'. Such durability might also have been initially held against them by guild members, who feared a loss in revenue from a fall in demand for replacement frames or repair work.

Nevertheless foreign imports, which in the late 1660s included a sudden glut of copper frames from France, were another of the company's bugbears, and those found to be selling unapproved overseas wares faced similar penalties. The manner and zeal with which its wardens and officials enforced its rules make them seem like prohibition-era G-men. They are forever off raiding premises and smashing up illicit eyewear with the righteousness of temperance campaigners discovering stills of bootleg moonshine. 'At the shop of Mr. John Hyefield two dozen of French spectacles set in white copper frames. The glass of them was broken by consent' runs a typical account of a search, this one undertaken on 29 April 1669 by the company wardens Mr John Radford and Mr John Verney. Further entries in the company's records seem to suggest that haberdashers such as Elizabeth Bagnall were rather frequent offenders. And often doubly so. For not only did they stray on to the spectacle makers' turf by selling specs in the first place, they also confounded the offence by peddling substandard products, as this entry, again detailing the exploits of Messrs Radford and Verney in 1669, illustrates: 'They found in Mr. Jekyll's shop a Haberdasher two paire of Spectacles being looking glasse ground only on one side, which by consent were rased over.' Intriguingly, quite a few weavers also appear to have had a side hustle in grinding watch glasses – something the company's attack dogs were dispatched to stamp out.

The company's aims, though, were noble enough. They were merely attempting to ensure the integrity of their trade and prevent shoddy spectacles flooding on to the market. After all, the company's own spectacle makers had to serve a seven-year apprenticeship before being able to practise. New apprentices were usually engaged at sixteen (a fee of a guinea had to be paid to take on trainees under that age) and therefore didn't obtain 'the freedom of the company' until they were twenty-three. Providing, of course, they'd learnt the art of spectacle making to their master's satisfaction. Each master was allowed only a single apprentice, though a second boy might be taken on towards the end of the first's training period. The engagement of any staff outside of such apprentice schemes was considered a serious offence, and attracted heavy fines of up to £5. Law documents cite the example of William Spencer, a spectacle maker in the Minories who in 1668 was fined £3 for employing his own son Thomas as an unbounded hand on the sly. 'Contrary to the ordinances' Thomas was found to be neither 'An Apprentice' spectacle maker nor to have served the mandatory 'Seaven yeares to the same Trade', and so Spencer senior was ordered 'no further' to employ him at 'the Trade of Spectacle-Making or anything thereunto belonging'.

If the Worshipful Company took great pains to police who could and could not make and sell spectacles, what might today be termed customer service often left much to be desired. There were still no eye tests, and purchasers were mostly left to select their spectacles for themselves. Such guidance as there was came from categorising the spectacles by the age the makers considered most suitable. Although the Spanish oculist Daza de Valdés had first attempted to establish a more formal system of numbering lenses by their varying strengths in 1623, trade adverts for John Marshall, our leather-frame-vending spectacle maker on Ludgate Street, some seventy-one years later still boasted of the ease of buying glasses from his shop because 'he doth set the age of the person on the frame ... as some people age 30 take glasses for 60 or 70. He does this to prevent mistakes, as some people have injured their eyes by buying the wrong frames.'

The difficulties in this period of obtaining a suitable pair of spectacles, or receiving adequate medical treatment for all but the most basic eye complaints, are more than borne out by the experiences of Samuel Pepys.

## A sight for sore eyes

A man with a wandering eye in more senses than one, Pepys abandoned his diary on 31 May 1669 convinced he'd go blind otherwise. It's tempting to wonder whether this foremost chronicler of his age might have stuck at it if he'd been better served by the spectacle makers and oculists he'd consulted before then.

He was just thirty-six. His journal had been kept doggedly, if furtively by candlelight and at the end of his working days, for the previous nine and a half years. Written in the then standard Shelton's system of shorthand deployed by clerks of Pepys' generation, it was only ever intended for his eyes only. As an added precaution, and lest it be read by his wife Elizabeth, passages touching on his extramarital dalliances with and/or opportunistic pawing of serving girls, tavern barmaids, and the daughters, wives and mothers of friends and colleagues (variously undertaken in their places of residence, work, leisure, at theatrical entertainments, in horse-drawn transport and even during religious worship) were completed in the loving tongues of Spanish, French and Latin.

There are those who contend that the problems Pepys later suffered with his eyes could have been the result of a syphilitic infection. And such a theory can't be discounted entirely. Syphilis was rife in Restoration England. The disease was no respecter of class or creed either, it infected prostitutes and aristocrats alike, although perhaps hitting aristocrats who visited brothels disproportionately hard. And since most aristocrats, in the spirit of those times of anti-puritan rebellion, did this with abandon, the disease was pretty widespread. The libertine and poet John Wilmot, Earl of Rochester, has become practically the historical poster boy for the disease in this epoch. Alongside 'ravenous chancres' on his penis, inflamed eyes and the eventual near complete loss of sight were among the symptoms of syphilis to have afflicted Rochester, whose nose also became so rotted by the disease he took to wearing a false one contrived of silver. In correspondence from 1671, a protracted absence from court was blamed on the fact that his 'eyes could endure neither wine nor water'. Similarly Pepys would devote passages of his diary to the continuing difficulties he was experiencing with eye strain and sore and weeping eyes. As the years progressed, he reported headaches and an increasingly painful sensitivity to certain kinds of light. All of which could potentially point to syphilis.

The diary also reveals that in 1664 Pepys feared that his mortally ill brother Thomas was dying from syphilis – the public shame of which he seems more concerned about than the imminent demise of his unmarried younger sibling. Thomas, who was socially awkward on account of a stutter and had made something of a hash of their father's tailoring business and got into debt, was already something of an embarrassment to the diarist.

That Pepys is so concerned about ailments, his own and those of other people, is ultimately what makes it unlikely that he himself had syphilis. Having undergone an excruciating operation for the removal of a bladder stone the size of a snooker ball, the diarist writes constantly about his bowel movements. He is unsparingly frank in describing any urinary matter and the many enemas and purges he subjected his system to. Yet there's little in the diary to indicate he caught so much as a dose of the common clap, let alone the hardly less common syphilis. But his eyes did trouble him. He sought the advice of learned friends and physicians and acquired spectacles from the shop of the most celebrated spectacle maker of the day. A spectacle maker who was not only a member of the Worshipful Company but also its master at that time. Despite this, Pepys received perhaps the worst advice possible and was sold glasses that modern optometrists calculate would have been wholly inappropriate for his condition.

No single diagnosis or prescription quite fits all of the various symptoms he describes, some of which are either arcane or vague and frequently both – not entirely surprising when they hail, as they do, from an era when educated men thought the body to be governed by four humours and spoke of its functions and malfunctions accordingly. And carrying a hare's foot to ward off colic, as Pepys did for a while, was considered a sensible medical precaution. But there are certain clear and persistent issues. One in particular is his difficulty with reading and writing for any length of time – an activity that eventually became so exhausting and physically painful he was unable to read or write for more than a few minutes. This coupled with watery eyes, redness and an increasing inability to tolerate light from candles or even the glare off sheets of paper has led optometrists to conclude that Pepys was most likely hypermetropic, or long-sighted. There is some suggestion that he probably had a slight astigmatism as well, a defect caused by an unevenly curved cornea, which would only have exacerbated his difficulties. Especially since this defect remained uncorrectable in Pepys' lifetime.*

The first time Pepys recorded a problem with his eyes in the diary

---

* As we will see, it wasn't until the nineteenth century, following the work of Sir George Airy, that a correcting lens for astigmatics was finally developed. Airy was the Royal Astronomer at Greenwich, a place that Pepys, as the great reformer of the Royal Navy and the effective founder of its naval college, had known well.

was on 25 April 1662, when he surmised that too much alcohol might have been the cause: 'I was much troubled in my eyes, by reason of the healths [libations] I have this day been forced to drink.' And who knows, he could have been right on this occasion. At the start of that year Pepys had taken a solemn oath to leave off both play-going and drinking wine. Though he would drink as much ale and beer as before, and having already succumbed to wine by February, he was finally to give up the oath as a bad idea in September. But indulgence after a period of abstemiousness can lead to rather severe hangovers.

Pepys, however, was never able to be abstemious for very long. And as his eyes from now on became a much more persistent issue, booze, or as often as not the beer he drank, was often held to be the culprit. On 24 July 1665, he records, for instance, 'Only, for want of sleep, and drinking of strange beer, had a rheum in one of my eyes which troubled me much.' In May the following year he complained that his right eye was 'sore and full of humour of late' and stated that the cause was 'my late change of my brewer and having of 8s[hilling] beere'. A month later he maintained that 'the drinking of some strong water' had set his eyes off again. A further change of brewer was advanced in the hope of remedying the situation. But to no avail, because in December 1666, Pepys was – amusingly enough, given the brewers' former membership of the same guild – to beat a path to a spectacle maker. This visit was undertaken rather interestingly to acquire a pair of 'green spectacles' – a colour, as already noted, thought to be beneficial to the eyes since Roman times, if not before.

'I did this evening', he dutifully records on 24 December 1666, 'buy me a pair of green spectacles, to see whether they help my eyes or no.' Sadly, in the very next line he reports, 'Then to the office and did business till my eyes began to be bad', suggesting that the green spectacles were not, on a first go at least, quite the panacea he'd hoped for. He would nevertheless persevere with them for a time and subsequently experimented with viewing theatrical performances and reading with the aid of an odd assortment of binocular tubes. His lack of vanity at using such implements in playhouses speaks of his commitment to the dramatic arts. Or at worst, his unwavering desire to see appealing ladies on stage at any cost, despite earlier oaths to the contrary.

At work, however, in the rooms of the Naval Board in Seething Lane, whose oak-panelled gloom was only barely dispelled by the flickering candles used to illuminate the office on working days that often stretched late into the night, Pepys increasingly availed himself of a clerk. In the tradition of Pliny the Elder (another naval man and government functionary) and countless other officials and bureaucrats in the centuries before spectacles, Pepys dictated letters and had reports read to him by an office boy to rest his eyes. And at home in their only marginally less gloomy quarters in the same complex, his wife was similarly tasked with reading to him to avoid any further unnecessary eye strain. The diary he continued, for obvious reasons, to maintain himself.

On 18 October 1667, however, he sought the services of the most famous spectacle makers of the day, John Turlington. Turlington, dubbed 'the first ... celebrity optician' by Neil Handley, curator at the Museum of the British Optical Association, was the son of a founding member of the Worshipful Company of Spectacle Makers. His father, also named John Turlington, was a signatory of the original petition sent to Charles I in 1628. Held in the highest esteem by his fellow spectacle makers, John Jr would serve as the company's master between 1665 and 1668 – a period when all of its earliest records (aside, miraculously, from its charter) were incinerated in the conflagration of the Great Fire of London. But as fate would have it, on the day when Pepys visited Turlington's shop in Eastcheap, the master himself was out and the diarist was attended to by his daughter instead. According to Handley, in this era it was 'common for wives and daughters to be active in spectacle makers' shops' and they 'often took over the business on the death of the proprietor' and were 'admitted to the Freedom of the Company on that basis alone ... The first woman admitted in her own right was Lucretia Clarke in 1699, who nevertheless qualified by patrimony.' When the first woman who was a complete outsider was admitted, alas, is a date unknown. And unfortunately for Pepys, on this occasion Turlington's daughter was to give him terrible advice.

As set down in the diary, Pepys bought not one but 'two new pairs of spectacles' from her that afternoon, accepting the recommendation that he would get the most 'help' and the greatest 'ease' from 'very young sights', i.e. spectacles with concave lenses for short-sightedness. A fortnight later he was back, one unsatisfied customer with a bone to pick with 'Turlington, the great spectacle maker' himself. Turlington, though, was to double-down on his daughter's prescription. On 4 November 1667, he not only urged Pepys to stick with 'young ones' but warned him against 'old spectacles' by telling the diarist quite emphatically that 'nothing' could 'wrong' his eyes more than 'reading glasses'.

Pepys at this point was only thirty-four years old, so it's probable that both father and daughter thought him too young a candidate for the 'old spectacles' with convex lenses they customarily dished out to the presbyopically challenged middle-aged. Yet if contemporary diagnoses are correct, these were exactly the type of glasses he most likely needed to aid his long-sightedness, though underlying conditions, an astigmatism or problems with convergence, could still have troubled him. But concave spectacles would almost certainly have made matters far worse. We know that he did eventually obtain reading glasses. In a later journal known as the Tangier Diary, a record of his voyage in 1683 to Morocco with the Admiral of the Fleet Lord Dartmouth to help oversee the winding up of England's ill-fated North African colony, he writes about packing what are now deemed these 'indispensable spectacles' for the trip. (Pepys, now fifty, would also by this point have aged into presbyopia, which tends to afflict naturally long-sighted people sooner in any case.)

The Tangier journal is about the closest Pepys ever came to keeping a regular diary again after the abandonment of his log in 1669. His ocular shortcomings leave us all the poorer for the lack of Pepys' inimitable personal insights into events such as the Third Anglo-Dutch War and the Glorious Revolution of 1688, events that he had a front row seat for, but for want of decent spectacles failed to write about. But the art of spectacle making was to become rather more scientific from now on.

# 4

# Taking Sides on the Margins

Pepys died at the age of seventy in 1703, living just long enough to see the arrival of London's first daily newspaper. Though by the time the first edition of the *Daily Courant* was printed by Elizabeth Mallet of Fleet Street in 1702 he was residing in what was then the Surrey countryside, ill health having caused him the previous year to repair with his books and housekeeper nurse (and possibly lover) Mrs Skinner to the house of his friend and former clerk Will Hewer in splendidly bucolic Clapham. After his death, newspapers and scandalous gossip sheets such as the *Tatler*, initially established in 1709, flourished in the city's coffee houses, venues Pepys himself had once frequented, though their numbers were to increase in this new century. In 1726 the Swiss noble César de Saussure noted that in London even quite ordinary 'workmen habitually' began 'the day by going to coffee-rooms to read the latest news', and with more people than ever squinting at print with clearer heads and sharper minds, the demand for spectacles rose in tandem.

An engraving by William Hogarth (and displayed on the College of Optometrists' website) of the mathematician and astronomer Martin Folkes, and Joseph Addison, the poet, essayist, editor and Whig politician, sitting in Button's Coffee House in Covent Garden in around 1720 illustrates that correlation. Button's was the base of Addison's weekly paper the *Guardian*.

Would-be contributors could submit letters, stories and limericks via a lion-headed letter box affixed to the coffee shop's wall, and this hive of louche London literary life was frequented by the likes of Jonathan Swift and Alexander Pope as well as young men availing themselves of the prostitutes in the neighbourhood's bordellos. Hogarth is thought to have designed the letter box, and in this picture Folkes is found holding a pair of nose spectacles in one hand, while on the table in front of him lies a smouldering long-stemmed pipe, what look like a further pair of spectacles, and a parliamentary news sheet bearing the headline 'Votes of the Commons'.

It was now, at long last, that the solution to the problem of keeping spectacles in place, a problem Folkes was evidently wrestling with and which had bedevilled wearers since their creation, was finally found. The answer now appears so obvious as to be almost unbelievable. But it was not until the 1720s that some bright spark, most likely a spectacle maker in London and a member of the Worshipful Company, and quite possibly having woken up and drunk some coffee, realised the potential usefulness of ears – and spectacles with side pieces arrived.

This being the story of spectacles there are, as ever, rival claimants to this innovation. A French spectacle and mirror maker called Marc Thomin, for one, who by the 1740s (or most probably a good decade before that) was proffering 'spectacles with silver and steel arms which hold onto the temples and do not hinder breathing'.

Dates, too, remain contested. A Tudor-era oak screen at St Peter's Church in Wormleighton, Warwickshire, is adorned with the head of a noble-looking man wearing possibly a crown and round granny-style spectacles that have what appear to be side arms. Though his long flowing locks, which add a touch of John Lennon circa the White Album to the carving, conceal his ears entirely, making it impossible to say for sure. There is also an intriguing grave in Kirkliston outside Edinburgh in Scotland. On a headstone erected to the memory of Margaret Shield and dated 1727 there are two carved pediments each bearing, instead of the more common grinning skulls of death, heads wearing spectacles with what again look like side pieces. The appearance of this sepulchral imagery in a then relatively out-of-the-way location would seem to imply that their invention must have occurred earlier than is otherwise documented.

But as it stands, we know that by 1728 or 1730 (when they are specifically mentioned in trade adverts), if not slightly earlier, Edward Scarlett was offering what he called his 'temple spectacles' to the world. These are, in the words of Neil Handley, 'the first eyewear', essentially the first spectacles that could be donned like a piece of clothing. And indeed Scarlett's spectacles were made to be worn in combination with another item of headgear, an item that no person of quality in Georgian London was without in public: a peruke, or powdered wig. The vogue for wigs in England, which first caught on in the court of Charles II, following French aristocratic fashions, was another by-product of syphilis. Along with sores, rashes and blindness, the disease also causes patchy hair loss. Pepys, once again pondering the damage the diarist's syphilitic brother Tom might do to his own reputation, wrote on 14 March 1664 that 'If [my brother] lives, he will not be able to show his head – which will be a very great shame to me.' A wig, often scented with lavender or orange to throw off the smell of rotting flesh beneath, was therefore capable of hiding a multitude of sins. Since deteriorating eyesight was another symptom of syphilis, Scarlett was clearly on to a winner with his 'temple spectacles', the side pieces of which ended in metal spiral rings, usually covered in soft velvet for added comfort, that rested on the temples rather than over the ears, and would not ruffle the curls of a wig. Later models in this mode by other spectacle makers would have longer pronged sides that, hatpin-style, could be plunged into the wig to keep the spectacles securely in position.

As well as pioneering the breakthrough spectacles with side pieces, Scarlett is credited with first introducing the practice to Britain (at least) of numbering lenses according to their focal length (in English inches) rather than by the age of their intended wearer. His trade cards maintained that he 'Grindeth all manner of Optick Glasses [and] makes spectacles after a new method, marking the

Focus of the Glass upon the Frame, it being approv'd of by all the Learned in Opticks as [the] Exactest way of fitting different Eyes'.

Apprenticed to Christopher Cock of Long Acre in 1691, Scarlett had obtained the 'freedom' of the Worshipful Company of Spectacle Makers in 1705 and served as its master in 1721-2. He traded first at the Old Spectacle Shop in Dean Street near St Anne's Church, Soho, and later together with his son (also called Edward) at the Archimedes and Globe in Macclesfield Street only a few hundred yards further down the road, in what is today Chinatown. St Anne's was then a comparatively new parish church. It had only been consecrated in 1686, to serve the needs of the area's growing population of Huguenots, the Protestant immigrants from France who came to England fleeing religious persecution in the aftermath of the Catholic French king Louis XIV's revoking of the Edict of Nantes, which had granted them freedom of worship, the previous year. William Maitland, the Scottish merchant and antiquarian, would subsequently write of St Anne's that 'Many parts of this parish so greatly abode with French that it is an easy matter for a stranger to imagine himself in France.' By 1711, when the population of the vestry of St Anne's was put at 8133, 40 per cent were calculated to be French. Scarlett's trade cards were as cosmopolitan as the district he worked in, their text printed in English, French and Dutch. Though the Dutch translation, apparently, leaves a lot to be desired.

His cards also bore the royal crest and proclaimed his services to the Prince and Princess of Wales, the future King George II and his queen consort Caroline of Ansbach. Scarlett would update his cards upon the prince's succession in 1727. Prior to that, however, the Hanover-born George, having quarrelled with his father, had spent a decade living in semi-disgraced exile from court as Scarlett's near neighbour in Soho, although in rather higher style, the royal couple occupying one of London's grandest mansions, Leicester House, in what remained the still leafy Leicester Fields. During those years the prince and his wife attended services at St Anne's Church.

Another resident of Scarlett's Soho, and a frequent guest at the

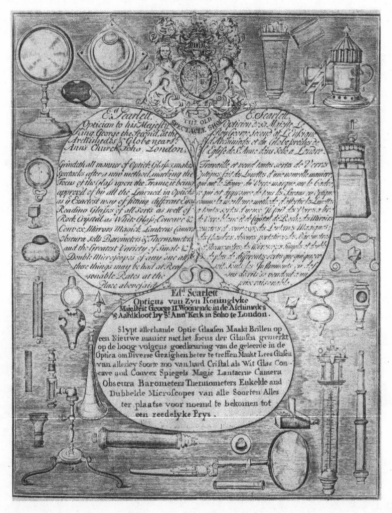

Edward Scarlett trade card, circa 1728–30.

prince and princess's salons in Leicester House, was the formerly reclusive Cambridge don turned Master of the Royal Mint and president of the Royal Society Sir Isaac Newton. The falling-apple-dodging discoverer of gravity lived at 35 St Martin's Street just off Leicester Fields, his house kitted out with a rooftop observatory stocked with telescopes of his own design.

Newton, whose scientific reputation was first made by a paper on colour and the refraction of light through a prism and the invention of a powerful type of reflecting telescope (the prototype fitted with an alloy mirror he personally cast and ground), often described himself as an optician. But in the same way that an expert in mathematics is called a mathematician, the title for him meant a person skilled in the science of optics, not a maker or seller of optical instruments.* By the 1730s and 1740s, however, this latter (and modern) sense of the word was increasingly common, especially in France (if spelt *opticien*), having become analogous, etymologically speaking, to something like physician for a supplier of medical treatments.

Scarlett, ever conscious of European trends, was billing himself as an optician in his adverts and on his trade cards from possibly as early as the 1720s. The title would not, however, appear in the records of the Worshipful Company until December 1756. It was then that a certain John Berge was listed in an account of a Court Meeting as an apprentice bound to Peter Dollond, a member of the guild described officially for the first time as 'an optician'. Berge itself is a surname originating from the province of Gaul, suggesting that the trainee was likely of French, Belgian or Dutch extraction. As indeed was the case with his master, whose family name would come to be associated with optical equipment and spectacles for the next 250 years. Its final eradication from Britain's high streets only occurred in 2015.

## From silk to spectacles

Peter Dollond's own devoutly Protestant grandfather Jean was a silk weaver originally from Normandy, though that name, most likely a corruption of 'D'Hollande' or 'of Holland', hints at an earlier migration from the Low Countries. Like many other industrious Huguenots, Jean Dollond sought refuge among fellow émigré craftsmen in Spitalfields on the eastern border of the City of London at the end of the seventeenth century.

---

\* The Worshipful Company records one London spectacle maker operating in premises 'at the sign of The Sir Isaac Newton'.

For his son John, born in 1706, silk never held quite the same fascination for him as science, where whole new horizons were opening up. Previously incalculable calculations were being made in mathematics thanks to Newton's and Gottfried Leibniz's invention of calculus. The heavens and oceans and faraway lands could be scanned, charted and navigated with the help of Newtonian reflective telescopes and object-glasses, and the secrets of biology and botany pored over with sharper compound microscopes. As extant houses in Princelet Street attest, the high windows of Spitalfields weavers' attic and upper-floor workshops were designed to help maximise the amount of light needed to complete their intricate loom and needle work. John Dollond may well have spent his earliest working days framed by such fenestration, each glance up from the bench leading him to gaze out through the panes of glass and contemplate the great sky above, piquing an interest in optics and astronomy that would obsess him from adolescence on. At fifteen he was designing and constructing his own sundials having already undertaken largely autodidactic studies of Latin, Greek, anatomy and geometry. But with a wife, his own workshop and by 1731 a son Peter (baptised that February at the French Protestant church in Threadneedle Street) to support, his optical obsessions were to remain a strictly amateur pursuit for the next two decades. Though in the true sense of the word, his tinkering with lenses in dedication to the advancement of telescopic instruments was undertaken with love and devotion rather than for obvious financial gain.

As a member of various scientific societies, including the London Mathematical Club, whose meetings at the Monmouth's Head in Spitalfields he began attending while still an apprentice in his teens, John Dollond knew or corresponded with some of the most eminent authorities in the field. In his friend and sometime rival John Bird, a much admired instrument maker on the Strand trading at the sign of 'The Sea Quadrant', he had an example of a former silk weaver who'd taken the plunge and gone pro. Yet Dollond remained in textiles and urged his son Peter to do the same. The boy reluctantly commenced his apprenticeship as a silk weaver at the age of thirteen in 1744. However he would never take up the craft professionally. As a definite chip off the old block, having been raised amid his father's hobbyist enthusiasms, Peter threw himself instead wholeheartedly into all things optical and was by 1750 to be found running a shop on these lines in Vine Street in Clerkenwell.

It must have done well enough because just two years later, the twenty-one-year-old Dollond persuaded his forty-six-year-old father to join him in the enterprise. The pair entered into a formal partnership in 1752 and took new premises to the west at Exeter Exchange off the Strand. There Dollond and Son 'at the sign of the Golden Spectacles and Sea Quadrant' established themselves as distinguished makers of innovative astronomical and navigational instruments as well as, of course, spectacles. With their micro-meters (an improved version of a heliometer or astrometer, a device for measuring the position of the sun and other heavenly bodies in the sky), sextants and revolutionary achromatic (colour-free) lensed telescopes they attracted the custom of the likes of Captain James Cook and the Astronomer Royal Nevil Maskelyne. No further thoughts were devoted to silk looms.

In 1761, flushed with the success of his inventions and the plaudits they had brought him from the profession at large, John Dollond was honoured with a medal by the Royal Society and appointed Optician to King George III, who'd only recently suc-ceeded his grandfather (and the now late Edward Scarlett's great patron) George II. Alas, on the evening of 30 November that year, while reading a book about the moon, whose orbit and cratered surface his devices now allowed astronomers to study with greater ease and in far more detail than before, he suffered a stroke that left him speechless and he died only a few hours later.

## Temple pieces

Another significant figure in the Worshipful Company of Spectacle Makers in this era, and a glass grinder Dollond himself sought out during his amateur years, was James Ayscough. The company's master in the year Dollond and son initiated their partnership, Ayscough is thought to be the first person to use the term 'achromatic' in a printed advert for his wares. Like his peers, and operating from a shop on Ludgate Street (now Hill) at the sign of the Golden Spectacles and Quadrant, Ayscough made and sold a huge variety of optical goods including magic lanterns and opera glasses, along with instruments such as thermometers and barometers. But for the story of spectacles, his special contribution was to improve on the concept of sides, greatly extending their length from the mere temple pieces of Scarlett and adding additional hinges, to make them 'double-jointed' so they could be folded halfway along. The final bendy end bits in some instances might then be tucked, and even be tied together, behind the head.

Ayscough claimed that the enormous advantage of his swing-sided spectacles was that they would 'obviate all the objections made to the common spring spectacles, as they neither press upon the nose nor the temples; the complaint against these being the pressure they cause on that place, which stops the circulation of the blood, and thereby occasions to many people violent head-aches'.

Memorably described as 'the exceptionally energetic son of a Wiltshire clergyman', Ayscough was to publish at least two slim volumes on spectacles where he set down, chapter and verse, his own personal gospel of spectacle wearing. With titles almost as long as the tomes themselves – *A Short Account of the Nature and Uses of Spectacles: In which is recommended a Kind of Glass for Spectacles preferable to any hitherto made use of for that Purpose* and its sequel from 1752 *A Short Account of the Eye and Nature of Vision, Chiefly designed to Illustrate the Uses and Advantages of Spectacles, Wherein is laid down Rules for chusing Glasses proper for remedying all the different Defects of Sight* – these books were, like many of their kind in this period, not much more than thinly glossed catalogues for products he manufactured. Plugging, for instance, a nice line in lenses, he offered what nearly a century earlier might have suited Samuel Pepys. They were 'a little ting'd with blue' and said, apparently, to 'take off the glaring Light from the Paper and renders every Object so easy and pleasant that the tenderest Eye may thro' it view any thing intently without pain'.

This was, after all, the tireless London of Samuel Johnson, and a great age for pamphlets and tracts of all stripes: literary, religious, political, scientific, satirical and/or salacious. The Grub Street of the day was, at least according to the scrofulous Lichfield-born scribbler's own dictionary, 'much inhabited by writers of small histories, dictionaries, and temporary poems'. These dog-eat-dog hacks for hire kept an insatiable reading public stocked with items to meet the highest and lowest of autodidactic tastes.

The symbiotic relationship between hack and specs is perhaps further illustrated by a pair of Ayscough-style swing-sided spectacles believed to have belonged to Johnson himself that are held in the British Optical Association Museum in London. The good Doctor, having contracted scrofula (then known as the King's Evil) at the age of two, most probably from drinking infected cow's milk, suffered nearly as badly with his eyes as Pepys.

Johnson's problems with his vision, though, were compounded by a host of other physical and psychological ailments, among them deafness, obesity, dyspepsia, flatulence, heart failure, gout, insomnia, mania, depression and possibly Tourette's syndrome. Excessive weight is thought to explain the extraordinary wide angle of the swing-hinged sides of this particular pair of spectacles; their side pieces appear to have been expressly designed to pivot out like pond skaters' legs to accommodate Johnson's massive, fleshy face. Or someone with an equally gargantuan head, as the museum's curator Neil Handley concedes ownership has yet to be conclusively established. They certainly look the part, anyway.

## Margins and double spectacles

But in 1749, just as Johnson was moving into a house at 17 Gough Square in whose upper-storey rooms he would devote the next six years to completing his lexical masterwork, an optician and instrument maker, shortly to open a shop just around the corner on Fleet Street, would publish a dictionary of his own. The second edition of Benjamin Martin's 560-page *Lingua Britannica Reformata or a New Universal English Dictionary* would, in fact, be in the shops nearly a full year before Johnson's effort was finally finished, a task the latter dictionarist was only able to complete with the aid of six amanuenses. And retailing for a mere six shillings against the £4 10s eventually demanded for Johnson's, Martin's dictionary was well received, running to two editions. But the arrival in 1756 of a comparatively cheap (ten shillings) abridged single-volume version of Johnson's opus killed it stone dead. Relegated to a footnote of lexicological history, Martin's book is almost entirely forgotten today. As largely is the man himself.

Yet at the time of his death in 1782, Martin was acclaimed as 'one of the most eminent mathematicians of the age' and 'a philosopher who was an honour to his country'.* An inventor recalled not unfondly by horologists for a weight-driven table clock, an optical instrument maker, a peripatetic public lecturer and the editor of the *General Magazine of Arts and Sciences*, his written and commercial output was prolific, if bordering on the incontinent. Martin churned out essays, treatises, text books and self-aggrandising broadsides and promotional pamphlets for each of the multitude of products he launched. Algebra, the orbits of comets, electricity, artificial magnets, trigonometry, maps, globes, microscopes and telescopes are all subjects tackled across his sprawling published works. Along, of course, with the English language itself.

As an instrument maker and optician, though, with premises on Fleet Street, he would be responsible for devising some of the most distinctive – if, it has to be said, preposterous – spectacles ever made. Spectacles whose specific virtues he naturally touted in

---

* Shortly after his death, a painting of a bewigged Martin was acquired by the Museum of Curiosities in Lichfield, Johnson's birthplace. This establishment, which pre-dated the British Museum by several years, was founded in the home of the eccentric antiquarian, surgeon and apothecary Richard Greene. Greene was a relative of Johnson. The literary lion, if initially rather sniffy about his kinsman's endeavour, gradually warmed to the project and donated to the collection an axe, a lance and an ink stand he'd used when compiling his dictionary. The whereabouts of Martin's portrait are now unknown and only an engraving of it, which was published in 1785 in an issue of the *Gentleman's Magazine*, a journal to which Greene himself was also a regular contributor, survives.

print in a 1756 dispatch entitled *An essay on Visual Glasses, vulgarly called spectacles, wherein it is shewn that the common structure of those glasses is contrary to the rules of art, and very prejudicial to the eyes; the nature of vision in the eye explained, and glasses of a new construction proposed.* Copies of this twenty-eight-page tract could be obtained from his shop.

Martin was born of farming stock in 1704 in the village of Worplesdon in Surrey, then a predominantly rural county, and despite its proximity to London much of it only tangentially connected to the capital by stagecoach. He almost certainly worked as a plough boy when young. But then so too did Robbie Burns and the nabob Sir William James of the East India Company. And Martin, similarly, had his sights set on getting off the land and making something of himself. Especially after having had, as an early reviewer put it, his 'head altogether turn'd to mathematicks and philosophical speculations'.

Working hard on his studies after the hard graft of the day, he was supposedly finally able to leave the fields after receiving a bequest of £500 from a relative. By the 1730s he was married and running a school in the Sussex cathedral city of Chichester. It was here that Martin first ventured into the optical trade with a small shop and also began to write and publish books. His assault on the capital's spectacle scene would not come until nearly twenty years later, with much of the intervening decades spent writing countless more books and touring the country giving apparently reasonably well-remunerated talks on natural and experimental philosophy.

By the time Martin opened his London shop in either late 1755 or early 1756 'at the sign of Hadley's Quadrant and Visual Glasses' on Fleet Street, and only a stone's throw from both Samuel Johnson's Gough Square home and the offices of the Royal Society in Crane Court, Martin was well into his fifties. Like most people of that age, presbyopia had set in. And in the *Visual Glasses* essay Martin explained that it was the need to wear reading spectacles himself that eventually drove him to develop what would become known as his 'Martin's Margins'. Since, he wrote, 'I now used them myself, I resolved at once to have a pair as perfect as my skill in Optics and the form and make of the eye could direct me to construct'.

In the pamphlet, Martin went on to castigate existing forms of reading glasses on three grounds. Firstly, their lenses were in parallel, whereas they should point to the object to be viewed. Secondly, they let in two or three times as much light as necessary, leaving the eyes 'weak and watery'. And thirdly, 'good definition' was hard to achieve, as the lenses in these spectacles allowed light of all colours to pass through them.

His solution was make spectacles whose lenses converged at an axis for normal reading distance. A not entirely unreasonable move. But his belief that too much natural light was 'prejudicial to the eyes' resulted in him blocking off part of each lens with 'an annular piece of horn', the effect of which was to lend his spectacles their peculiar doughnut-shaped appearance, with an additional occluding outer rim surrounding the lens itself. Furthermore, those lenses were tinted violet. This colour scheme derived from Newton's misguided thesis that light was made up of molecules of physical particles rather than rays. Violet, as the smallest, was deemed the least harmful to the eye in Martin's reading of 'the divine geometer's' ocular rainbow.

This vogue for coloured lenses was also one shared by Ayscough, who in his earlier pamphlet had maintained that 'It has been found that common white glass gives an offensive glaring light, very prejudicial to the eyes, and on that account, green and blue Glasses have been advised though they make every object appear with their own hue ... I was induced to make trial of the new kind of glass and of a greenish cast ...' Nevertheless, Martin dismissed green lenses as vulgar, as was his wont.

His 'Visual Glasses', or 'Margins' as they have since become more widely known, were treated with contempt by London's spectacle-making establishment. But this was not to prevent the more unscrupulous of its members (and plenty more outside the company) from copying the design in response to demand. His own catalogues contain frequent warnings to customers to beware of cheap imitations. Would-be purchasers are expressly told to

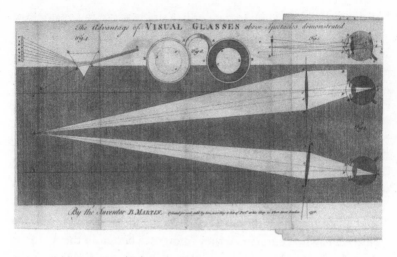

Benjamin Martin's Visual Glasses, 1756–8.

guard against peddlers and hawkers who, it was maintained, were attempting to pass their knock-off versions as Martin originals by scratching the initials 'BM' on to their frames. Such logo fakery implies that there was a market for designer glasses over two centuries before Calvin Klein and co. got in on the act.

It might also be argued that Martin's Visual Glasses were no better optically than any other spectacles then available – something that holds true for some of the pricier branded frames of today. But in Martin's case it is questionable what, if any, benefits accrued from the elaborate combination of shading rings and tinted lenses that was the trademark feature of his range, images of which graced all his catalogues. An oversized replica pair, alongside a Brobdingnagian quadrant, hung above his Fleet Street shop as the sign.

An inventory from the sale of Martin's effects following his death in 1782, an ending speeded on by a failed suicide attempt prompted by bankruptcy, revealed that he held some 500 ready-to-go pairs in stock, along with a large number of unmounted lenses and unglazed frames. These quantities were a testament to the importance of the line to his (sadly, in the end, slumping) bottom line. Their sheer ubiquity, thanks to numerous imitations, also ensured that while to date only a single surviving example of Scarlett's temple spectacles has come to light, hundreds of 'Martin's margins' are still with us, held in various states of decay and repair by museums and collectors around the world.

Novelty is certainly a factor in their contemporary value as antiques. On eBay, as of January 2021, lensless pairs in iron sell for around £250 a pop, silver ones for over £400. It probably also explains their improbable popularity when they were young and new. But it is plain that even then, plenty of those who tried them questioned their worth. Part of Martin's essay even addresses itself to those souls who have dissed his Visual Glasses or failed to appreciate the subtle boons they brought to the weary-eyed. To customers who complained they 'didn't see better' in them or find them 'easier on the eye' than ordinary glasses, or that they made little difference when it came to viewing in painful light, Martin merely urged patience, suggesting that time would out and rewards accrue to those who persevered with them.

According to the Worthing-based retired ophthalmic optician and antique spectacle collector John Dixon Salt, who owns four pairs of Martin's Margins, the general consensus among the profession today is that they were little more than 'a marketing scam'. In the past, he says, 'some have suggested [that the design] might have "helped" in reducing "the thickness and weight" of the lenses', which would be 'true of very high-powered lenses, but the lenses [in Martin's Margins] were not sufficiently large enough to a make a real difference. Nowadays', he adds, 'we have high refractive lenses to reduce the thickness and can also use lenticular lenses that resemble a fried egg, having the power only in the central part. But the central optical zone used now is still larger than the whole lens size in Martin's time.'

If Martin's Margins were of dubious optical merit, another style of spectacle developed at this time continues to be worn to this day, if inevitably in slightly more refined forms: the bifocal, spectacles fitted with lenses comprised of two halves of differing magnification, the bottom usually set for reading and the upper half for distance. The person often cited as their inventor is that founding father of the American republic Benjamin Franklin, who from the late 1750s spent seventeen years in London acting as a lobbyist cum agent for the English colonies of Pennsylvania, New Jersey, Massachusetts and Georgia.

Conceivably, the kite-flying advocate of lending libraries and the inventor of lightning rods could have purchased a pair of Martin's Margins had the mood taken him. Hypermetropic (long-sighted), Franklin wore spectacles almost constantly in later life, a fact commemorated in official portraits and satirical cartoons. The latter representations of the man who was to promote the turkey as the republic's national bird tended to err on the owlish. The long nose and lank-over-the-ears hair standing in for beak and wings – you get the picture. Indeed it is the peculiarity of one pair of specs he is depicted wearing in a political cartoon from 1764, a pair of specs that do have a certain bifocal look about them, that some believe proves Franklin must have invented them. But his prolonged period in London from 1757 to 1775 (with a brief stint back in the US in 1762-3) overlapped almost exactly with the heyday of 'Martin's Margins' and corresponded with his eyesight deteriorating with age.

Throughout this time he lodged at 36 Craven Street near Charing Cross, only a few doors down from the current location of the British Optical Association Museum at the College of Optometrists. An oil painting believed to be of Franklin wearing spectacles (though rather basic round metal nose numbers) dating from 1777 is another of the museum's holdings.

This, though, was Franklin's second spell in what remained at that point not just the capital of England but also America. He'd first visited London as an ambitious, downright precocious young printer in 1724. During this brief original stay, he wrote and published a pamphlet, 'a little metaphysical piece ... entitled *A Dissertation on Liberty and Necessity, Pleasure and Pain*', and made the acquaintance of Sir Hans Sloane, the secretary and future president of the Royal Society, selling him 'a purse made of asbestos, which purifies by fire' – as you do.

Franklin had to come to London largely to obtain printing kit – which reflected a broader trading relationship between the home nation and its North American colony. By and large, raw materials and crops such as tobacco, cocoa and sugar cane flowed out of America and the Caribbean. Meanwhile, manufacturing and the selling on of finished goods remained the preserve of the mother country. This arrangement meant that early settlers in America were entirely dependent on spectacles from England.

Over a decade after his first sojourn in London, and by then a successful entrepreneur and the publisher of the *Philadelphia Gazette* and the phenomenally profitable American annual *Poor Richard's Almanack*, Franklin was engaged in their sale in the Pennsylvania Colony. Adverts for 'just imported' English spectacles ('to be sold by B. Franklin') appeared in the pages of his *Gazette* in 1738.

But his interest in spectacles would take on a new dimension when he possibly commissioned some of the first pairs of bifocals. 'Possibly' is the operative word here. The idea of split-lensed spectacles was mooted as early as the 1680s by Johann Zahn. A monk and inventor from Würzburg, Germany, among Zahn's other far-sighted ideas was the camera, whose potential possibilities he outlined in 1685 in his comprehensive survey of optical instruments *Oculus Artificialis Teledioptricus Sive Telescopium*, 140 years before the French inventor Nicéphore Niépce finally worked out a way to fix a photographic image on paper. Or very nearly, anyway. And a not dissimilar length of time would elapse before Zahn's split-lensed spectacles became a reality, the route to their realisation no less littered with potential claimants on their eventual invention as the camera.

One contender is Samuel Pierce, a London optical instrument maker reputed to have supplied Benjamin West, the Pennsylvania-born historical painter to the court of George III and the second president of the Royal Academy, with a pair of 'Divided Spectacles' in around 1770, the period when West was composing his famous study of the Battle of Quebec, *The Death of General Wolfe*. Sir Joshua Reynolds, also reported as wearing bifocals by some biographers, has been cited as another of Pierce's possible customers.

There is, however, little to support either of these claims and a good deal of speculation around whether either painter wore bifocals as such.

Another optician in the (split) frame is Peter Dollond, who, depending on who you believe, was either already making glasses along these lines or made some for Franklin. As Hugh Barty-King, author of *Eyes Right*, the official biography of the Dollond & Aitchison firm, delicately puts it, 'there is a tradition (*unsupported by evidence*) that he anticipated Benjamin Franklin in the invention of bi-focal spectacles'. My italics are for emphasis, but this is not the most fulsome of endorsements by any standards. He does, however, go on to quote at length from a letter Franklin sent from France to his friend George Whateley on 23 May 1785 in which Dollond is mentioned by name in relation to what the American called his 'double spectacles':

> By Mr Dollond's saying that my double spectacles can only serve particular eyes, I doubt he has not been rightly informed of their construction. I imagine it will be found pretty generally that the same convexity of glass, through which a man sees clearest and best at the distance proper for reading, is not the best for greater distances. I therefore had formerly two pair of spectacles, which I shifted occasionally, as in traveling I sometimes read, and often wanted to regard the prospects. Finding this change troublesome, and not always sufficiently ready, I had the glasses cut and half of each kind associated in the same circle. By this means, as I wear my spectacles constantly, I have only to move my eyes up or down, as I want to see distinctly far or near, the proper glasses being always ready.

By now serving as America's first ambassador to France, which had supported the colonists' revolutionary cause with financial, military and naval aid, and residing in the suburb of Passy, just outside Paris, Franklin went on to explain how his double spectacles helped his mission in the country. Being able to wear a single pair of spectacles with two types of lenses, he writes, was 'particularly convenient ... the glasses that serve me best at table to see what I eat not being the best to see the faces of those on the other side of the table who speak to me; and when one's ears are not well accustomed to the sounds of a language, a sight of the movements in the features of him that speaks helps to explain, so that I understand French better with the help of my spectacles'.

John Adams might have wished Franklin was less easy at *tables françaises* with his new glasses, since after visiting Paris the future second President of the United States would lambast Franklin for wasting his time on 'incessant dinners and dissipations' and not doing enough diplomatic work. In France, and due to his advances in the field, Franklin was also affectionately known as the 'Electric Ambassador', leading Adams to a further grouch that here it was 'universally believed' that the American revolution had been accomplished singlehandedly with a wave of 'his electric wand'.

Franklin returned to America in July 1785, after eight and a half years in Passy, and he was on his deathbed by the time news of the first stirrings of the French Revolution reached him in 1789. He responded to such dispatches enthusiastically; some of its initial instigators were, after all, known to him personally, and claimed inspiration from Franklin's ideas of scientific progress and political liberty, while more than a few of the most able revolutionaries on the ground would prove to be French military veterans who'd supported the Americans in their battle against the British. Franklin died on 17 April 1790, with little inkling of the terrors to follow. In Paris, the great man's death was announced to the revolutionary National Assembly by his friend Honoré Mirabeau, and a vote that mourning should be worn for three days in Franklin's honour was carried almost unanimously.

## Incredible quizzers

Of all the incidents that ensued in the aftermath of the storming of the Bastille, perhaps the one that might have confused Benjamin Franklin the most, at least as a man of science and self-consciously modest dress – even in French courtly company he appeared *sans perruque* and wearing a simple coat of a brown fustian material – was the eventual adoption of so-called quizzing glasses by a young generation of politically radical French dandies.

Once Edward Scarlett or quite possibly Marc Thomin in the Francosphere had finally solved the issue of keeping spectacles in place with side pieces, it might have been reasonable to assume that all other styles of glasses and optical aids would slip into obsolescence. Yet by a perverse logic, the very fact that such spectacles gave their wearers free use of both hands and were therefore most readily adopted by those engaged in work needing ten digits' worth of easy action put a black mark against them. Particularly in aristocratic circles, where anything that smacked of trade was beyond the pale. The wearing of spectacles since their very inception in the Middle Ages had, as we've seen, almost always been commonly associated with physical and even mental weakness, and medical opinion for centuries more often came down strongly against their extended use into the bargain. The result of these prejudices was to produce a marked preference for hand-held optical aids, like those once used by our old friend Pope Leo X when out hunting, among the most affluent of European society into the late eighteenth century.

Where the wearing of spectacles might be frowned upon at court balls and gatherings, a modest lens (or two) fixed to a decorous handle elegantly hewn in a precious metal could be wielded discreetly like a fan and was as much an ornament or a piece of jewellery as an optical aid. Now, come the French Revolution, such devices were deemed irrevocably emblems of the ancient regime. That connection was played up by Pressburger and Powell in their 1946 film *A Matter of Life and Death*. Marius Goring appears as the celestial emissary Conductor 71 dispatched to retrieve a British airman, played by David Niven, shot down over the English Channel and bound for heaven but accidentally mislaid en route to the afterlife by a rather earthly fog. Goring's Conductor is a heavily affected and thickly accented French aristocratic coxcomb who 'lost his head' in the Terror and whose foppish sartorial accoutrements include a crook-ended candy cane-like walking stick and a dinky quizzing glass attached to a ribbon around his neck, this part of his anatomy also swathed in a thick, elaborately tied linen scarf.

Yet such a get-up could equally mark the Conductor as an aged member of *les incroyables* – the youthful French fashion sub-cult of the later revolutionary period. This style tribe (and their female counterparts, the *merveilleuses*) was first classified in a caricature by the artist Carle Vernet in December 1796. Although later acclaimed as a depicter of cavalry-heavy Napoleonic battles, equine subjects in full snort and rearing-front-legs mode, and horse-related sporting scenes, Vernet initially 'found his vocation' in creating 'pitiless' studies 'of the idiocies of his contemporaries', as the *Benezit Dictionary of Artists* succinctly puts it. And those contemporaries, after the fall of Robespierre in 1794, rebelled against Jacobin austerity by purposefully adopting a libertine costume of bizarrely overblown excess. Young men wore their hair in artfully tousled dishevelment and grew long sidelocks nicknamed *oreilles de chien* (dog's ears). Around their necks they wore massive white-linen cravats, while fine legs and other masculine assets were shown off in tight pantaloons. The figure-hugging cuts of these strides aimed to convey something of the nobility of antique nudes, just as the diaphanous dresses sported by their opposite numbers the *merveilleuses* aped 'classical' draperies of Greco-Roman statuary. But enormous importance was placed on the *tout ensemble* and an outfit hardly thought complete without the appropriate accessories.

Canes, riding crops and quizzing glasses came high on that list for the look went beyond the clothes to encompass a manner of gestures and an exaggerated mode of speech and turns of phrase. Their habit of exclaiming 'C'est incroyable!' ('That's incredible!') in a pose of astonished lisping disbelief at each and every snippet of news or political gossip supplied Vernet with the title of his first cartoon – and that phrase was soon applied collectively, if usually derogatorily, to this generation of flaming creatures (the similarly ironic simpering of 'merveilleuse' – 'marvellous' – among the dashing *jeunes filles* the source of its feminine equivalent). Vernet's cartoons were to define the zeitgeist, spawning prints, plays and

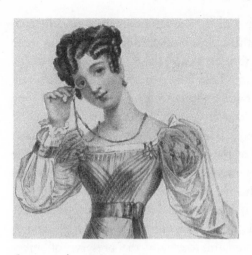

Quizzing glass.

a journal named in honour of these readily mocked young meteors, who embraced the label as a badge of pride and continued to express their dissent for prevailing political orthodoxies in flamboyant style. That Vernet's first satirical study featured a pair of young bucks, one campily inspecting his stylish acquaintance through a quizzing glass, resulted in this optical aid becoming almost a full-on fad, something akin to a high-fashion hula hoop for the 1790s. Even Napoleon in his imperial phase would come to use a hand-held two-lens scissored quizzer to inspect battle plans and maps.

In Britain, the quizzer would become most readily associated with the original Regency dandy, George 'Beau' Brummell. As a man whose motto was 'clean linen, plenty of it, and country washing', Brummell was fastidious to a fault. His daily toilet reputedly took five hours and he was said to polish his boots with champagne. That Brummell should prefer to survey the world with haughty froideur through the lens of a small gold quizzing glass – an instrument that he'd hold with a daintiness so overdone it bordered on the aggressively threatening, between thumb and forefinger, and which was attached to a silk ribbon around his neck – seems almost too predictable. Inevitable.

Although a quarrel with the Prince of Wales and mounting debts would force Brummell to flee to France in 1816, where he was to spend the remainder of his life (coming, before his bitter end in an asylum in Caen, to lose yet more money, any interest in his appearance, and finally his mental faculties), he had fed the trend, and quizzers were only to rise in fashionability in England.

Minor variations to this style would produce both the lorgnette and the monocle. The former was a pair of spectacles that folded neatly into a handle and whose lenses, once unfurled like a fan, could also be bent over one another to form a single magnifying glass; the first spring-loaded version was patented in London in 1825 by Robert Bretell Bate, an optician at the Poultry later to serve as the master of the Worshipful Company of Spectacle Makers. The latter was a small round glass on a chain or ribbon that could be held in the eye socket for a certain amount of time. Although its invention is often credited to the eighteenth-century Prussian aristocrat and antiquarian Philipp von Stosch – and in Hollywood movies it remains eternally the preserve of spike-helmeted, heel-clicking Bismarckian generals and Red Baronesque World War One flying aces – the monocle seems to have caught on first in England. According to the optical historian J. William Rosenthal they only took off in the German-speaking world after the Austrian optician Johann Friedrich Voigtländer, inspired by examples he'd seen in English aristocratic society, began producing monocles for his well-heeled clients in Vienna at the beginning of the nineteenth century.

That quizzers and monocles, especially, were being adopted by the young as a matter of style rather than optical need alarmed many medical practitioners, who warned against the potential dangers such lenses could pose to the eyes of these trend seekers. In 1824, one London physician, Dr Kirchiner, maintained that 'A single glass set in a smart ring is often used by trinket fanciers merely for fashion's sake, by folks who have not the least defect in their sight and are not aware of the mischievous consequences of such irritations. This pernicious plaything will most assuredly in a very few years bring on an imperfect vision in one or both eyes.'

A piece in the *National Advocate* headed 'Vision and Fashion' and published in that same year expressed particular concern about the use of monocles by women:

we now perceive ladies and misses, with eyes perfectly good, and sometimes very handsome, in constant use of eye glasses [monocles], which, set in a gold case, and suspended by a gold chain from the neck, look very pretty and finical. Now, what is the effect of trifling with this delicate organ?

The habit of using one eye for a glass, necessarily weakens and impairs the other, which not being kept in operation, becomes weak and torpid. So that, long before use or nature render the eye weak, both become decayed in strength, and then glasses are indispensable. Fashion, it is true, is very arbitrary; but fashion should never be unnatural. Ladies may wear white instead of black – feathers instead of wreaths – they may have long or short waists – wear high or low shoes – these are caprices of fashion, but it is torturing to nature to use a glass to good eyes – to compress the waist by cords and corsets to the size of a wasp, driving the blood to the head, and checking free respiration – or leaving off flannel in cold weather, to preserve a genteel shape. If dame fashion is not kept under due subjection, our ladies will die of naked elbows, and grow blind by using eye glasses.

The Paris-based journal *Hygiène de la Vue*, meanwhile, warned of the possibly ageing effects of monocles, writing in 1847 that 'Of a hundred persons who use this little square piece of glass which they hold in place only by making faces, 90 surely could do without it. The only result is that they make themselves vulnerable to myopia at the same time they prematurely develop crow's feet, the despair of so many women.'

Monocles would come and go, enjoying periods of revival over the next century, notably in the 1910s, when a whole new generation of hard-partying bright young things chose to adopt this now antique style of optical aid to emphasise their frivolous modernity, much as the *incroyables* had done with their quizzers before them. But rather like Vauxhall Pleasure Gardens, perhaps because the quizzing glass was so synonymous with the wicked decadence of the gouty old Regency era, it was doomed not to survive too long into the more puritanical Victorian period.

Nevertheless, Benjamin Disraeli, the leader of the Conservative Party and future Prime Minister of Britain, continued to use one until at least 1863. That March, however, he attended the marriage of the Prince of Wales to Alexandra of Denmark in St George's Chapel in Windsor Castle, and having taken his quizzing glass with him to better observe the proceedings, raised the instrument only to find himself staring straight at Queen Victoria. The monarch did not appreciate being spied upon at her own son's wedding, and Disraeli, mortified beyond belief by his breach of protocol, 'did not', as he later confessed, 'venture to use' the 'glass again'.

But by then, in any case, the wheels of industry had turned and spectacle making, like everything else, had entered the steam age. Speed, efficiency and self-improvement were to be the watchwords of this epoch, and there would be little time for fripperies once beloved of tousle-haired French popinjays.

# 5

# Steam-powered Vision

In the hazy swirl of the watery blues, warm golds and creams of J. M. W. Turner's *Rain, Steam and Speed*, the funnel of the Great Western Railway locomotive thundering across the bridge at Maidenhead looks as tall and jet black as one of Isambard Kingdom Brunel's top hats. An enigma of this almost overfamiliar but still uncanny masterpiece, a picture often cited as the first significant railway painting in the history of art, is that for all the steam flying about, the funnel itself is pretty smokeless. Certainly no fat plume issues from its cast-iron spout. Where almost everything else is a blur, the engine is like a jackknife cutting across the canvas. Nothing the picture conveys is going to get in its way. Just ahead of it a small brown hare (once painted out) darts for cover – Mother Nature's most light-footed creatures outpaced at last by man's infernal machines.

The picture was painted and exhibited at the Royal Academy in 1844 when Turner was sixty-nine and Gladstone's Railway Regulation Act had just been passed – a wide-ranging piece of legislation that left the possibility of the nationalisation of the railways open and compelled companies to provide at least one train a day at a cost not exceeding a penny a mile. Like many of the artist's late paintings it was met with bewilderment by the majority of critics and his contemporaries. Even Turner's most loyal champion John Ruskin, who'd been mesmerised by the dizzying colour and light of his earlier canvases, was horrified by *Rain, Steam and Speed*, though arguably more by its frighteningly contemporary subject matter than its execution. But the singularity of Turner's vision, particularly in such mature work, with its confounding use of fiercely evaporating imagery, blazing scarlets and yellows and subdued browns and blues, caused immense speculation about his eyesight.

In 1872, just over twenty years after Turner's death, Dr Richard Liebreich, a distinguished German ophthalmologist then serving as the head of ophthalmology at St Thomas' Hospital in London, gave a lecture at the Royal Institute 'On the effects of certain faults of vision on painting', with particular reference to Turner. Liebreich was seeking to offer a medical explanation for the presence of certain colours and tropes in his paintings. He put forward the theory, subsequently published in a book, that the blurred shapes and luminous fogs to be seen in Turner's riper canvases were the result of a cataract that caused the diffusion of light in his visual field. The lecture was greeted warmly by the magazine *Nature* which declared that Liebreich had 'successfully vindicated the title of physical science to extend its researches into the domain of art criticism by applying optical laws to painting'. Others, however, were to protest that during his lifetime and after it (when contemporaries, associates and family members had been widely canvassed for reminiscences about the great painter), no one had ever mentioned him having a cataract. But this faith in science to provide answers and Liebreich's retrospective deductive, diagnostic approach are tellingly representative of the major shift in intellectual thinking of the Victorian age. The age that was also to give us Sherlock Holmes, the creation of Arthur Conan Doyle (himself, of course, a failed ophthalmologist), who argues in *A Study in Scarlet*, the 1887 story in which Holmes made his literary debut, that in solving problems 'the grand thing is to be able to reason backwards ... analytically'.

In the case of Turner's eyesight, though, a pair of round tortoiseshell spectacles with jointed metal sides and lenses with a modest correction for myopia, along with a magnifying glass and snuff box, were among his posthumous effects. In 2003 these artefacts went up for auction at Sotheby's, while two further pairs of spectacles also purported to belong to the artist and once owned by Ruskin were put on display at Tate Britain. Stepping into the role of Liebreich this time round was the consultant ophthalmic surgeon James McGill who also advanced a diagnosis of untreated cataracts, adding colour blindness and worsening short-sightedness, a slight astigmatism and presbyopia into the list of optical afflictions suffered by the painter. But in depicting the world as he saw it, no matter how impaired, Turner's genius, as McGill acknowledged, was in supplying a means for everyone to see it differently. Perhaps more clearly if anything, and at a moment when technology was making it both harder and easier to see well, with machines simultaneously bringing cheaper mass-produced spectacles and better optical aids and swathing daily life in insanitary thick black smoke.

Travelling on trains, though, opened up whole new vistas, recasting space, distance and motion. In accelerating the pace of industrialisation, they would quite brutally bend the physical environment to their will, leaving iron rails and brick archways where there might have been open meadows, hills and dales, and coating everything in their path in a film of smoke and soot. Even time itself wasn't safe. The Great Western Railway's programme of standardising all the clocks on its lines in 1840 heralded the end of Britain's hotchpotch of different regional time zones, where Plymouth, for example, lagged a whole twenty minutes behind London. The wrought-iron rigour of railway timetables eventually led to the nation running to the strict tempo of Greenwich Mean Time.*

Time in this newly industrialised society was money; labour, like travel, mechanised; and factory workers' output measured against the ticking clock. Samuel Smiles, the first biographer of railway pioneers George and Robert Stephenson and whose austere doctrine of striving and self-improvement was to become

---

* As Simon Bradley points out in *The Railways*, such differences were actually 'a sign of sophistication rather than backwardness' and 'the culmination of scientific clock-making and astronomical observation', the latter aided by finer spyglasses and telescopes that allowed local variances to be calculated so precisely.

the mantra of the era, would list 'punctuality, and the orderly employment of time' among the virtues that any ambitious working man (he didn't consider women) had to cultivate to achieve success. Along with diligence, industriousness, thrift, cleanliness, self-discipline and self-control.

And being able to make out the station clock and read the small print of the *Bradshaw Railway Guide* soon became as vital a part of daily life as keeping abreast of the latest dispatches, say, from the Crimea or Afghanistan in *The Times* – the newspaper itself purchased from a W. H. Smith on the station. For this very reason opticians such as the late Victorian London firm of Aitchinson & Co. advertised widely on railway stations, their large enamel signs bearing the logo of an owl accompanying the slogan 'Are your eyes right? If not, consult Aitchinson & Co.' The company also advertised on the front of London omnibuses to catch the attention of the millions of Mr Pooters tootling to and from work from the metropolis's expanding rings of suburbs.

The Duke of Wellington is said to have worried that locomotives would encourage the lower orders to move about. Others were more concerned about the health hazards of travelling at such speeds. Writing on the issue in about 1840, one physician named Dr Granville touched on the potential negative effect on the eyes, maintaining that 'Being wafted through the air at the rate of 20 or 30 miles an hour must effect [sic] delicate lungs and asthmatic people, movement of rail trains will produce apoplexy; and the sudden plunging into darkness of a tunnel and emerging as suddenly cannot fail to make work for the oculist and it has never been doubted that the air in such tunnels is of a vitiated kind.'

Whatever damage dipping in and out of dark tunnels could have caused train passengers, their eyes were definitely at risk from airborne matter. Carriages offered little or no protection against passing flies and birds, or flying hot cinders, flecks of soot and sparks from the wheels on the rails. Responding to this deficiency, spectacle makers began manufacturing special 'eye-preserver' or railway (railroad in the USA) or traveller's glasses. These were D-shaped (or four-lensed) spectacles with folding lenses, sometimes opaque or tinted, at the sides, to keep out smuts and shade the eyes. Previously this style of spectacle had been worn by those with damaged corneas or other sensitivities.

A widely worn, less expensive alternative to the D-type of railway glasses were simpler protective spectacles, somewhat like swimming goggles, with eye-cups with small oval tinted lenses surrounded by a fine blued-steel wire gauze and with a cord that connected the eye-cups and fastened behind the head, which were sold 'to keep off flies, dust &c., glare of light and cold draughts or wind'. Preserving goggles with just wire eye-cups of this style were standard issue to workmen and railway workers and especially train firemen, to help save their eyes from motes and hot fragments of coal and coke and whatever else came flying at them as they stoked the engine's furnace.

There is an interesting circularity in the mining of coal and the steel wire used to make these types of goggles and increasingly also spectacles. Until Sir Humphry Davy created his safety lamp in 1815, the extraction of coal from the bowels of the earth had been an exceedingly dangerous enterprise. Aside from the obvious difficulties of tunnelling and preventing shafts collapsing, miners forging underground often encountered pockets of gases such as methane, what was called 'firedamp', and carbon monoxide, which were either highly flammable or could cause asphyxiation, and sometimes both. The Davy Lamp supplied an early warning system, the flame on its wick burning higher and bluer when these gases were present. A key feature of its design was that the flame was shielded by a fire-arresting wire mesh gauze. And wire was yet another product whose manufacturing would come on in leaps and bounds thanks to industrialisation, when steam-powered looms, at first deployed in the textile industry, supplanted waterwheel-driven wire drawing machines. Because more coal could be dug, thanks to the Davy Lamp, more wire could be made more quickly, especially after refined mild steel that was easier to draw into wire came along in the opening decade of the nineteenth century, which was immediately used to produce cheaper spectacle frames.

The injuries that could be sustained while engaging in industrial

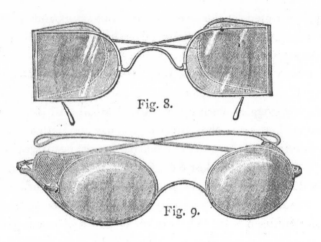

Fig. 8.

Fig. 9.

Railway glasses, illustration by Robert H. F. Rippon.

labour could be horrific. The perils of not wearing protective spectacles are illustrated by the case of William Ball, a puddler and shingler at the Coalbrookdale Company's Horsehay foundry in Shropshire for forty years, who had to leave the ironworks after being blinded in one eye by a stray piece of molten metal. Ball, however, was to become a famed wearer of thickly lensed D-shape spectacles in the wake of the accident, as many lithograph portraits and etchings of him show, during the brief period when he became one of early Victorian England's odder celebrities. The miniature and the massive, from General Tom Thumb to Jumbo the elephant, seemed to have held a peculiar fascination for our nineteenth-century forebears. Although only 5 feet 9 inches in height, Ball weighed 40 stone and his chest measured 75 inches. His waistcoat was so big, it was claimed, that 'three men could be buttoned into it'. After appearing as 'The Shropshire Giant', 'The Largest Man in England' and under the pseudonym 'John Bull' at county fairs and other rowdy shows, he came to national prominence when he was invited to present himself at the Great Exhibition, Prince Albert's jamboree of trade and industry in Hyde Park in 1851.

Journeying to London by train, Ball was too large to occupy

any of the standard passenger seats and had to be housed in the guardsman's carriage for the length of the journey. While apparently 'falling victim to thieves' and hating almost everything about London, this obese man in D-spectacles was to take his place amid the 15,000 exhibits from more than forty countries, including the Koh-i-Noor diamond and the first gas stove, under the canopy of Joseph Paxton's exhibition hall. 'The Crystal Palace', as it was christened by *Punch*, was a Cinderella's slipper of a building assembled from prefabricated modular sheet glass and wrought-iron columns. Its panes were supplied by Chance Brothers of Spon Lane, Smethwick. Established in 1824, the company became one of the most significant manufacturers of glass in the nineteenth century, glazing Charles Barry and Augustus Pugin's gothic Houses of Parliament and the face of the tower clock ('Big Ben'). Their Smethwick works churned out coloured, crown, plate and optical glass, including lenses for spectacles, sunglasses and around 2000 lighthouses.

A vaulting symbol of a brighter, lighter future, and put up in the year of the abolition of the window tax after concerns that typhoid was spreading in ill-ventilated miasmic rooms, Paxton's palace was as spectacular as almost anything inside it. Which also included some of the earliest examples of spectacles with wire hook-curled side pieces, marketed as hunting or riding glasses.*

At the time of the exhibition the opticians Thomas Harris & Sons of Great Russell St, wishing to cash in on the event, advertised

---

* Forty years later, Dollond & Co. were to unleash 'Spectacles for Horses' on the world, these equine goggles specially lensed to 'remedy shying and promote high-stepping', as adverts for them noted. The company appeared willing to take any ridicule in their stride, observing that 'No doubt, many may smile at the idea of Spectacles being used by horse-trainers, but it must not be lost sight of that Science has done much in the past which was previously ridiculed – and that much is still to be accomplished no-one will deny.' *Brewer's Phrase and Fable* of 1870 also relates that 'Bar'nacles' was then a slang term for reading glasses, 'so-called because in shape they resembled the twitchers used by farriers to keep under restraint unruly horses during the process of bleeding, dressing or shoeing. This instrument formerly known as a barnacle, consisting for two branches joined at one end by a hinge, was fixed on the horse nose.' The name was possibly a corruption of *binocles*, or 'double eyes'.

a visual aid (probably an opera glass, though they did also mention their range of 'crystal spectacles') called 'Harris's Exhibition Glass' said to be '(portable and powerful) made expressly for viewing the Contents of the Crystal Palace' and 'admirably adapted for looking at the Paintings in the Royal Academy's Exhibition'. Visitors to either, they maintained, 'should not be without one'.

Wellington, whose pessimistic predictions that hordes of the unwashed would trash the exhibition failed to materialise, rode and hunted throughout his long life. He even kept a scratch pack of sixteen foxhounds during the Peninsular War campaigns and as a young man sometimes hunted up to three days a week. The Iron Duke was, as his military colleague, friend and biographer George Robert Gleig would write, 'very proud of his eyesight'. Which, in Gleig's version of events, 'continued to be remarkably good and clear to the last'. He went on to maintain that there was 'no doubt that the Duke could, at eighty-three years of age, read in the open air a well-written manuscript without using spectacles'. Gleig was a soldier, a gentleman and a man of the cloth, so it would be unjust to doubt his word. Here, however, he seems to have chosen his words rather carefully, for the statement allows plenty of wriggle room for Wellington to have used spectacles indoors when landed with far less well-written manuscripts. Which is precisely what he did do, and only out of vanity chose to avoid wearing his glasses in public wherever possible. And never when in the saddle.

A pair of Wellington's spectacles from the early 1840s, with a document handwritten in ink authenticating their provenance, was auctioned by Christie's in 2016, in a sale that also saw a slice of Queen Victoria's wedding cake and a leather wallet once owned by Napoleon (and gaudily embossed with gilt imperial-crowned Ns and looking not unlike some knock-off Louis Vuitton bag) come up for grabs. The spectacles had 'round lenses and folding wire sides with arrow-shaped ends (one arm broken)', and came with 'a dark-red leather, gilt-tooled embossed' case bearing the name of the firm of Jones at '62 CHARING CROSS' inside and a gold X on either side outside.

Most striking, though, is that the Iron Duke's frames were of blued-steel wire. Blueing involved tempering and treating the steel to create a hard oxide film on the surface to prevent it from rusting. It might be expected that someone of Wellington's rank – he had twice served as Britain's Prime Minister – would be more likely to have worn gold rather than less costly blued-steel spectacles. But blueing originated in gun-making in the late eighteenth and early nineteenth centuries, possibly lending blued-steel spectacles a kind of no-nonsense military cachet. They were judged suitably U (in Nancy Mitford's terminology) to receive a thumbs-up in *Good Society*, a guide to etiquette published eight years after Wellington's death, which maintained that 'If spectacles are necessary they should be of the best and lightest make and mounted in gold or blue steel.'

Wellington, along with Napoleon and Queen Victoria, was a customer of the Prussian-French clock maker Abraham-Louis Breguet. Described as the Leonardo da Vinci of horology and the genius who invented the wristwatch and made the first carriage clock for Bonaparte, Breguet was also one of the first people to use blued-steel for hands and screws in timepieces because it wore better than gold. Blue hands continue to be a rather showy feature of the luxury watches produced under the Breguet brand name these days, and which retail for six-figure sums. Though now they are made in the Vallée de Joux in Switzerland rather than in Paris, as they were in Breguet's lifetime, and for nearly 200 years.*

On both sides of the Channel the professions of optician, spectacle maker, clock maker and jeweller continued to overlap; the inventory of a typical Victorian optician also contained chronometers, barometers, thermometers and other instruments, and in 1844 watch and clock makers W. Loof of Tunbridge Wells boasted of the patronage of Queen Victoria and her mother the Duchess of Kent, selling 'Spectacles, Eye and Reading Glasses' alongside 'a large and superior stock of Watches, Clocks, Timepieces, and Jewellery of every description' and 'Sheffield plated goods'. As we shall see,

---

* Although Breguet had been born in Neuchâtel, which today is in Switzerland but then was Prussian territory.

such casual business arrangements would eventually persuade the opticians to up their game and professionalise to see off dabblers cannibalising their trade.

## Like clockwork

But it was the presence of so many clock makers in and around Geneva and the rich deposits of iron in the Morez valley that led to almost all of France's spectacle making becoming concentrated on the French side of the Jura mountain range in the 1820s. Even today the Haut-Jura town of Morez claims the title of 'the eyewear capital of France' and maintains that it alone accounts for 55 per cent of the total output of the country's spectacle industry, with '88% of the 10 million frames' turned out there every year continuing to be manufactured in metals. Plastic ones, meanwhile, are the speciality of near regional neighbour Oyonnax, which seemingly adds a further 25 per cent to the national frame-making tally.

The story of how this mountainous borderland country on the eastern fringes of France, covered with snow for five months of the year, ended up as such a Mecca for Gallic spectacle making revolves around one man: Pierre-Hyacinthe Caseaux. A farmer who tended land and raised cattle in a tiny rural hamlet outside Morez, Caseaux by all accounts occupied himself during the long and chilly months of winter, as many of his ilk did, making nails from iron wire. Morez lies on the river Bienne whose strong currents had powered local ironworks for centuries, and nails formed an essential component in the construction of the area's traditional houses, which are faced with wooden weatherboards tacked on to keep the brutal conditions at bay.

At some point in the 1790s, when Caseaux was approaching his fifties and probably suffering from age-related presbyopia, he acquired a pair of spectacles in Geneva, the nearest place where glasses of any quality could be bought. And as a city where the Protestant reformer John Calvin spent his final years in the sixteenth century, goldsmiths and jewellers had stealthily moved into clock and spectacle making as a means of assuaging their Christian consciences and keeping in profit. By some mishap or other, the frames on Caseaux's Swiss spectacles got damaged. He improvised, setting the surviving lenses in a replica fashioned out of twirled pieces of leftover iron wire. The resulting frame was convincing enough for him to experiment further and take a more advanced prototype to a jeweller-optician in Geneva, who reacted positively and ordered some for his shop. From here the Jura glasses industry was born, and by 1846 there were a hundred spectacle makers working in Morez. Caseaux's younger partner Jean-Baptiste Lamy continued the business on the elder man's retirement, and in Morez in the 1880s Lamy's heirs built the most advanced hydroelectric-powered glasses-making factory in nineteenth-century France. By which time spectacle making and the manufacture of steel, which was also used for casks by local vintners of Jura wine – a regional tipple comparable to Burgundy – were almost the only games in town.

Steel wire frames, as the author of *Good Society* had noted, were admired for their lightness. But some of the first attempts to create an even lighter frame by removing the rims entirely had already been initiated on the Continent by the Viennese optician Voigtländer, who in around 1820 constructed a pair of spectacles that Paxton would surely have admired, where the lenses and bridge were formed from one single piece of glass. If incredibly inconspicuous and surprisingly modern-looking, they were far too fragile to be practical.

Another Austrian called Waldstein advanced the design and produced a version in the 1840s where the metal bridge and sides were pinned into the lenses, and this enjoyed commercial success and was widely imitated. Though again, they were easily damaged and their wearers had to be able and willing to fork out for repairs in addition to the cost of the spectacles themselves.

A slightly cheaper and less fragile alternative was the new breed of thinner wire frames that arrived in the 1860s thanks to newer precision tools that allowed grooves to be cut in the edges of the lenses. In this way a rim of a far finer steel wire could be threaded into the lenses, creating an even more discreet frame.

These were frames typically advertised as 'invisible'. A catalogue for the Bristol-based opticians and spectacle makers Dunscombe from 1875 lists 'Invisible Steel Spectacles ... Designed principally for short sight', and maintained that with 'Dunscombe's Lightest Invisible Steel Spectacles, the frame weighs but a few grains'. Equipped with 'Hook sides to fasten behind the ear' and 'mounted with Finest Brazilian Pebble Lenses' they were priced at one pound, five shillings and sixpence but cost only fifteen shillings with 'Lenses of Finest Glass'. Also available were 'Dunscombe's Elastic Blue Steel Spectacles' with 'Finest Brazilian Pebble Lenses', yours for just ten shillings and indicative of the use of tensile steel wire for frames.

## Totally wired

But the most high-wire act of this era was the pince-nez. A form of eyewear that dispensed with side pieces and other standard means of support and named from the French for 'nose-pincher', it first appeared in around 1840. They succeeded in capturing the popular imagination all over Europe and in America and were thought quite smart, in all senses of the word, by both men and women. Sir Arthur Conan Doyle was to place a pair at the heart of his 1904 Sherlock Holmes mystery 'The Adventure of the Golden Pince-Nez'. First published in the *Strand Magazine*, where Holmes had made his debut, the story, which features one-time Russian anarchists, has the Egyptian-cigarette-smoking 'consulting' sleuth solving the murder of a factotum to an elderly professor, who died still clutching in his hand the aforementioned spectacles. In a bravura show of his deductive powers, Holmes, after inspecting the pince-nez for just a few moments, hastily scribbles down a complete description of the assassin they should be looking for, even concluding that the killer, who he claims is 'a woman of good address, attired like a lady' with 'a remarkably thick nose' and 'eyes which are set close to either side of it', 'has had recourse to an optician at least twice during the last few months'. Though more weirdly he also maintains, against plenty of evidence to the contrary of a fairly active optical trade at the time, that 'since opticians are not very numerous, there should be no difficulty tracing her'.*

Damned more recently by the optician and historian Ronald J. S. MacGregor as 'fragile, unstable, uncomfortable' and offering 'poor centration for a pair of lenses' in comparison with spectacles with side pieces, perhaps what ultimately appealed to the Victorians about the pince-nez was its contemporary ingenuity. With their piano-wire construction and elastic sprung bridges, and all parts machine-tooled, they were practically wearable tech. A steampunk spectacle, sprung and cantilevered as majestically as an airship. Bendy enough in some iterations to be folded up, they were often termed 'folders', their lenses sliding neatly over one another, and allowing them to be tucked discreetly into a waistcoat pocket. When next needed they could be fished out, sprung back into shape and easily restored to the face. Often worn on a decorative chain or a fancy ribbon, pince-nez appeared in a bewildering array of rim-shapes and varieties – the Canadian Folder, the Boson Clip, the Perfection Folder and the Improved Imperial Guard (sold as 'the best and easiest adjustable eyeglass guard in the market') – and manufacturers outdid themselves promising ever more comfortable and efficient clips to keep them on the wearers' noses.

There were, nevertheless, certain prescriptions that, at least to begin with, pince-nez were ill suited to. Keeping the lenses at the appropriate axis to treat astigmatisms was one particular difficulty that wasn't solved until a suitably complicated rigid frame

---

* The pince-nez's associations with the Victorian bourgeoisie and their false consciousness ensured that the ship's doctor Smirnov in Sergei Eisenstein's 1925 Soviet agitprop movie *Battleship Potemkin*, a fictional account of the failed first Russian revolution of 1905, appears in a pair. Smirnov uses his pince-nez to inspect the ship's ration of maggot-ridden meat, which is shown in all its festering glory by Eisenstein in a close-up through their lenses, and which the doctor blithely declares safe for consumption by the already ill-nourished sailors. In an equally famous sequence towards the film's end, when Tsarist forces conduct a massacre on the Odessa Steps, a grandmotherly woman in pince-nez is shot through the eye – signalling, far from subtly, her failure to see how evil the ancient regime truly was.

christened 'the Astig' was arrived at in the latter years of Victoria's reign. Although the condition itself hadn't even been identified until the beginning of the nineteenth century.

Astigmatism, like myopia and hypermetropia, is a problem of refraction that can affect both the short- and long-sighted. It's caused by an abnormal curvature of the cornea or lens. Effectively the eye is more egg-shaped than spherical which results in the blurring and distortion of images regardless of the distance of the viewer from them.

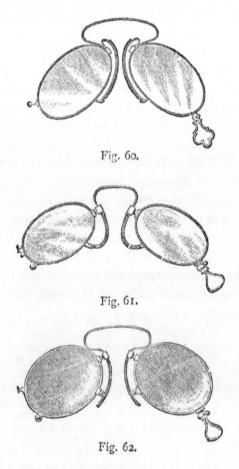

Fig. 60.

Fig. 61.

Fig. 62.

Pince-nez, illustration by Robert H. F. Rippon.

One of the first descriptions of this problem appeared in a lecture in 1801 by Thomas Young, the Quaker physician and polymath who helped decipher the Rosetta Stone and came up with the 'double-slit experiment' to demonstrate the interference of light waves. Young, who suffered with the condition himself, analysed the problem in reference to his own poor eyesight and explained he was able to correct it by looking obliquely through his glasses. Seemingly he didn't quite see the full significance of his observations. Over twenty years would pass before the mathematician, astronomer and Cambridge don George Biddell Airy turned his mind to the matter, after he had become troubled by 'a malformation in his left eye' that seems to have come on in 1825 in addition to his already pronounced myopia.

As the future Astronomer Royal and someone who'd spend much of his life looking at the stars through lenses, he similarly found relief by angling his spectacles. He worked out that 'the rays of light coming from a luminous point and falling upon the whole surface of the pupil' did 'not converge to a point at any position within the eye' but converged 'in such manner as to pass through two right angles to each other'.

Airy consequently set about calculating the focal powers needed to correct this optical aberration. He then designed a cylindrical lens that could bend the light into focus, and had one ground to his specification by a man named Fuller in Ipswich. Overwhelmed by the results, he presented his findings in a paper to the Cambridge Philosophical Society in which he wrote enthusiastically, 'I have found that the eye which I once feared would become quite useless can now be used in almost every respect as well as the other.'

The optical trade was swiftly in on the act. By 1828, cylindrical lenses for astigmatism were already being imported from England and sold (and soon after that manufactured) in Philadelphia by the Scottish-American family firm of McAllister, whose patriarch John McAllister Sr had arrived in America from Glasgow shortly before the Revolutionary War and is saluted as the 'founder of the profession of opticianry' in the country. However, the earliest known optician on record in the States is a woman: 'the widow of

Balthazar Summer' was in 1753 advertising in the *New York Gazette* as a 'grinder of all sorts of optic glass'. But as the optical historian J. William Rosenthal has argued, since the demand for optical goods was to remain 'too small to support a local industry' and lenses were 'high-value, low-bulk durable goods easily imported from low-cost production centres in Europe', America continued to 'import the bulk' of its optical goods until well into the nineteenth century. Rosenthal suggests that the War of 1812, which disrupted trade with Britain, might have stimulated those like McAllister to begin making their own frames and later lenses. But the most significant factors in America becoming much more self-sufficient would be the influx of new skilled immigrants, accompanied by a growing public and professional interest in science and technology.

## American eyes

McAllister Sr died in 1830, the year John Jacob Bausch, one of the two men said to have introduced the pince-nez to the United States, was born in Württemberg, Germany.

Bausch was among the so-called Forty-Eighters, a whole generation of mostly young and progressive Germans, Czechs and Austro-Hungarians who emigrated to America following the failure of the revolutions in their native lands that year. Bausch, who'd served an apprenticeship in the optical trade under his older brother learning how to grind lenses and make spectacles in metal, horn and tortoiseshell, was to endure a horrendous storm-ridden forty-nine-day crossing of the Atlantic by sailing ship. After arriving in New York in April 1849 he moved upstate to Buffalo, only to find himself in the middle of a cholera epidemic. Pushing on to Rochester, he took a dollar-a-day job as a turner in a wood shop and met another thoughtful young German lad called Heinrich (later Henry) Lomb, just a couple of years older than himself and originally hailing from Hesse-Kassel. They became fast friends.

After Bausch lost parts of two fingers on his right hand in a buzz-saw accident, Lomb supplied financial support for his injured compatriot. The pair, partially in lieu of that debt and with an

additional $66 worth of backing thrown in, became business part-
ners when Bausch established an optical goods shop, the only one
in western New York, with, supposedly, 'a tray of optical blanks
and some miscellaneous horn frames'. Soon, however, Bausch was
offering homegrown 'European-style' spectacles with steel rims for
$1.50, silver ones for $2 and gold for $9. And by around 1855 Bausch
& Lomb were selling pince-nez to the American public. Brigham
Young, the Mormon pioneer and founder of Salt Lake City, Utah,
was among the stateside devotees of the style.

While Lomb enlisted and went off to fight in the American
Civil War for the Unionist cause in 1861, Bausch remained in
Rochester and had a fateful encounter with a hulk of vulcanised
rubber on the local streets.*

Patented by Charles Goodyear of Naugatuck, Connecticut, in
1844 and named after Vulcan, the Roman god of fire, vulcanised
rubber was the new miracle material of the mid-nineteenth century. The potential of natural rubber, the gooey sap bled from
trees in Brazil, as a malleable waterproof material had already been
recognised by Charles Mackintosh who invented the rubberised
cloth his name remains synonymous with in the 1820s. But wider
applications of rubber, and its liquid form latex, were stymied by
its unfortunate habit of melting in warm weather and cracking in
the cold. It was only when Goodyear, after experimenting with
the stuff for over ten years, combined it with sulphur and heated it

---

* Though accounts differ, Abraham Lincoln, who is thought to have first
acquired glasses for reading in Chicago from the oculist Dr John Phillips in
the early 1850s, is reported to have donned spectacles to deliver the Gettysburg
Address on 19 November 1863. Recalling this momentous speech in 1891, the
journalist John Russell Young wrote, 'From an ancient case he drew a pair of
steel-framed spectacles, with bows clasping upon the temples in front of the ears,
and adjusted them with deliberation.' Young's description seems to tally with
a pair of particularly ingenious pocketable folding spectacles that the President
is known to have owned, though Lincoln's pair were in gold. Manufactured by
Burt & Willard – a partnership between John Burt of Hartford, Connecticut,
and William W. Willard of Syracuse, New York – these 'folders' were in their
words 'So constructed as to allow the folding together of the glass frame and
the short temple bows and cups, forming one of the most convenient and snugly
portable spectacles for use and for the pocket ever before invented or used.'

up that a durable substance was found – one that was quickly put to use making tyres, boots, shoes, balls, piping, mats, and now, thanks to Bausch, spectacle frames. Bausch & Lomb began offering vulcanite rubber spectacles, cheaper and lighter than horn, in 1866. The company purchased sheets of the stuff; once heated up, the shapes of the frames were punched out with a hand-operated press.

But the influx of technically proficient émigrés from Europe and a more fractious relationship with England in areas of trade, combined with a greater national demand for spectacles as ever-expanding armies of Bartlebys with (from 1873 onwards) Remington typewriters bashed out the invoices and letters needed to keep the economy and western progress going, produced a more self-sufficient local optical industry in America. Where imported English frames could sometimes cost several dollars, American manufacturers were able to reduce the price of steel frames to a dollar, and vulcanite frames in Philadelphia were advertised for as little as ten cents a go.

On both sides of the Atlantic, though, frames and lenses were to become sophisticated factory fodder by the end of the century. Mass-produced to a range of specifications, spectacle parts and lenses of varying prescriptions were now capable of being precision-engineered to be interchangeable. The protectionist monopolies once enjoyed by the Worshipful Company of Spectacle Makers were distant history; free trade was king while Victoria reigned. And in a laissez-faire economy where shopping was on the brink of becoming a leisure activity with the arrival of the first department stores, such as the Bon Marché which opened in a purpose-built steel-framed building in Brixton in 1877, such modular eyewear presented retailers with opportunities. Jewellers, chemists, fancy goods shops and even ironmongers could carry stocks of frames and lenses that could be assembled while customers waited.

More worrying for traditional opticians and spectacle makers in England, though, was the installation in the 1890s by the Automatic Sight-Testing & Optical Supply Company of do-it-yourself eye-testing machines in (or just outside) branches of W. H. Smith at railway stations. Like the What the Butler Saw kinetoscopes that prefigured cinematic motion pictures, these were penny-in-the-slot, peer-in-the-viewfinder, crank-the-handle devices. But instead of being presented with a sequence of flickering images of bashful young ladies coyly undressing in their boudoirs, the rail passenger looked through the eye-holes at a test-type and used the handle to scroll through a series of numbered lenses until it was legible. They then wrote down the numbers of the lenses required on an order slip that was deposited in a slot in the machine. Spectacles or 'folders' were promptly made up with the appropriate prescription and could either be posted out or collected in person from the firm's West End showrooms at 65 & 66 Chancery Lane, Holborn. Boastfully advertised in 1892 as 'No Better Glasses for the Preservation of the Eyesight can be supplied even at £100 per pair', they cost two shillings and sixpence 'in Case complete'. Which works out at about just over a tenner at modern-day prices. The optical profession would respond to such disruptive entrepreneurial interlopers by further professionalising itself.

# 6

# Assessing the Profession

As might be recalled from Samuel Pepys' encounters with the Turlingtons, opticians and spectacle makers hadn't historically engaged themselves much with eye tests. The notion of testing a patient's sight and selecting bespoke lenses was really another nineteenth-century phenomenon spurred on by medical science and the establishment of dedicated ophthalmic hospitals. What would become the Royal London Ophthalmic Hospital or Moorfields Eye Hospital, the first hospital in the world devoted to eye diseases, opened in West Smithfield in 1805, around the time of the Napoleonic Wars, as the London Dispensary for Curing Diseases of the Eye and Ear. Its remit shrank to the eyes alone after its founding director John Cunningham Saunders confessed to having

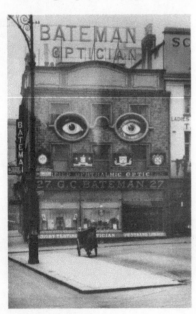

Bateman's Opticians,
East Street, Brighton.

had 'little success in curing diseases of the ear' to its board of governors. Saunders died in post in 1810. The next year, though, the hospital's surgeon, Benjamin Travers, began teaching courses in ophthalmology. In 1816, when Travers published his textbook *Synopsis of the Diseases of the Eye*, three Americans, Edward Delafield, John Kearny Rogers and Edward Reynolds, enrolled on the course. On completing their studies and returning to the States, the first two men established the New York Eye Infirmary and the latter joined a colleague in Boston to found the Massachusetts Eye & Ear Infirmary, both institutions modelled after Moorfields.

But it was in continental Europe that the study of the eye received one of its greatest boons, when in 1851 Hermann von Helmholtz, the associate professor of physiology at the Prussian University of Königsberg, invented the ophthalmoscope.

Helmholtz had been fascinated by the luminosity of the eye, the ways in which light entering the pupils seemed to be reflected back, and sought to capture it as a means of looking into its internal workings. He spent some eight days knocking up a prototype, made of cardboard, spectacle lenses and a glass from a microscope. With this astonishingly crude contraption he nevertheless became the first person to look at a living retina.

In a letter to his father, the headmaster of a Potsdam gymnasium who'd encouraged him to study medicine, Helmholtz spelt out the significance of the discovery he'd made using

a combination of glasses through which it becomes possible to illuminate through the pupil the dark background of the eye, and to do so without applying blinding light and simultaneously to see exactly all details of the retina, indeed even more exactly than one sees the exterior parts of the eye without enlargement ... One sees the blood-vessels most elegantly, the branched arteries and veins, the entrance of the optical nerves into the eye etc. Until now there was a series of extraordinarily important eye diseases that combined together under the name 'black star', a terra incognita, since neither in life nor, for the most part, in death did one learn something about the changes

in the eye. Thanks to my invention the most specialised investigation of the interior structure of the eye will become possible.*

Helmholtz published a forty-three-page pamphlet outlining the
workings of his ophthalmoscope. But perhaps more importantly
for its widespread acceptance he also embarked on a two-month
tour of German-speaking universities in August and September
1851, an itinerary that took him into Austria and Switzerland,
along with brief excursions into France and Italy, all of which
proved that seeing really was believing. The ophthalmoscope
accrued immediate converts everywhere it went. And as a non-
invasive examination tool it also became the go-to healthcare
device of the wealthy unwell seeking answers to their ills and the
opportunity to enjoy specialist attention in their drawing rooms,
spas and private clinics. None of which should denigrate its
unrivalled importance in the diagnosis of ocular health.

If the eyes, as Shakespeare had expressed it, were windows to
the soul, then the ophthalmoscope gave doctors, perhaps for almost
the first time, a fighting chance to play God when trying to save
people's sight. Or at the very least a better means of figuring out
what had gone wrong.

Recalling the period before Helmholtz's invention, John
Whitaker Hulke, a surgeon at Moorfields who was born in 1830,
remarked that in his 'earliest student days the ophthalmoscope
was unknown and errors of refraction were so little understood
that a small tortoiseshell case, which could easily be carried in
the trousers pocket, containing half a dozen convex and concave
spherical lenses, was held to comprise a sufficient stock for every
trial'. According to Margaret Miller, biographer of the British
Optical Association, in this period oculists and ophthalmologists,
at least in Britain, 'regarded themselves primarily as medical men
and considered the fitting of glasses below their dignity'.

---

* Another digression, but haunting to reflect on the video for 'Blackstar', a track
from David Bowie's final album of the same name, in which the singer appeared
with bandaged eyes with beads standing in for pupils.

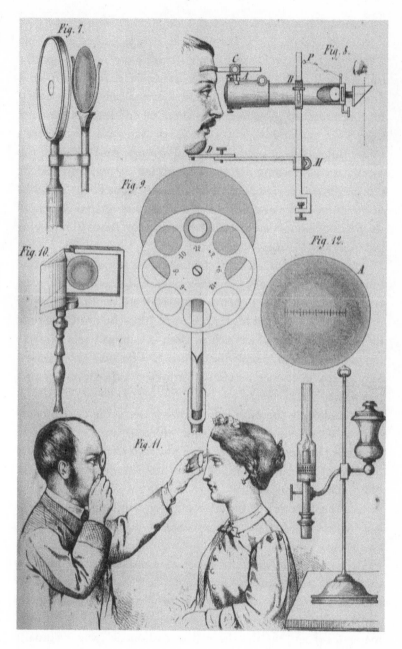

Ophthalmoscope in action.

Some of Moorfields' surgeons, such as Alfred Smee who gave a series of lectures at the hospital that were published as a book, *The Eye in Health and Disease*, a revised edition of which appeared in 1854, still held against prescribing spectacles for certain conditions (myopia in his case) unless it was absolutely necessary. Having observed, however, that labourers and soldiers were not short-sighted while bookish types were, Smee was to propose a causal link between occupations and myopia. And while he was mostly against dishing out glasses to all but the most myopic, he did, nevertheless, invent an optometer – a device that could be fitted with a range of different lenses that were rotated in front of the patient's eyes – that he hoped would aid opticians in supplying the most suitable prescriptions.

This was more in line with thoughts about glasses on mainland Europe, where in the 1850s ophthalmologists such as Carl Ferdinand Ritter von Arlt, the Bohemian professor of ophthalmology at Prague University, and his former pupil Albrecht von Graefe and his assistant Richard Liebreich in Berlin, were to begin promoting glasses as an invaluable therapeutic tool for optical physicians. Something, in essence, as vital as surgery or other more invasive treatments.

Far and away the most important figure in the development of optical prescription at this time, though, was Dr Franciscus Cornelis Donders, the professor of physiology at the University of Utrecht who in 1858 established the first eye hospital in the Netherlands. Donders was also the first person to offer a clear distinction between hypermetropia (long-sightedness) and the age-related presbyopia and to suggest how prismatic lenses might cure squints, often the result of congenial hypermetropia. His 1864 book *On the anomalies of accommodation and refraction of the eye with a preliminary essay on physiologic dioptrics* became a set text for ophthalmic surgeons and progressive opticians alike, and Donders' advocacy of lenses that were measured in one-metre focal lengths that he called a 'dioptric' was eventually adopted almost universally. Donders' other and perhaps most magnificent contribution to the field of optics was to ask his colleague Herman Snellen in 1860 to come up with a chart to test patients' eyesight.

Snellen's first attempt featured an arrangement of variously sized symbols – circles, squares, plus signs and so on. Dingbats, essentially. Superficially these seemed to offer something universal. The illiterate, for instance, might still have been able to relate what they could see. But actually describing exactly what in hell the blurry dots and half-formed circles dancing in front of them were proved too difficult for most patients. Few of the symbols enjoyed the same level of immediate recognition as letters of the alphabet; illiteracy was, in any case, on the brink of extinction by then in the Netherlands: 90 per cent of Dutch men would be classed as literate by 1875. Realising his mistake, Snellen returned to his drawing board, and the now-familiar style of eye test chart with its descending lines of ever smaller letters was born.

An early customer was seemingly the British Army, which purchased Snellen charts in 1863. Its ranks just then were being augmented by legions of Volunteer Rifle Corps. These were grassroots units of amateur musketeers formed, often by patriotic college men and lower-middle-class clerks and artisans, amid fears of another conflict with France and drummed up by a national campaign spearheaded by *The Times*. The eye tests would therefore have helped to weed out some of the more hopeless shots rallying to calls to serve the empire.

## The Browning motion

On civvy street, however, the methods used and the quality of eye tests generally available were to continue to vary from practice to practice and shop to shop. In 1860, the Scottish ophthalmologist John Soelberg Wells had joined Moorfields as a clinical assistant after studying and working in Berlin under Albrecht von Graefe. From von Graefe, Wells inherited ideas about how glasses might be used to treat patients, and soon after his arrival the hospital appointed its first official optician, Thomas Doublet, a near neighbour of Smee's in Finsbury Square. Wells had consistently railed against what he termed 'unscientific opticians' and in 1862 wrote a book, *On Long, Short, and Weak Sight, and Their Treatment by the Scientific Use of Spectacles*, in which he damned the profession for doing more harm than good, stating that 'The proper and scientific choice of spectacles is indeed of great importance to the public, and I have no hesitation in saying that the empirical, haphazard plan of selection generally employed by opticians, is but too frequently attended by the worst consequences, that eyes are often ruined which might by scientific and skilful treatment, have been preserved for years.'

His suggestion was that doctors themselves should conduct sight tests and issue prescriptions that the opticians would then prepare. But there were opticians who were serious – and scientific – about their craft who believed that they needed to become much more like doctors and undergo some form of training before they were allowed to issue members of the public with spectacles. One of the most vocal on this matter was John Browning.

Marrying at least three times and living to ninety-four years of age, Browning packed a lot into his long life. The possessor of a full-flowing soup-catching beard for much of that time, he fulfils the Victorian ideal of a restlessly curious and astonishingly productive entrepreneur, inventor, scientist and occasional author. Descending from a line of nautical instrument makers from Kent, Browning studied both medicine and chemistry before joining the family firm and transforming it into one of the most forward-thinking manufacturers of scientific instruments in Britain. From the company's factory in Minories and later on the Strand, Browning designed, and his sixty-strong staff made and marketed, barometers, ophthalmoscopes, spectroscopes, microscopes, cameras, field and opera glasses, and electric lamps. He counted William Henry Fox Talbot, the Royal Greenwich Observatory and Her Majesty the Queen as clients and installed the first electric light in London at the Guildhall for an official banquet to honour the visiting Shah of Persia in 1873.

But the profession he gave to census takers and which appeared on the plates affixed to the backs of his brass cameras was 'master optician'. His contribution to the field of eyewear would include an especially rugged D-shaped protective spectacle with a nickel frame and extra thick lenses of Brazilian quartz that was aimed at cack-handed blood sports enthusiasts and advertised as 'shot-proof', with an 'improved "non-pressure" Canadian folder' with 'light springs fitted with tortoise-shell nose pieces'.

In 1883 he published *How to Use Our Eyes and How to Preserve them by the Aid of Spectacles*, a book whose first print run sold out in three weeks and which by 1889 was already on to its seventh revised edition. One of the new chapters added was on 'Ladies' Veils' and whether they were 'beneficial or not to the eyes'. Answer: it all depended on the type of veil, apparently.

Browning, as perhaps might be expected, was a man of trenchant and sometimes peculiar opinions on all things ocular. The book is studded with illustrations that offer visual support to a long catalogue of dos and don'ts that range from the correct way to wear spectacles to the position to adopt when sitting reading at the fireside with your cat. While he is amused to note that one of his middle-aged clients realised that spectacles would be required after 'becoming Bradshaw blind' (after the railway timetable), one of Browning's particular bugbears was those who read while travelling by train, one missive against mixing literature with locomotion headed 'How to Blind Yourself: Reading in a Railway Carriage'.

But he was to take particular aim at what he called the 'quacking of spectacles' by the unqualified and the unscrupulous, and misleading trade advertising:

Do not believe that any loudly puffed spectacles can be of special service to you. There is a skill, of course, required in making good lenses of fine optical glass or Brazilian pebble; but there is more skill required in suiting the spectacle to each person's requirements. How can this skill, only to be acquired by knowledge combined with great experience, be possessed by every watchmaker, chemist, jeweller, or ironmonger who buys a dozen pairs of spectacles and writes up that he is a PRACTICAL OPTICIAN?'

Despite having attended the Royal College of Chemistry himself, Browning calls out chemists for sharp optical practices, accusing them of acting as shills for manufacturers by circulating pseudo-medical pamphlets in their names promoting the health merits of certain spectacles that the public are unaware are printed up by the glass makers themselves. Even lower than chemists, watch makers and ironmongers, in Browning's eyes, are the barkers who sell spectacles and folders, 'which of course have magical properties according to their vendors, at exhibitions, fancy fairs and bazaars'. Outrage rising – you can almost hear the hairs in his beard bristling at the thought of the impertinence of it all – he adds: 'The dealers in these spectacles actually take hold of people by the shoulders and put the spectacles or folders on to their faces before asking leave to do so. If these are to be the opticians of the future, then the necessary qualities for a successful optician will be a face of brass, lungs of leather, the tongue of a Cheap Jack.'

Inevitably enough, the best kind of opticians were the ones in his own image who did as he did. In the chapter labelled 'Browning's Method of Testing the Sight', the master optician revealed that he used three main instruments: an optometer, a width measurer for working out the distances between the pupils, and a set of Short-Sight Test Lenses, which look like a six-pack of lorgnettes stuffed in the one handle. He nevertheless becomes rather coy about his 'Method', maintaining that 'I cannot, however, give the method I adopt in using these instruments, because it varies with the varying condition with the sight of the applicants.' Reproduced, however, are examples of Jaeger tests, i.e. test-types of varying font sizes and instructions on the distances from which they should be legible, and so forth.

The book ends with a highly apocryphal-sounding story intended to ram home the dangers posed by sloppy sight tests. Browning recounts that a man with inflamed eyes came to see him having been prescribed glasses that were far too powerful for his myopia. When asked how his optician, located 'in one of the leading thoroughfares of London', tested his eyes, Browning is aghast to hear the details. This so-called optician merely handed the man 'a trayful of spectacles' and left him to try them on in turn until he alighted upon a pair with which he could see the weathercock on the spire of the church a 'quarter of a mile off'. Once these were found, the job was done and the patient was advised to 'wear them constantly'. Fuming on the man's behalf, Browning complained that 'Short of putting this gentleman's eyes out with hot irons, it would have been difficult for the optician to do anything more likely to deprive him of sight.'

By now Browning was not alone in feeling that opticians needed to up their game. If even once-lawless village pursuits such as football now had formal rules, governing bodies and, as of 1888, a league of professional teams, how could eyes continue to be tested by mostly unaccredited individuals with little knowledge of optics?

James Aitchison was a Londoner of Scottish stock with blue eyes, all the more piercing for being narrowly spaced together, and a bushy moustache waxed at the ends and tended as carefully as topiary. In 1889, at the age of twenty-nine, he became so disgusted with the slack methods at the High Holborn opticians he'd been apprenticed to that he left to found his own practice to engage in 'more scientific ways of assessing eyesight'.

Setting up on Fleet Street, a thoroughfare already dominated by newspapers and publishers, and billing himself as a 'Consulting Oculist Optician' who had 'made the Eyes and the Science of Optics as applied to Spectacles his special study', Aitchison offered glasses for as little as a shilling a pair, though his average price was two shillings and sixpence, and initially imported much of his raw materials from Germany. Within six years he had three shops, the grandest on the Strand near the Savoy Hotel and equidistant from Whitehall and the offices of government, the publishers on Charing Cross Road and Longacre in Covent Garden, and the theatres and restaurants of the West End.

Like his near neighbour, Aitchison possessed strong and odd opinions on defective eyesight. Perhaps most controversially, he believed that uncorrected eye conditions could lead to criminality and even murder.

## The case of the Lambeth poisoner

This theory was reinforced following Aitchison's involvement in treating a patient, Thomas Neill, for a pronounced squint with eyeglasses. Unbeknown to him, Neill was wanted for the murder by poison of a prostitute, Matilda Clover, in the Lambeth Road. The killer, dubbed 'The Lambeth Poisoner' by the gutter press, had in fact studied medicine at McGill University in Canada and at the University of London. Never qualifying, he appears to have suffered a nervous breakdown and developed both a dependency on opiates and a hatred of what was then referred to as 'the fairer sex'. Posing as a medic and calling himself Dr Neill Cream, he'd arrived in London in 1891 fresh from serving a ten-year prison sentence for second-degree murder in America after poisoning another woman. His squint had featured prominently in police photographs that were circulated on both sides of the Atlantic. He was therefore anxious to have it corrected. Staying in the Anderton Hotel on Fleet Street, Neill had beaten a path to Aitchison's nearby door.

The moustachioed optician was more than happy to aid someone who appeared educated and interested in the latest advances of optical science. They discussed which lenses and frames would best cure the defect. Two pairs of gold-framed glasses were prescribed, and these spectacles, bearing the name of Aitchison stamped on their sides, were delivered to Neill's hotel.

After Neill's arrest and the discovery of this branded eyewear, the optician was subpoenaed to confirm his client's identity. The trial concluded on 21 October 1892 with a guilty verdict and the homicidal faux doctor was sentenced to be hanged. On the scaffold the condemned man claimed to be Jack the Ripper, only adding to the notoriety of the case. But five days before the execution Aitchison wrote to *The Times* arguing that long-standing, untreated hypermetropia in Neill's left eye was a likely contributing factor in his criminal behaviour. The strain of unconsciously trying to overcome the defect since infancy, he argued, had done him 'an incalculable amount of harm'. For years he would have been plagued by 'headaches and nervous pains'. These ailments, exacerbated by study, Aitchison maintained, had probably precipitated the collapse and subsequent lapse into addiction, the opium taken, in effect, as a form of self-medication (to use the current phrase) to stave off the symptoms actually caused by his faulty eye. All of which, he believed, could easily have been 'obviated if his eyes had been corrected in early childhood'.

It's an extreme case, obviously, but to argue that someone's quality of life and therefore their life choices might be adversely affected by an eye condition that has caused them pain for decades has a certain logic about it. But in the 1890s, arguments about criminality and the inheritance of genetic conditions such as eye defects often slipped uncomfortably easily into discussions of eugenics, and breeding out such tendencies. Aitchison held that glasses should be prescribed as early as possible as a preventative measure to stop problems, ocular or psychopathic or a combination of both, developing later in life.

On these grounds, and to avoid early eye strain, he confessed in an interview in 1894 to being 'strongly opposed to educational overpressure' in childhood, 'especially when, to school lessons, severe home work' was added. But Aitchison was among those opticians who lobbied for more study and formal qualifications for his own profession to improve standards. With a group of distinguished opticians, he would go on to establish the Optical Institute, a society that met to discuss training. It looked into the possibility of creating a school 'devoted to the instruction of workmen in the scientific instrument trades and the higher education of optical designers'. That dream was not to be realised, but Aitchison would raise funds to support evening classes in optics at other institutions and cajoled the industry into providing prizes and scholarships. This, though, was by then a boom period for what had become known as 'technical education' in Britain.

Its cause had been championed since the 1860s by the German-born iron-master and Liberal MP Sir Bernhard Samuelson. While there had been Mechanics' Institutes where budding engineers and artisans from poor backgrounds wishing to 'improve themselves'

had been able to acquire 'useful knowledge', there was nothing to match the technical schools flourishing in Germany and
Switzerland (where, incidentally, by the end of the nineteenth
century the finest optical glass was manufactured, and specifically
in Jena). Samuelson headed up a Royal Commission on 'Technical
Instruction' in 1881. Its findings, published in 1884 – along with
the arrival in the interim of the Polytechnic on Regent Street, a
'trade school' offering day and evening classes in commercial and
technical subjects, established by philanthropist Quintin Hogg –
resulted in the passing of the 1889 Technical Education Act. This
piece of legislation provided for public funding of adult education
by local authorities, and specifically for schools offering 'instruction in the principles of science and art applicable to industries, and
in the application of special branches of science and art to specific
industries or employment'.

## Opticians by association

On-the-job apprenticeships remained the norm in most industries, including the optical trade, where technically the seven-year
spectacle makers company rule still applied. But some firms, such
as J. Raphael & Co. of Clerkenwell and the Anglo-American
Optical Company of Hatton Garden (and Nassau, New York),
had already begun offering more advanced courses and saw the
benefits of technical education. The latter company had been
founded by Stanley Druiff, a jeweller, clock maker and 'wholesale
and importing optician' who'd first gone to the United States in
around 1881 to procure fountain pens, watches and glasses to sell
for a profit back home. The spectacles, it emerged, did best of all
back in Britain. Within ten years, Druiff had overseen the creation of the company's own dedicated school of optics in London.
It offered training in refraction and sight-testing for salesmen of
spectacles and issued certificates and diplomas for efficiency. It
was run along the lines of the Polytechnic and offered courses by
correspondence or in person in classes or by private tuition. 'We
guarantee', promised the school's press adverts, 'that providing the

student' gave 'sufficient time and attention to the subject taught', they would then make a 'thorough Refractionist'.

The march towards the 'professionalism' sought by Aitchison and Browning received another boost in 1891 when Charles Hyatt-Woolf provided the industry with its own trade journal, *The Optician*. Once described as 'a cultured gentleman of Fleet Street', Hyatt-Woolf seems to have held down almost as many jobs as the former Chancellor of the Exchequer George Osborne, most of them in the inky-fingered realm of journalism and with a technical brief. Editor in his time, and often at the same time, and from the same offices on Fleet Street, of *Popular Science Siftings* and *The Instrument World*, he also published an optical dictionary and a volume on nutrition and diet entitled *Food Frauds and Foods that Feed*.

It was in the pages of *The Optician* on 13 August 1891 that Hyatt-Woolf published a proposal calling on the Worshipful Company of Spectacle Makers to organise the education and examination of opticians, providing them with a certificate and officially recognised qualifications. The proposal was all but ignored by the guild, which like most livery companies had by that time become much more of a social and philanthropic entity that held good dinners with plenty of speeches, finished off with port and cigars, than the trade body of old (though it would belatedly come round to the idea and go on to offer qualifications of its own). Frustrated by the lack of response, Hyatt-Woolf and a group of like-minded opticians that included John Browning, Robert Sutcliffe of Rochdale and Bristol's Matthew Dunscombe formed their own organisation, the British Optical Association (BOA), in February 1895. With offices at 17 Shaftesbury Avenue, it started building a lending library and instigated its own educational and learning programmes and examinations for opticians, the first of which were held in Liverpool in January 1897. Exams were held in London later that year, in July, in the Anderton Hotel on Fleet Street where Thomas Neill, Aitchison's murderous patient, had stayed.

Robert Sutcliffe, a committed railer against 'the loose and dangerous method ... of purveying ready-made spectacles by a process largely of self-selection', was to serve as the BOA's first secretary.

Assisting him in this role was his son John, who'd go on to make himself almost indispensable to the association. A talented contra-bass player, choirmaster, conductor and the director of a Lancashire operatic company, Sutcliffe Jr had originally been set on a musical career. At twenty-one, however, he seems to have been persuaded that optics offered a steadier line. He took classes in medicine at Owens' College in Manchester and at the Manchester Royal Eye Hospital before joining his father's practice. But he soon branched out on his own with premises on the coast at Blackpool. This once genteel Lancashire bathing place was then swelling into a lively working-class seaside resort, and one whose rather distinguished cultural offerings, enhanced by the recently opened Opera House in the Winter Gardens, must have held their appeal for a music lover like Sutcliffe. He seems to have already been offering classes in optics in the town, by correspondence, prior to the formation of BOA, but he appears to have seized upon the organisation as something of a lifeline and a means for him to break out of merely practising in the provinces.

Sutcliffe was to remain at the association for over forty years, becoming its first official instructor and finding an outlet for his literary side as the editor of its house journal, the *Dioptric Review*. Though he did plot an alternative career in progressive politics, standing unsuccessfully for the Labour Party in a seat in Liverpool in the 1929 general election. In an almost comically cruel ending for someone who'd devoted his entire life to better sight and was pernickety about lighting, he died shortly after retiring from the association in a road traffic accident in 1941 during a wartime black-out.

Sutcliffe drove the creation of a museum at the association when in 1901, the year of Queen Victoria's death, he received a substan-tial donation of old spectacles. It wasn't until 1914, however, when the BOA moved to a new home in the medieval legal chancery of Clifford's Inn Hall off Fleet Street after a lengthy, if temporary, sojourn in Piccadilly, that its burgeoning collection of spectacles and optical instruments, mostly antique but some modern, were able to be housed in display cabinets suitable for public viewing.

This new museum was scheduled to open in 1915 but the outbreak of the First World War saw the association's facilities and Sutcliffe's considerable energies diverted to support the war effort.

## Gas, mud and blood

The declaration of war on Germany at eleven o'clock at night on 4 August 1914 was greeted with dismay by many who'd believed a conflict with a nation with which Britain shared close ties of kinship, culture and trade could be avoided. While relations between the countries had been strained since the Boer War by a naval arms race as the Kaiser had sought to equip his country with a modern battleship fleet to rival the Royal Navy's, Britain remained heavily reliant on German imports. That dependency was at its most pronounced in the optical trade. Some 60 per cent of England's optical glass came from Germany and the factories of Carl Zeiss, Ernst Abbe and Otto Schott in Jena, with an additional 30 per cent sourced from Parra Mantois in Paris and only 10 per cent manufactured at home, most of that coming from Chance Brothers, the Smethwick firm who'd glazed Paxton's Crystal Palace.

On 7 August, just three days after war had been announced, *The Optician*, no doubt expressing a sentiment common across the industry, announced its regret at the outbreak of hostilities. 'Many Germans', it stated, 'have worked year after year side by side with our own people in the wholesale trade, and upon terms of cordial friendship with them. The testimony of these men, both here and in Canada and the USA, is that there is no such thing as Anglophobia on the part of the German democracy.'

The hope that the conflict would be a brief gentlemanly skirmish was shared on both sides. It was officially the position of glass makers Chance Brothers who assured the British government that they'd meet any military needs but resisted calls to increase their production.

Although the British had more recent experiences of warfare, its South African campaign had been waged in a style Wellington could have just about recognised, with a cavalry, pith helmets, buglers and scouts. There were no aeroplanes, tanks or mustard gas; only the barbed-wire ringed 'concentration camps', khaki uniforms and the involvement of Lord Kitchener hinted at the horrors in the trenches to come. But then, just as in the interim period mass-produced petrol-powered motor cars had rendered horse-drawn cabs obsolete, so the First World War would be fought by industrially scaled mechanised means – machine guns rather than bolt-action rifles, and chemical weapons rather than cavalry charges. And as Christmas slipped by and the war continued with the mud of Flanders and France running with blood as the death tolls rose with every passing month, there was a dawning realisation that optical glass would play a far greater role in this conflict than in any that had preceded it. From gun sights, field glasses and gas masks to pilots' goggles, aerial reconnaissance cameras and submarine periscopes, it was to be a vital component of what H. G. Wells in the spring of 1915 termed the 'scientific war'.

That June, the only recently formed Ministry of Munitions' Optical Munitions and Glass Department brokered a 'public-private partnership' agreement with the previously recalcitrant Chance Brothers to increase and massively expand the range of military-grade optical goods it produced. The company went on to excel itself and by 1918, according to the economic historian Stephen Sambrook, was able to provide 'virtually everything that had been obtainable from Schott in 1913' and much more that had hardly been dreamt of then.

During the first year of the war roughly a third of all volunteers had been rejected as unfit. In August 1914 recruits had to be between nineteen and thirty-eight years of age and of a minimum height of 5 feet 6 inches with chest measurements of 34 inches. But in the face of mounting casualties these requirements were relaxed throughout the war, ages eventually rising to forty-five and heights shrinking down to 5 feet. Also overturned were measures of ophthalmic fitness, with previously ineligible myopic and hypermetropic men now deemed eligible for service.

And in January 1916 Sutcliffe was tasked with setting up the Army Spectacle Depot at the British Optical Association's HQ in

Clifford's Inn Hall to supply glasses for conscripts – a mammoth operation that would see some 290,000 pairs of spectacles issued to British soldiers over the course of the war. Sutcliffe was assisted by an extensive staff of women and four Royal Army Medical Corps opticians and their work continued with officers in the field. The functional wire-framed round spectacles that were prescribed were capable of being worn under gas masks. German opticians, meanwhile, came up with even neater military glasses that dispensed with metal side pieces in favour of goggle-like cloth and leather ties to the back of the head. More tragically, though, the depot soon found itself increasingly tied up with offering ocular prosthetics for injured men returning from the trenches. The depot's fitting set typically contained 150 different types of glass eye, and some 22,000 eyes are estimated to have been distributed around the country. And perhaps because of Sutcliffe's associations with manufacturers in the area, Blackpool would become the hub of its Artificial Eye Department, and remains to this day the home of the National Artificial Eye Service. Sutcliffe was given an OBE for his contribution to the war effort.

When America entered the war in 1917, Bausch & Lomb, like Chance, was called upon to make up the shortfall in optical glass, and was soon managing a ton a day and by the end of the year supplying the General Munitions Board with 70 per cent of its optical needs. That same year, and despite the political turmoil of the Russian revolution and the battles at Ypres, Hollywood nevertheless supplied the world with its first bona fide spectacle-wearing movie star in the shape of Harold Lloyd, who provided the world with something to laugh about despite themselves.

# PART TWO
## 7

# Taking Hollywood in Horn-rims

The double L Welsh name of Lloyd bites the
foreign tongue that tries to say it and local
substitutes once were common. This, however,
fails to explain why, up to a few years ago,
I was known in Great Britain as Winkle. It
appears to have had something to do with the
glasses, but just what was never successfully
explained to me.

HAROLD LLOYD,
*An American Comedy* (1928)

As the silent cinema comedian Harold Lloyd was to recall in his autobiography, the round horn-rimmed spectacles that became his on-screen trademark were 'found in a little optical shop in Spring Street, after scouring Los Angeles'. Yet these glasses, which were to become as familiar to audiences the world over as Charlie Chaplin's bowler hat, moustache and cane, were the third pair he'd tried on.

The first, drawn from the prop department of Hal Roach's Rolin studio in the old Bradbury Mansion, a ramshackle turreted Queen Anne-style chateau in Downtown Bunker Hill (and nicknamed Pneumonia Hall by its movie-making inhabitants for its appalling draughts), were too heavy.*

The rims of the second pair he unearthed were too large. They obscured his eyebrows and restricted the range of possible facial expressions, and in silent movies the waggle of an eyebrow could make or break a scene, an agile face doing the work of countless lines that could not yet be said on screen. The decision of Lloyd's contemporary Buster Keaton, 'The Great Stone Face', to deliberately limit his expressions as much as possible was an exception that only proved the general rule. We notice what he's not doing. But we have to be able to *see* he's not doing it too, as Lloyd patently understood.

Lloyd was twenty-four when he stepped into that shop on Spring Street and finally alighted, like Goldilocks and her porridge, on that third and perfect pair – a fateful purchase that was to transform his career and do no harm to the sale of horn-rimmed glasses either.† Spring Street was then the centre of Los Angeles' financial district and dubbed 'the Wall Street of the West'. It was home to the city's earliest skyscrapers, the place where in 1898 Thomas Edison's assistant James H. White filmed the first ever moving pictures of Los Angeles, thirty seconds of flickering, scarcely moving horse-drawn traffic and lots of men in hats. Lloyd would go on to shoot the daring finale to perhaps his most famous film, the clock-face-climbing, vertigo-inducing *Safety Last!*, on the roof of the Marchmont Bank on the same street.

Lloyd was to prove an extremely astute businessman. Abstemious when it came to alcohol and with a clear head for figures, he spent cannily, controlling the production and retaining,

---

* Roach and Lloyd had started out as extras, both appearing with the future director Frank Borzage as the three eunuchs attending the birth of Samson in Universal's 1914 portrait of the hairy biblical Hercules.

† Lloyd, like many Hollywood performers, had been exempted from military service in the Great War – his essential contribution to morale once America had entered the war in April 1917 taking the form of the missing and long since considered lost patriotic movie *Kicking the Germ out of Germany* (1918) and his comic output at large.

or obtaining, the rights to the bulk of his output, and accordingly suffered none of the financial hardships endured by peers like the sadly bibulous Keaton. But the greatest investment he ever made was the seventy-five cents he paid for those spectacles.

Blessed with good eyesight, Lloyd did not, in 1917, need corrective glasses. (He was, however, nearly blinded two years later when a promotional photography session went horrifically wrong and what was believed to be a fake bomb prop unexpectedly exploded, taking with it the index finger and thumb of his right hand and causing injuries to his eyes and face.) The spectacles he wore on screen throughout his heyday were lensless to avoid any glints from studio lights, though a pair with clear glass were retained for public appearances. A deception that probably fooled no one – certainly not readers of *Photoplay*, who in January 1920 were treated to a profile of the actor by Anabel Leigh headed 'Specs Without Glass' – and perhaps only underlined the degree to which Lloyd's film spectacles were a costume, a disguise. No more real than the cat's-whisker moustache he'd previously glued on for his debut cinematic comic character, the hapless stove-pipe-hatted Willie Work; or the one he sported for his more popular and equally ludicrously moustachioed successor, the Chaplinesque Lonesome Luke, an antic clown whose clothes were as short and tight as Charlie's tramp's were baggy and oversized.

Without his glasses, Lloyd could pass unnoticed. As he would confess to his ghostwriter, Wesley W. Stout, 'With them I am Harold Lloyd, without them a private citizen. I can stroll unrecognised down any street in the land at any time without the glasses, a boon granted no other picture actor and one which some of them would pay well for.' So confident was Lloyd of this anonymity that while he was in New York in 1927 filming scenes for *Speedy*, his last full-length silent movie, the star bet its director Ted Wilde that he could walk down any two blocks in the city that Wilde cared to nominate without being recognised. It was a wager Lloyd won, the comic successfully sauntering glasses-free along 41st and 43rd Street at 4 p.m. on a typically bustling afternoon in the Big Apple, without a single Manhattanite batting an eyelid.

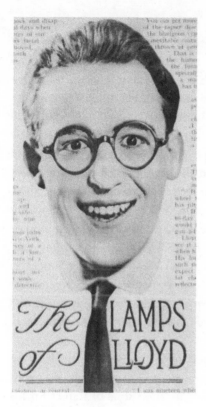

The use of a pair of glasses as a piece of comic costume was hardly original. Jesters were not infrequently depicted with spectacles in Dutch paintings and engravings in the late fifteenth and early sixteenth centuries. The anomaly of Lloyd's spectacles as comic devices is that they were never deployed to any great anti-authoritarian or anti-intellectual ends. Arguably they were never especially comic as such, certainly not in comparison with the big shoes, spindly canes and twirled moustaches that until then largely demarcated characters on the silent screen as funny (and not least his own previous efforts). 'You always had to have a moustache if you were

Harold Lloyd, movie magazine clipping, 1920.

with [Mack] Sennett,' George Harris, a performer who worked at Keystone in those early days, stated in 1980, wryly amused, some sixty-five years on.

But many of the situations in which Lloyd was filmed wearing spectacles, on the football field and in full team kit in movies like *The Freshman*, are deeply and often surreally comic and yet played deliberately straight so that their ridiculousness passes almost unnoticed. The viewer accepts the idea that Lloyd will compete in a college football match in spectacles – and get pummelled into the pitch by jocks in the process and surface triumphant with his glasses in place – because he is never seen without them at any other time. In the boxing ring, in bed asleep, at Santa Monica beach, in the swimming pool ... time after time, in one-reeler, two-reeler and full-length features, Lloyd was to emerge with his glasses on and intact, no matter what other madness had ensued, the action at odds with his sober appearance. To remove the glasses would be to lose the character. He didn't and couldn't exist without them. For the same reason, and with the same results, decades later Woody Allen was to appear in anachronistic 1970s horn-rims in Napoleonic period-set *Love and Death* and as a spectacle-wearing robot in the sci-fi comedy *Sleeper.* These cinematic instances are taken at face value precisely because they, like Lloyd's glasses character's sporting turns, were in keeping with Allen's on-screen comedic persona rather than any period or setting he might supposedly be inhabiting. Charles Hawtrey, too, wore the same round-rimmed glasses whether playing Seneca in *Carry on Cleo* – a spoof of the sword-and-sandal epic *Cleopatra* – or a Tudor courtier in *Carry on Henry* – the bawdy comedy franchise's response to *Anne of the Thousand Days*, another period drama starring Richard Burton.*

Nevertheless, and as is often said, timing is everything in comedy, and Lloyd was the right man with the right idea and, perhaps most importantly of all, the right style of frames for his moment. For his horn-rims were not made of horn, or natural tortoiseshell, but a form of plastic – and practically the same material as the highly inflammable celluloid his movies were shot on. The film stock's incendiary nature resulted in the loss of several irreplaceable prints of his earliest pictures in a fire in a

---

* By contrast, however, when Lloyd came to make *Grandma's Boy* in 1922, a movie he came to hold in particular esteem, the actor put on square-shaped period spectacles and mutton-chop sideburns to play his own grandfather in sequences set in the American Civil War. Curiously, this may possibly have triggered a revival of the style as several American spectacle makers launched so-called 'Colonial' frames the following year. The movie, however, also contains a prologue detailing Harold's character's bullied childhood, the child actors playing Harold as a toddler and a school boy clearly identified by their oversized round glasses – something Woody Allen would imitate in the flashback scenes of *Annie Hall*, where Jonathan Munk, playing nine-year-old Allen alter ego Alvy Singer, wears an exaggerated version of the comic's horn-rims.

storage vault at Lloyd's 15-acre Beverly Hills estate, Greenacres, in 1943. The fire very nearly claimed the life of the actor himself, when he came close to being overcome by fumes while attempting to rescue many priceless, smouldering canisters of film from the inferno.

## Dreams in celluloid

A scarcity of billiard balls is often cited as one of the key factors in the evolution of plastics in the late nineteenth century. This table and cue game and others like it became all the rage in America in that period and the number of regular players continued to grow as the century marched to its end and a new one dawned. One of the many doomed enterprises embarked upon by Lloyd's Mr Micawberish father, James Darsie 'Foxy' Lloyd, was a pool hall and luncheon counter in San Diego. This establishment was purchased in 1911 in the belief it was a sure-fire bet with the $3000 compensation money from an injury caused by a brewery's drunken truck driver. The business, situated 'fifty-feet off the main travelled path' for trade, as Lloyd ruefully recalled, failed, but it did at least serve to bring the young would-be actor to California.

Forty years earlier, however, the preferred material for the balls to play such games as billiards and pool remained ivory, which was expensive and becoming increasingly difficult to obtain in sufficient quantities since it involved the tracking down and mass killing of wild elephants in Africa and Asia. Few then had great qualms about the slaughter of innocent animals for sport or to provide the raw material for a popular indoor pastime capable of being played in evening dress while supping brandy and smoking cheroots. But the hunt for something cheaper and easier to come by motivated the New York billiard table manufacturers Phelan and Collender in 1868 to offer a prize of $10,000 to anyone who could produce a viable synthetic alternative. Enter billiards buff and inventor John Wesley Hyatt of the Hyatt Billiard Ball Company (later the Albany Billiard Ball Company) whose experiments with cellulose nitrate and camphor resulted in an easily fabricated and versatile thermoplastic he christened celluloid. As a billiard ball substitute this substance, alas, had its shortcomings, not least its potential for combustion. Hyatt recalled that he received 'a letter from a billiard saloon in Colorado' whose patron wrote to inform him that if the balls struck one another at force, they sometimes produced minor explosions like a sparking cap gun. While the owner professed to 'not caring so much about it', a notable down-side was that on these occasions 'instantly every man in the room pulled out their pistols'. Alternative recipes using combinations of fibre pulp and gum shellac and other primitive plastics with little or none of the volatile cellulose nitrate frequently turned out to be safer options for billiard balls for the time being. But celluloid's commercial potential was rapidly grasped, initially for costume jewellery and picture frames, and then for knife handles, fancy goods, collars, cuffs and dickeys, dentures, hair combs, piano keys and, of course, spectacle and sunglass frames – along with film stock.

It was in the 1880s that the Reverend Hannibal Goodwin, rector of the Episcopal Church in Newark, New Jersey, first con-ceived the idea of substituting rollerable strips of celluloid film for photographic glass plates. This notion, clearly heaven sent, was arrived at while the Reverend looked into ways of making stereopticon slides of religious imagery for his church lectures. 3D photography, as it happens, was to become an enthusiasm of Lloyd's following his retirement from on-screen acting, glamour shots of a swim-suited Marilyn Monroe something of a speciality. But without Goodwin's celluloid innovation there may never have been a movie industry to start with. That the business in America became based on the west coast, in and around Los Angeles, was largely the result of movie makers seeking to evade patents on the process held by Thomas Edison in New Jersey. Edison and his associates in the Motion Picture Patent Company, such as Eastman Kodak in Rochester, New York, often sought to enforce their patents by mob-handed force. California was a long way from New Jersey, and its judges and lawmakers far less friendly to Edison and the interests of a cabal of eastern companies whose claims on the intellectual property rights of film production many way out west chose to deem stifling to local competition and ruled against on anti-trust grounds.

That the land, to begin with, was cheap, cattle were more numerous than cameras, labour was plentiful, and the weather was warm and sunny and conducive to shooting outside nearly all year round were added bonuses. But the light had the knock-on effect of encouraging its first generation of stars to don sunglasses to protect their eyes from the light.

## Sunnier days for shades

There had been glasses with tinted lenses for as long as there had been spectacles, the idea of screening out bright sunlight with an emerald or coloured stone, as we've seen, pre-dating spectacles and going back as far as Ancient Rome if not before. But it wasn't until the turn of the twentieth century that scientists in France and Germany came to understand the full extent of the damage ultra-violet light from the sun could do to the eyes. In response, French glass makers produced a greenish-yellow tinted glass known as 'Euphos glass' that held some hope of limiting the transmission of these harmful rays, and this was widely used in sunglasses and goggles for driving in the Edwardian period. Between 1911 and 1913, however, the distinguished octogenarian English chemist, physicist and former spiritualist Sir William Crookes succeeded in creating a new type of glass that blocked out ultraviolet light and paved the way for the development of modern sunglasses.

Crookes was inundated with offers from opticians and optical manufacturers who saw the potential for the lenses in sunglasses and spectacles. 'Crookes Lenses', promoted with a portrait of the bearded and bespectacled Sir William and with the claim that they brought comfort 'to Eyes of Age and the Eyes of Youth' by taking 'all sting out of glaring light', would be manufactured by Chance Brothers of Smethwick and marketed in Britain by Wingate Opticians of Wigmore Street, London. In 1913, the American

Optical Company of Southbridge, Massachusetts, snapped up the rights to his lenses for the United States, ensuring that 'Crookes' became as much a brand-name byword for sunglasses across the Atlantic as Hoover for the vacuum cleaner. When in 1922 import duties forced this New England firm to devise an anti-UV lens of their own, the New York firm of Bausch & Lomb picked up the option and began manufacturing 'Crookes' sunglasses which they suggested could even be worn after the summer had passed 'to relieve the eyes from the glare of indoor lighting during the dull afternoons and long evenings of the winter season'.

The timing of Crookes' invention was propitious because far more people would want to wear sunglasses from now on. And *want* rather than *need* is perhaps the operative word here because this wider desire to wear them would not be entirely unrelated to their adoption by Hollywood stars and the rich and famous. Though the promotion of 'heliography' or sun therapy, peddled as a treatment for tuberculosis by the likes of Swiss physician Dr Auguste Rollier at the turn of the century, didn't hurt either. Such medical prescriptions did their bit to transform sun-seeking into a healthful pursuit, putting desert resorts such as Palm Springs and summering on the French Riviera on the map for affluent (rather than merely ailing) Americans. This in turn called time on the Victorian idealisation of the pallid as interesting, and helped to push the suntan into vogue – and, thanks to Coco Chanel, eventually on to the pages of *Vogue*.

For spectacle makers and those engaged in the new and widening fields of plastic manufacturing in the opening decades of the twentieth century, the rising interest in sunglasses presented enormous opportunities. Suddenly here was a type of glasses that, far from being conjoined with the stigma of physical defects, was thought of almost entirely in terms of fame, glamour, wealth, health, athleticism and desirable sun-dappled international destinations. No one minded wearing sunglasses. Famous people went out of their way to wear them, after all. And if you wore them, then who knows, other people might think you were famous too. Or so some of the logic probably went.

The trend for shorter hair for women would also inadvertently help spur the production of plastic frames for spectacles and sunglasses. Though there is a noticeable synergy between shorter, salon-styled hair and plastic frames. Both were thought sleeker, cleaner and more hygienic than anything that had gone before. The bob – that quintessential helmet-shaped hairstyle of the Flappers – was popularised by the American ballroom dancing star Irene Castle. Castle had her long hair cut into what was dubbed 'the Castle Bob' in 1915 – the same year she appeared, newly shorn, with her husband and hoofing partner Vernon in the semi-biographical silent feature *The Whirl of Life*.

At that point in America, Leominster in Massachusetts had become the predominant centre for the manufacturing of celluloid products. The majority of its plants were turned over to making the decorative combs that women up to that point had used to tame and pin up the tresses of their long hair. So many, in fact, that Leominster was popularly known as Comb City, though its involvement in hair products pre-dated the invention of celluloid. But faced with a massive fall-off in demand for combs as thoroughly modern Millies hacked off their hair in imitation of Castle and Hollywood's Colleen Moore, many local companies diversified into making plastic frames for glasses, and Samuel Foster, a former employee of the Viscoloid Company, one of the biggest celluloid-makers in Leominster, went on to establish the firm of Foster Grant and would pioneer the production of injection-moulded plastic sunglasses in the city.

Capable of being manufactured at scale and far more cheaply than natural tortoiseshell though it could be coloured to look just like the real thing, or in even more arrestingly shaded versions of it, the celluloid horn-rimmed spectacle frame itself was as emblematic of modernity as the cinema and seal-sleek bobbed hair. Relatively easy to repair and comparatively inexpensive to replace, here was the spectacle as a wipe-clean paradigm of early twentieth-century efficiency. These were positively Fordian, mass-produced glasses for go-getters and, in that period, worn predominantly by the young, their elders and betters still wedded to wire pince-nez, sidelocks and floor-length skirts. All of which appears to have influenced Harold Lloyd, who remembered that when he came to choose his on-screen spectacles 'the vogue of horn-rims was new, and it was the youth, principally, that was adopting them . . . and the suggestion of youth fitted perfectly with the character' he 'had in mind'.

Four years before Lloyd first donned his round plastic horn-rims, the *Kansas City Star* newspaper, for instance, reported on the emergence of this type of spectacles. Its writer maintained the style was a continental import to America from Vienna that had arrived in about 1908 – not long, incidentally, before the Austrian father of psychoanalysis Sigmund Freud paid his one and only visit to the United States. The look apparently took until 1910 to reach Kansas. Here in this Midwestern state of decidedly sober tastes, one that voted in favour of the prohibition of intoxicating liquors in 1880, these horn-rims had been considered pretentious and an affront to sensible dress. To begin with, wearers, like the boater-hatted in late September, ran the risk of open ridicule in public or worse. But the *Star*'s columnist noted with alarm that such glasses were increasingly being worn around town with a perverse sort of pride that bordered, to their mind, on the offensive. 'And now', the article went on, 'comes an age of glorying in infirmity. The average human person, instead of being ashamed that his eyes are on the blink, actually seems to be proud of it. He gets his pre-scription done up in owl-like round lenses the size of twin motor lamps. And he has these framed in bulky tortoiseshell, imitated in celluloid. Wearing them, he looks as wise as a tree full of owls and as conspicuous as a red-headed man at an Italian picnic. He is perfectly shameless about it.'

F. Scott Fitzgerald's debut novel, *This Side of Paradise*, a heavily autobiographical bildungsroman published in 1920 but partially looking back to its protagonist Amory Blaine's time at the fictional St Regis prep school and Princeton before the First World War, identifies a particular college type of that era, 'the slicker' – a sort of proto-nerd to the jockish 'BIG MAN' who similarly wears horn-rims as a status symbol. 'The slicker', Fitzgerald writes, his description in terms of dress matching almost exactly Lloyd's glasses character, 'was good-looking or clean-looking ... He dressed well, was particularly neat in appearance, and derived his name from the fact that his hair was inevitably worn short, soaked in water or tonic, parted in the middle, and slicked back as the current of fashion dictated. The slickers of that year had adopted tortoise-shell spectacles as badges of their slickerhood, and this made them so easy to recognize that Amory and Rahill never missed one.'

Lloyd, if then obviously piggybacking on an existing trend, was nevertheless to increase the appeal of horn-rims exponentially. At the height of his fame in the 1920s, Lloyd's movies were bigger box-office draws than those of either Charlie Chaplin or Buster Keaton. Distributed internationally by Pathé, the French company whose early Parisian film farces supplied the template for Hollywood's first slapsticks, Lloyd was a familiar face to movie-goers around the globe. In 1925 the French newspaper *Le Temps* explicitly mentioned Lloyd, observing that he sported 'heavy eye-pieces as buoyantly as a cavalry officer manoeuvring his troop', in a piece on the current vogue for eyeglasses that it suspected was 'in great part' down to the 'American influence':

> An attentive observer of our fashions, M. de Trévières, has char-
> acterised the present generation as the 'tortoise-shell-spectacle
> generation'. Spectacles, indeed, are a very significant peculiarity
> of our time. One might believe that the post-war humanity
> were composed wholly of the near-sighted, the far-sighted and
> the astigmatic. A fashionable youth must now shave his face,
> carefully plaster his hair back, leave off his hat, and protect his
> eyes with two aggressive lenses like automobile lamps – such is
> the synthetic portrait of the Americanized European ...

But what made Lloyd's films so universally popular was that the glasses character was an identifiable everyman – somebody's son, kid brother, cousin or sweetheart. He was also a fairly credible romantic lead rather than a slightly creepy vagrant who seemed to prefer the company of underage girls. One with an enviably high success rate with the ladies for a spectacle wearer too: Lloyd lost the dame to a rival in just two out of some 200 glasses films, a pattern set from the outset by the character's debut *Over the Fence* (1917), a one-reeler where Lloyd played an impoverished sales assistant in a gentlemen's outfitters who gets the girl after being mistaken for a baseball sporting ace.

Proof that he was truly on to something with these spectacles came when Lloyd had to seek out a second pair. After wearing them for a year and a half, and 'guarding them with my life' as he later maintained, the first frames broke from the inevitable wear and tear of producing one-reelers at a rate of almost one a week. In desperation he patched them up with paste and spirit gum but after three months the actor had no choice but to seek out a fresh pair. Adamant about retaining the exact same style of frame and seemingly unable to find replacements in Los Angeles, he sent them to Reynolds, an optical goods manufacturer in New York, to produce duplicates. The company shipped twenty pairs 'tailored to the measure of the old faithfuls', as Lloyd put it. But they also returned his cheque. The free advertising the films had provided for tortoiseshell rims, an enclosed note explained, 'still left them in his debt'. The firm got the gig to do all Lloyd's spectacles from then on.

Another spectacle maker, one of the biggest in the States, which most likely also reaped some of the benefits of Lloyd's boost to horn-rims, was the American Optical Company, those canny purchasers of the US rights to Crookes lenses. For only months before *Over the Fence* came out, AOC launched what would become one of the most successful styles of horn-rimmed spectacles ever made: the Windsor.

## Regal-sounding round rims

Established on the banks of the Quinebaug River at Southbridge, Massachusetts, just over 30 miles south of the celluloid epicentre of Leominster, the AOC traced its roots back to the 1830s when

William Beecher, a Connecticut-born jeweller who'd settled in this New England town, started making spectacles. In the well-worn corporate lore, Beecher turned his hand to glasses in disgust at the poor quality of those available at that time, America then being still quite dependent on Europe for the bulk of its optical goods. Southbridge was also home to one of the country's first cutlery-making factories, the Quinebaug powering the mills of the Henry Harrington plant that produced knives but also surgical equipment and firearms. This local expertise in steel making resulted in Beecher and Robert Cole, his apprentice but later head of the firm, advancing affordable steel-framed glasses over imported items, alongside classier numbers in silver and gold, to gain a significant proportion of the American market. Southbridge would become such a major manufacturer of optical equipment in the States that it was christened the 'Eye of the Commonwealth'. The AOC's premises were to swell into a whole complex named Lensdale with over 2000 employees. The firm under the stewardship of the Wells family and trading under the brand name Wellsworth would in 1905 expand to open a London office at 39 Hatton Garden to supply its wares across Europe – a trade that, if its newsletters are to be believed, seems to have held up during the First World War. In the aftermath of the conflict the firm, exemplifying the paternalistic instincts of major manufacturers of the period, would build model accommodation for a portion of its employees.

In July 1917, against an understandable background of anti-German sentiment three years into a war during which London and other parts of Britain had suffered bombing raids from German Zeppelin airships and biplanes, the British royal family changed their name from the House of Saxe-Coburg and Gotha to Windsor. Their new and unimpeachably British name was chosen after the Berkshire town and its castle, a fortress dating back to Norman times that had served as an official royal residence since the reign of Henry I in the twelfth century.

By chance it was in that very month that AOC unveiled its new Wellsworth Windsor spectacles. Whether this was intended to demonstrate solidarity with America's new allies is hard to say. But the company would go on to lend its support for the American war effort by supplying the US military with two ranges of practical white metal wire frames with hook-ended sides, the basic 'Liberty' for the grunts and a more refined 'Victory' for officers. They also backed US and Allied forces in Europe with optical units in the field. ('You cannot do your full duty to your country without good eyesight' was one of the firm's wartime promotional slogans.)

The Windsor, however, was a civilian spectacle. And a classy one too, definitely aimed at the more aspirational end of the American market, its regal title suggestive, if anything, of a nodding acquaintance with the recipients of the civil list gleaned from the *Tatler*. Or the location of properties for sale in the pages of a well-thumbed copy of *Country Life*.

Three years after its introduction Wellsworth were explaining the origins of the frame's name with a tale as tall and historically dubious as a swashbuckling Douglas Fairbanks picture. 'When King Arthur chose a place to summon his Knights of the Round Table,' stated one ad with blithe indifference to the standard mythological puff about Tintagel, 'he selected a beautiful spot called WINDSOR and the Windsor Round Tower still stands.' Just to further confuse things geographically, a gold-filled line of Windsors was named 'Canterbury' in 1929.

As a style, the Windsor arguably was something of a hybrid, old and yet new, perhaps a bit like the British royal family, then adjusting to their less Hanoverian appellation and estrangement from German cousins. A round white metal wire style of glasses, almost granny-like in shape, but with rims coated in 'a wine-colored' plastic material that, as they maintained, rendered them 'up to the minute in style and design'. Some of their advertising aimed more squarely at women – though the style appears today notably, encouragingly, unisex and was adopted by both men and women – argued that they were 'as fashion fun as a Poiret frock'. This was a reference to the French couturier Paul Poiret known in America as the King of Fashion and saluted for liberating women from corsets and petticoats with his Asian-influenced designs and daring promotion of 'lampshade' silhouetted tunic-dresses in the 1910s.

Strikingly in 1922, the year Harold Lloyd consolidated his status as box-office gold by breaking into feature-length movies, Wellsworth produced an 'All-Zyl appearance Windsor' having already unveiled the previous summer an 'All-Zyl Library R100 frame' – a round plastic style of spectacle that could easily have graced the actor's face in any of the glasses movies. Though so too could any pair of Windsors really.

Wellsworth were never bashful about their spectacles, being so bold in one press release as to maintain that its Windsors were 'STRONG, STYLISH and much BETTER LOOKING . . . than ordinary shell-rim styles' and that they aided youth, opposed age, improved looks and banished 'the tight little wrinkle around the eyes that come from trying to get along without glasses'. On what medical grounds these claims were made is probably anybody's guess.

The slickness of American spectacle ads was to be commented on by Aldous Huxley in *Antic Hay*, his acidic 1923 satire of London's bohemian demi-monde after the Great War. Discussing the power of advertising, Mr Boldero, the rapacious investor in a line of pneumatically seated trousers invented by Huxley's protagonist Theodore Gumbril, goes into rhapsody about their selling methods, telling Gumbril:

the most masterly examples I can think of . . . are those American advertisements of spectacles, in which the manufacturers first assume the existence of a social law about goggles, and then proceed to invoke all the sanctions which fall on the head of the committer of a solecism upon those who break it. It's masterly. For sport or relaxation, they tell you, as though it was a social axiom, you must wear spectacles of pure tortoiseshell. For business, tortoiseshell rims and nickel ear-pieces lend incisive poise – incisive poise, we must remember that for our ads, Mr. Gumbril. 'Gumbril's Patent Small-Clothes lend incisive poise to business men.' For semi-evening dress, shell rims with gold ear-pieces and gold nose-bridge. And for full dress, gold-mounted rimless pince-nez are refinement itself, and absolutely correct. Thus we see, a social law has been created, according to which every self-respecting myope or astigmat must have four distinct pairs of glasses.

The American Optical Company were masters of this art. They marketed their spectacles with original press campaigns and provided extra promotional material for window and in-store displays for opticians and printed cards for street cars to convey the Wellsworth frames and name to commuters on their daily rounds. They also reached cinema audiences with 'motion picture adverts' that were not unlike mini movies and starred known Hollywood actors in glasses-related dramatic scenarios. *Save Your Eyes* from 1917 employed the talents of the Irish-American actor Charles Wellesley, best known now for his turn in *The Lost World*, the silent forerunner to big-budget dinosaur extravaganzas such as *Jurassic Park* and based on a Conan Doyle novel. *A Two-Minute Tornado*, two years later, was described as 'an entertaining little comedy with a punch that will sell many an extra pair of Windsors', and featured Isabel Rea and Harris Gordon. The latter was the star of a 1915 adaptation of Oscar Wilde's *A Picture of Dorian Gray*; the former was a contemporary of Mary Pickford who played alongside Lionel Barrymore in *Under the Gaslight* (1914) but who seems to have vanished from movie making, and indeed recorded history, after about 1918, potentially making the Windsor commercial her final, if lost, film.

In April 1923, Wellsworth unveiled a notably hard-hitting national advertising campaign, one that combined a worthy enough public health message with the hard commerce of selling yet more Windsor spectacles, and got some flak for scaremongering. 'Death at the Steering Wheel' appeared in the same year that sales of the Ford Model T reached an annual peak of 1.9 million and a basic 'runaround' model with a hand-crank starter cost just $260 – Ford would freeze that price for the next three years putting

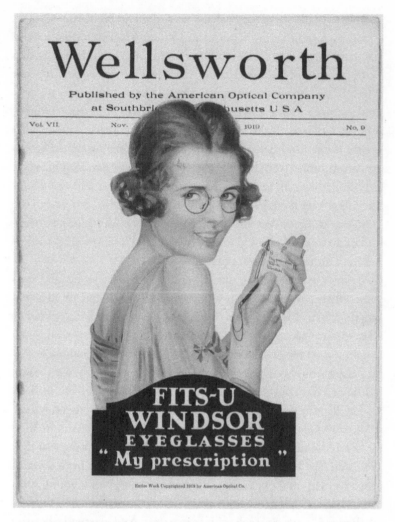

Fits U Windsor illustration, cover of *Wellsworth* magazine, November 1919.

a car within reach of the most modest budgets. The car was far from a purely urban phenomenon either, though more Americans would be living in cities than in the countryside by the end of the decade. In 1926 it was calculated that 93 per cent of farmers in Iowa owned a car. Ford himself had always promoted the Model T as the embodiment of homely rural America, a factor that meant the firm eventually lost market share as rivals General Motors, Buick, Cadillac, Chevrolet, Chrysler and Jordan began to produce more exciting vehicles with electric-starting motors and sleeker bodies with paintwork coloured other than black – thus speeding the Model T towards its retirement in 1927. But Wellsworth's ad, centred around a road accident with a guilty driver protesting 'Honest, I never saw her till she was nearly under' and the rejoinder 'He's worse than blind because he thinks he can see', touched on an uncomfortable truth. America's roads and its expanding network of country-spanning highways – just then being laid out under the US government's Federal-Aid Highway Act of 1921 and to the post-war military defensive plan by General John Pershing – were full of drivers who should never have been allowed behind a wheel without an eyeglass prescription.

The destruction of a shiny new Chevrolet (re-badged as a Butterfly Six to avoid offending its manufacturer and/or advertising their name) would be played for laughs by Harold Lloyd in *Hot Water*, released a year after Wellsworth's car-crash campaign. In keeping with Lloyd's other movies his lensless spectacles stay firmly in place throughout and the only impediment to the actor's vision while driving comes when a scarf worn by his on-screen mother-in-law flaps in front of his face, causing him to veer across the road.

It was Cecil B. De Mille who observed a common bond between movies and the motor car in the US, once stating that they reflected 'the love of motion and speed, the restless urge towards improvement and expansion, the kinetic energy of a young, vigorous nation'. Arguably both also finally compelled many visually challenged souls to seek out spectacles. And particularly after 1930 – only seven years after Wellsworth's 'Death at the Steering Wheel' campaign – when many states, among them Massachusetts, New York, New Jersey, Connecticut, Pennsylvania, Rhode Island, New Hampshire and the District of Columbia, introduced new tests requiring all motorists to possess at least 20/70 visual acuity and a 120° field of vision.

We might possibly have expected less negativity around wearing glasses for driving. When motoring was in its infancy, the first open-topped vehicles, shaped like bathchairs with belching stoves bolted on and chuntering along accompanied by thick clouds of exhaust smoke, compelled drivers to put on goggles merely to see where they were going and keep bugs out of their eyes. What was adopted out of expediency, along with some shapes of floppy cloth caps and cuts of heavy overcoats, became identified with the thrust of petrol-powered propulsion and in due course was thought racy, and finally even stylish. Wellsworth was not alone in producing lines of what were billed as 'Auto Spectacles' marketed at drivers. These were glasses with a certain, if largely by now superficial, protective element which could be fitted with clear, corrective or tinted lenses. Their 'Roadster' range of 'Clear Vision Spectacles' were, for instance, aimed at 'People of moderate means who want glasses to wear only occasionally for protection against sun glare or sharp winds'.

With America's total national wealth more than doubling between 1920 and 1929, even those of moderate means would have a bit more to splash around on consumer goods at five-and-dime stores and on new appliances like refrigerators and radio sets. Increasingly companies like Wellsworth, as Huxley noted, sought to frame spectacles in terms of an aspirational lifestyle and as a means of enhancing contemporary leisure activities.

## With a view to exercise

If the 1920s have become a byword for frivolity, excess, greater sexual licence, prohibition-evading speakeasies, jazz and dancing the Charleston and black bottom, thrills and entertainment were also sought in sports. Some were daring and deadly, like motor racing and skiing, and were enjoyed mostly vicariously, but others were fundamentally about taking health-giving physical exercise after the horrors of war and the flu pandemic. Women, in particular, only recently electorally emancipated, were now participating in games of all sorts, in far greater numbers than before the war. And at a juncture when figure-hugging, knitted costumes from the Jantzen Mill of Portland, Oregon, were changing 'bathing into swimming', and the American Olympic gold medallist Gertrude Ederle was on course to become the first woman to swim the English Channel, Windsor spectacles were being promoted with illustrations of bobbed-haired beauties in bathing costumes. How practical it might have been to swim in these glasses is perhaps something of a moot point.

Golf was another sport whose popularity with women was boosted by the success of Edith Cummings at the US Women's Amateur championship in 1923. Dubbed 'The Fairway Flapper' and the model for Jordan Baker in Fitzgerald's *The Great Gatsby*, Cummings was the first golfer and female athlete to grace the cover of *Time* magazine. Those wishing to emulate her and improve their own game could naturally avail themselves of Wellsworth's 'Sporting Glasses', which were sold with images of figures in golf gear and spectacles chipping balls with the self-assurance of trophy-winning amateurs at the Brookline Country Club.

Baseball, meanwhile, found a whole new audience after World Series games began to be broadcast on radio in 1921. Two years later, when there were estimated to be over 200 radio stations across the United States, Wellsworth paid tribute to this rapidly expanding media revolution with a luxury 'Radio Line' frame, the style 'Bevelled', or so the ad claimed, 'to reflect the beauty of gold', if also possibly in a nod to the edging of deco radio cabinets of the time. But the firm had already been selling a supposedly 'World Series winning' style of glasses on the strength of its benefits to live spectators of the sport. Adverts for these spectacles show a married couple sitting in a stadium enjoying a game. The man is holding a programme score card to which, thanks to his bifocals (or so the picture leads us to infer), he can cast a glance at close range while also surveying the action on the distant field.

Out on the diamond, of course, professional players in spectacles were rather thinner on the ground, hence Lloyd making hay with the notion of a four-eyed baseball star in his glasses character's debut *Over the Fence*, most of which was shot on location and in the breaks between innings of the East-West College charity game in Berkeley, California. Yet in the year of its release, 1917, the St Louis Cardinals possessed a spectacle-wearing pitcher of some repute in the shape of (Henry) Lee 'Specs' Meadows – only the second ever professional baseball player to wear glasses. The first, Will 'Whoop La' White, was a near-sighted pitcher for the Cincinnati Reds and the Cincinnati Red Stockings who'd hung up his glove back in 1886.

With memories of 'Whoop La' grown dim, Meadows, a spectacle wearer since the age of six, faced an uphill struggle, enduring, as one baseball commentator put it, 'jeers, taunts, and sneers' at the start of his career and from scouts, coaches, players and fans alike. Before being hailed as 'one of the most dependable rubber-armed hurlers' in the game, the pitcher was, as *Baseball Magazine* reported in 1915, 'regarded as a piece of comedy because he wore glasses'. That joke would wear off in the light of his on-the-pitch prowess, and the tall, dark and handsome, if speccy, Meadows would go on to front advertising campaigns for Lucky Strike cigarettes and Magic liniment. (Though not, as far as can be ascertained, any brand of spectacles.)

The Cardinals were to nurture the careers of two further spectacle-wearing baseball stars in the 1920s, George 'Specs' Toporcer and Charles 'Chick' Hafey. Hafey's kit bag was reported to have contained three pairs of spectacles of differing prescriptions, the player varying them as required when he headed off into the outfield or stepped up to the home plate to bat.

To this day Hafey remains one of only two players exalted to the Baseball Hall of Fame who wore glasses.* Hafey was to retire from baseball in 1938, the same year that Harold Lloyd withdrew from acting. It's fascinating to consider what possible effect Lloyd's on-screen persona may or may not have had on these few players, who were his direct contemporaries, and even those who came slightly later. Like the bespectacled Dom DiMaggio, younger brother to the more famous Joe, and known as the Little Professor throughout his career at the Boston Red Sox during the 1940s

---

* The other is Reggie 'Mr October' Jackson of the Oakland Athletics and New York Yankees who received the Babe Ruth award in 1977.

and early 1950s. Lloyd, after all, bowed out of the 1930s with the role of an Egyptologist in *Professor Beware* – that picture's failure with critics and punters only stiffening the actor's resolve to retreat behind the camera and into production.

In his heyday, though, Lloyd's glasses were never an impediment to his character in any sport or endeavour. His comedies brim with as many speeding cars, games and physical activities as Wellsworth adverts. Part of the glasses character's normalness was that he did things that average Americans in Midwestern cities like St Louis and Cincinnati did or wanted to do. Like playing baseball in spectacles.* As a portrait of the mores of urbanising and industrious middle America after the Great War, Harold Lloyd's comedies supplied a barometer of the optimism of their age. That he wears glasses is part and parcel of that great national myth then peddled by Hollywood and to an extent instantiated by many of its stars' personal rags-to-riches back stories, that anyone could make it in America. The country, in this reassuring narrative, was a level playing field and everyone had a sporting chance. Not even glasses could hold you back if you were determined enough. You could, as Lloyd did in *The Freshman*, triumph in the college football game and get the girl without having to remove your zylonite frames.

After the Second World War, Lloyd was coaxed into making what would prove to be his final picture by that maestro of screwball comedies Preston Sturges. The writer and director of *Sullivan's Travels* presented the reluctant star with a brilliant conceit: their movie together would explore the fate of Lloyd's character in *The*

---

* Cricket, a game that occupies roughly the same cultural space in Britain and across Commonwealth countries as baseball in America, has also had its fair share of bespectacled players: Roy Marshall of the West Indies and Hampshire; Charles Palmer, the diminutive captain of Leicestershire in the 1950s who began his career before the war at Worcestershire; Mike Smith, who captained England during the mid-1960s; the legendary West Indian batsman Clive Lloyd, whose eyes were damaged at the age of twelve when he tried to intervene in a school-yard fight; and the Yorkshireman Geoffrey Boycott, later to abandon his spectacles for contact lenses in the 1970s. More recently Jack Leach of Somerset and England was awarded spectacles for life by the Specsavers chain for his part in defeating Australia in the third Ashes test in 2019. The spin bowler was famed throughout the series for constantly cleaning his spectacles with a special cloth.

*Freshman*, catching up with him twenty-odd years after his stunning victory *con* spectacles on the football field. The resulting film, *The Sin of Harold Diddlebock*, which made creative use of match footage from the original movie, did little to burnish either of their reputations and was pulled on release in 1947 by Howard Hughes, the movie's mercurial backer. Hughes would spend the next three years re-cutting it and re-shooting only for it to meet with a similarly lukewarm reception from the public second time round.

As part of the original promotional work for the film, though, Lloyd, by then fifty-four and a spectacle wearer in daily life, was called upon to judge a beauty contest with a difference. Miss Spex-Appeal of 1947, held in Miami Beach, Florida, that February, found the one-time star of *Girl Shy* up to his neck in leggy lovelies in bathing costumes – but their most vital statistic in this contest was to be their spectacles.

# 8

# Bette Davis Eyes

A striking detail of the photograph of my parents' wedding that always enjoyed prime position on the lounge mantelpiece when I was growing up is that my father is not wearing his glasses. At their fiftieth anniversary party a year or so ago, I finally asked him about this and he claimed it was because my mother thought he looked 'better without them'. If so, my mother has therefore had to endure more than half a century with a man not looking his best, because throughout my entire life my dad has almost never been without his glasses. In every framed photograph of him in their house, the shape of his spectacles, moving from rather square horn-rims through to oversized golden aviators, spell out each passing decade as readily as the widening and narrowing of trouser legs, shirt collars and ties, and the changing-in-place of his thick hair and thin waist. But the idea that glasses reduce one's physical attractiveness runs deep – and until only recently applied doubly for women, as Dorothy Parker's notorious quip 'Men seldom make passes / At girls who wear glasses' attests. Parker came to hate this nine-word epigram, ruing the day she'd ever sent 'News Item' (as the piece was titled) to Franklin Pierce Adams at the *New York Herald Tribune* for inclusion in his regular column.

'News Item', though, owes its longevity to both its magnificent brevity and its encapsulation of a truth. A truth that, if not quite so universally accepted today, was widely taken as read in Parker's own time. Her voicing of it then might even be said to have led to others subsequently questioning its validity. But its outright rejection would be a long time coming. If indeed it has even come yet. A survey conducted by *Cosmopolitan* magazine in 2017 revealed that women wearing glasses on the dating app Tinder were 12 per cent less likely to receive a positive 'right swipe' than those without, the reason for this difference, according to the unnamed dating expert quoted in response to the survey by the *Daily Mail*, apparently down to the fact that 'seeing the iris gives us clues as to whether you can be trusted'. Rather than any societally ingrained and tacitly sanctioned bias against girls with glasses, say.

But when we talk about 'looking our best', the phrase, if more commonly referring to some kind of optimum physical appearance, can equally mean to see as clearly and accurately as possible. The means of doing the latter with the help of spectacles for the visually impaired, as we know only too well, is customarily believed to be at odds with the former. While the whole question of what ladies, at least of a certain class, could or should see only muddies the issue further. The late, great Poly Styrene of X-Ray Spex would comment in song that some people believed that 'little girls should be seen and not heard' but their own looking was just as circumscribed as their voices. As Camille Paglia, the feminist critic and provocateur, astutely commented in *Sexual Personae*, until the twentieth century 'a respectable woman kept her eyes modestly averted'. And the desirability, or expectation, of a certain selective blindness in the so-called fairer sex, in turn, made glasses a hurdle to attractiveness among a certain breed of men on the hunt for a mate. Their ideal candidate was, instead, someone decorous to *look at*. Ideally not a woman who'd look too closely into his affairs, in all senses of the word.

That historically women's bodies were widely proclaimed to be weaker and more feeble than men's contributed to the seventeenth-century Spanish ophthalmologist Benito Daza de Valdés arguing in 1628 that by logical extension they naturally possessed poorer eyes too.

The notion, however, that spectacles were peculiarly damaging to women's looks is a persistent one. In this book's introduction we met the optometrist Dr Norburne B. Jenkins who maintained in the pages of the American *Optical Journal* that glasses were 'very disfiguring to women and girls', and argued against them wearing them all the time or out in public, so long as prescriptions for home use were kept up to date. An advert for 'Ladies Eye Glasses' by the contemporary London opticians L. K. Leon & Co. of Piccadilly in the same year, 1900, boasted of their frames' ability to be worn, undetected, 'under a veil' and that they did not 'mark the most delicate skin'. While in the United States in 1918, the American Optical Company, of Wellsworth Windsor frame fame, vouched for the anti-ageing qualities of its range of 'Krypok' 'invisible' bifocals with the claim that 'Attractive women need not fear that the Krypok will add to their years'. They were clearly taken with the wording of this advert because in June 1921 they launched a whole campaign aimed at potential female customers under the banner 'Attractive Women Wear Wellsworth Glasses'.

A few months later, in the autumn issue of their trade newsletter, they spelt out their thinking behind the promotion, maintaining that

> It is because women have had the idea that glasses are not becoming that many of them have refused to wear them until the demand to do so has become more imperative. Even then, there are women who remove their glasses when they appear on dress-up occasions, because they think that they look better without them. These same women know they will have to pay for their folly the next day with a terrible headache, but still the glasses are placed aside. For this same reason women suffered agony and refused to consider the wearing of glasses even when their whole nervous system has been undermined because of their suffering from eyestrain.

But the slogan 'Attractive Women Wear Eyeglasses' is helping to overcome this prejudice and is teaching women that, after all, wearing glasses is just like the picking out of a certain style of becoming dress. Attractive women are starting to realise that there are glasses which really look well on them, and which add to their personal attractiveness and charm.

While the following spring the company proudly boasted that 'Wellsworth Windsors Win feminine favor', their efforts were perhaps already being hindered by the appearance of a new and wholly unorthodox eye exercise programme. One that promised the holy grail of 'better vision without glasses' and whose growing popularity just then threatened to lay waste to swathes of the spectacle industry.

## The Bates method

What made its emergence even harder for the optical establishment to swallow was that this system was not the brainchild of some outlandish quack. Nor the work of a deluded industrialist who subsisted on soaked wheat kernels and nursed megalomaniacal ambitions to replace all livestock with soya bean substitutes. No, this eye exercise regime was the work of one of their own – an ophthalmologist. And not just any old ophthalmologist either. For Dr William Horatio Bates had once been a luminary in the field. With degrees from Cornell and Columbia University's College of Physicians and Surgeons, he'd distinguished himself as an attending physician at Bellevue Hospital and the New York Eye Infirmary before going on to teach ophthalmology at the New York Postgraduate Medical School and Hospital. Wealthy, well married, widely respected and regularly consulted by his peers, Bates lived as gilded a life as any ophthalmologist probably could in America at the turn of the twentieth century.

But then on 30 August 1902, and in circumstances that defy belief, Bates, still only in his early forties, vanished from sight. All the ophthalmologist left behind was a letter to his wife. This missive, written in an uncharacteristically slapdash manner and boasting of all the money he hoped to earn, informed her he'd been unavoidably called out of town to perform 'some major operations . . . with Dr. Forche, an old student'.

Following a concerted search, one partially facilitated by the international league of Freemasons of which Bates had been an esteemed brother, some weeks later a man matching his description was finally identified as working as a medical assistant in the Charing Cross Hospital in London. His wife immediately embarked on the first steamer to Europe, but on being reunited with Bates in England found her husband had no recollection of her or his former career in New York. Briefly persuaded to spend some time with her recuperating under medical supervision in the Savoy Hotel, the ophthalmologist, after just a few days, gave his handlers the slip and promptly disappeared. His wife, despite scouring the globe, went to her grave heartbroken in 1907 having never seen him again.

Some eight years after his initial disappearance, however, a former colleague happened to be passing through Grand Forks, North Dakota – quite why is lost to history – and was astonished to discover his old friend running a small ophthalmology surgery in this backwater town of barely 12,000 souls. If he seemingly retained a portion of his medical knowledge, all other prior history remained a blank. The friend, nevertheless, encouraged him to move back to New York and the pair set up in practice together on the Upper West Side – a homecoming greeted enthusiastically by newspapers such as the *Herald Tribune*. Soon Bates resumed working as an attending physician, this time at the Harlem Hospital, where he met Emily Lierman, the woman who would become his second wife. But from an ophthalmic point of view Bates, much like Lenin in his sealed train from Switzerland to Russia, returned as a plague bacillus. The doctor who'd been at the forefront of modern optical science seemed to have undergone a complete volte-face, and now began to proselytise a peculiar system of eye exercises that went against all standard thinking.

Bates came to believe that 'our eyes do not fail us, we fail them'. In his view, almost all defects of vision were the result of emotional stress and strain and that conditions such as myopia, hypermetropia and presbyopia were not permanent disabilities determined by the fixed shape of the eyeballs or poor ability to accommodate, but temporary afflictions that with a will and a way could be corrected by relaxation and eye muscle-toning techniques. This was a kind of self-help course of callisthenics for the eyes. And Bates became a kind of anti-spectacles Samuel Smiles mounting a one-man crusade against eyeglasses, which he maintained 'did more harm than good' as they acted as a 'crutch' perpetuating errors of refraction without treating 'the underlying cause of the visual error'. In 1912, Bates' drive to rid America of glasses first became a matter of public debate when he fought a proposal to equip New York school children with spectacles. But it wasn't until five years later, when instructional lessons in what he called 'The Bates System of Eye Exercises' started to be printed in the magazine *Physical Culture*, that his theories reached a wider audience.

Launched in 1899 by the fitness fanatic, show-off, borderline charlatan and publishing impresario Bernarr Macfadden, a man who eschewed shoes and beds and whose personal regime included daily 6-mile walks with a 10lb lead bar and intermittent bouts of fasting, *Physical Culture* was close to the goop of its day. A best-selling font of wellness advice and organ of record for the rising cult of body building, it peddled dietary tips and work-out routines that ranged from the useful to the potentially harmful to a widening group of health-conscious Americans. Bates' eye exercises were an immediate hit with the readership, the magazine gaining subscribers with each issue they subsequently appeared in. Emboldened, in 1920 Bates self-published a book, *Cure of Imperfect Sight by Treatment Without Glasses*, which flew off the shelves, and it and a follow-up volume *The Bates Method for Better Eyesight Without Glasses* (published to even greater success posthumously in 1943) remain in print today, despite comprehensive and repeated debunking by eye doctors of almost all stripes. Thrown out of the American Medical Association for what they termed his 'unethical advertising', Bates was the subject of a Federal Trade Commission complaint in 1929 for making patently false and misleading claims. None of which seems to have stymied interest in his exercise regime, which following his death in 1931 gained its most eloquent advocate in the British novelist and thinker Aldous Huxley.

Huxley had been afflicted by poor eyesight since adolescence. Aged sixteen, the author of *Brave New World* had suffered an attack of keratitis (an inflammation of the cornea), possibly after contracting mumps, that left him nearly blind for eighteen months, during which time he learnt to read Braille and taught himself the piano by touch. Gradually he regained light perception in one eye and some of his sight in the other and was able to read normally again using a powerful magnifying glass and wore spectacles with ice-cube-thick pebble lenses at other times. The paucity of Huxley's vision, however, put paid to his dream of following a career in medicine. He turned instead to writing, producing at first verse and then novels, initially of a satirical (see *Antic Hay*) and later of a science-fictional bent, along with philosophical and political dispositions. Virginia Woolf, recalling Huxley's appearance in the 1920s when he was a valued member of her much-mythologised Bloomsbury circle of literary associates, commented that there was always 'a look of sightlessness in his eyes that reminded one of the blind seer'.

A decade later, and by that time living in California earning substantial sums dabbling as a Hollywood screenwriter, Huxley became acquainted with Margaret Corbett. Corbett was a Bates disciple who'd been tutored by the master himself and gone forth to spread the late doctor's gospel in Los Angeles where she counted (or at least claimed to count) several major movie stars as clients. Offering 'Natural Eyesight Improvement' and trading as 'an instructor of eyesight training', to fend off attempts by the Californian State Legislative to close her down for practising without a medical licence, her lengthy (and presumably reasonably well-remunerated) sessions with Huxley proved successful, as far as he was concerned. The writer gave up wearing his glasses and in 1942 wrote *The Art of Seeing*, an appreciation of Bates, if one with nearly as much to say about eastern meditation and Hindu mysticism (which he studied, almost simultaneously, as a disciple, along with Christopher Isherwood, of Hollywood guru Swami Prabhavananda) as the fabled method itself.

## All the single ladies

Notoriously, Bates himself relished whipping spectacles off new patients and smashing the offending articles in front of them, the clients seemingly then left to stagger, blinking and groping for the exit, with only their faith in his conviction that glasses were to their detriment to carry them out into the street and beyond. This method of ocular tough love is re-enacted almost exactly in the movie *Now, Voyager.*

A Bette Davis picture *par excellence* from 1942, it starred the actor as Charlotte Vale, a well-born but neurotic New England spinster who, through a course of analysis, the odd hour a day on a sanatorium weaving loom and the purchase of a complete new wardrobe, is transformed into a glamorous cruise-goer and potential marriage-wrecker. The new-look Miss Vale, wearing a sunhat broad enough to cause a solar eclipse, is first seen saunter-ing down an ocean liner gangplank. Her stylish clothes and the confidence with which she negotiates this walkway are in sharp contrast to Davis's opening moments in the movie, which the scene pointedly echoes.

Much like a crooner on an old dance band 78, it's some min-utes into the film before the leading lady finally appears. And the camera quite deliberately hangs back as long as possible, teasing us with fleeting glimpses of Charlotte's shoes (clompy, sensible lace-up Oxfords), stockings (thick and tea-brown-looking, even in black and white) and the hem of her housedress (shapeless and gaudily patterned) as she hesitantly descends the Vale family mansion's grand marble staircase, before revealing the true horror of the character's full ensemble. The viewer is primed to expect the frumpy worst, and the worst is what they get. The camera pulls back to show that Bette Davis was willing to suffer for her art. For not only is she wearing a low-waisted dress of sackish, untrammelled floral hideousness and her hair pulled back into a headache-inducing bun, her eyebrows are as thick and hairy as a couple of tussock moth caterpillars. And to top it all off, she has on a pair of thin wire spectacles of a like worn by Grandma Moses or the pitchfork-wielding farmer of Grant Wood's *American Gothic* painting.*

It is these spectacles, of course, that Dr Jaquith, a Walt Whitman-quoting psychoanalyst, will extract from Charlotte's face and snap in two at the bridge for good measure, the wire of the frame offering about as much resistance to the therapist as a spoon twiddled by Uri Geller. Portrayed by Claude Rains, the English actor who lost most of the vision in his right eye following a gas attack in the trenches of the First World War, Jaquith is the honey-toned, softly spoken voice of sanity; the calm eye of the emotional storm in a melodrama stoked by intermittent outbreaks of campily shrill histrionics and contorted declarations of fiery passion. The removal of Charlotte's glasses is the first step on the road to her metamorphosis. Jaquith breaks them on the brink of releasing her from his care at the sanatorium. And his shooing her out into the wild, like a bird with a broken wing nursed to health, eyewear-less but armed with a piece of paper bearing the Whitman poem 'The Untold Want' ('The untold want by life and land ne'er granted / Now voyager sail thou forth to seek and find'), is presented as one of the doctor's supreme acts of kindness.

The movie, whose ending doesn't conform to the usual Hollywood romantic norms, can be read as a search for female autonomy – a theme expressed far more explicitly in the original novel by Olive Higgins Prouty on which it was based. At the close of the picture, Charlotte opts, in effect, to remain 'an old maid', though she also gains a surrogate daughter. But fortunately for her, she doesn't look, or indeed feel, like one any more. She looks instead, and obviously enough, just like Bette Davis in her high prime. Those famous eyes, memorably described by film critic David Thomson as being 'like pearls too big for her head', and saluted in song by Kim Carnes, freed from any hint of spinsterly eyewear. For the film, for all its feminist credentials – and it

---

* Perhaps lest this opening be spoiled, it's telling that the original trailer to be screened in cinemas for the movie omitted any scenes with Davis as Charlotte at her dowdiest.

certainly has them – nevertheless conveys the idea that spectacles for women are the preserve of the ugly and left-on-the-shelf.

In the inter-war years, and in Britain in particular, the issue of left-on-the-shelf women – or what was dubbed 'The Problem of Surplus Women' – was to become a pressing concern to journalists and social commentators. If perhaps less so to the women themselves, who might have been relieved to be spared unwelcome matches and the stifling of freedoms enjoyed during the Great War itself. But following the slaughter of 700,000 British men, an already unequal distribution of Arthurs to Marthas was exacerbated: the 1921 census revealed that there were 1,702,802 more females than males in the population. While the bulk of those who died on the front were working-class men, the death rates among the sons of the landed and privately educated who signed on as junior officers were disproportionally higher. The British army lost some 17 per cent of its officers against 12 per cent of its ordinary soldiers. That this then left a swathe of upper- and middle-class 'gels' from decent homes potentially without suitable mates set alarm bells ringing among the great and the good and the hacks of Grub Street.

Vera Brittain, the novelist, nurse and pacifist campaigner whose fiancé, brother and two closest male friends were all killed in the war, expressed her own anxieties on this score in heartfelt verse. Her 1919 poem 'The Superfluous Woman' ended with the blunt, if resonant, question: 'But who will give me my children?'* Less sensitively, the *Daily Mail* pronounced surplus women 'a disaster to the human race' while running headlines that claimed 'Two Million who can never Become Wives' – a rounded-up figure that proved about double the eventual total. Although a decade after the census, half of the single women who were between the ages of twenty-five and twenty-nine in 1921 remained unmarried.

Infamously, women undertaking essential wartime work were

---

* The answer, in her case, was the political scientist George Catlin, whom she married in 1925. And one of those 'children' was the Liberal Democrat peer Shirley Williams.

among the first casualties of the peace. Those in jobs such as bus conducting, previously occupied by men before the war, were immediately let go, their posts to be filled by returning troops. But another consequence of the war was a formal adoption of marriage bars in the fields of teaching and nursing and in the civil service and certain other white-collar sectors like banking and insurance, many of which were not officially abandoned until after the following conflict. To marry, if you worked in these areas, was therefore not only to give up personal independence, but also the liberty to earn money and continue in a possibly cherished profession.

All of which, by a combination of a quirk of demographics and the grotesque inequity of labour laws, was to make the spinster an object of fascination in this period and beyond. Their single, if often emancipated, lives and modes of dress were reviled, mocked and, to a more limited extent, celebrated in newspaper editorials, cartoons, pamphlets, plays, novels, stories and films.

Not all spinsters wore glasses, of course. But if you encountered them only in the pages of contemporary novels or saw them on screen at your local Ritzy or Essoldo you could probably be forgiven for thinking otherwise.* *The Rector's Daughter* by Flora Macdonald Mayor, published in 1924 by Leonard and Virginia Woolf's Hogarth Press, is a classic of spinster literature, a poignant study of dashed hopes and unfulfilled passions underlaid with some biting social observations. At its opening, the novel's eponymous heroine, Mary Jocelyn, is 'a decline' of thirty-five resigned to 'mouldering along year after year' in the out-of-the-way East Anglian parish of Dedmayne. Here she tends to an aged and domineering father, the Virgil-loving Canon, in a crumbling rectory that until recently was also home to Ruth, a disabled sister in her care, and whose sudden death has left Mary feeling bereft

---

* The bespectacled teacher Cornelia Blimber in Charles Dickens' *Dombey and Son* is an even earlier example of the stereotype. Miss Blimber eventually marries another teacher at her father's school in Brighton, the shaven-headed Mr Feeder, B.A. After confessing to having had his 'eye on her' to Mr Toots, Feeder assures his one-time pupil that 'he don't object to spectacles'.

of affection. Shy to the point of awkwardness and so retiring in social situations that horsey members of the local country set speak over her as if she were 'empty air', the family cook is about the only friend she has. Seeking solace in books in a house teeming with the things (Bibles in every room – six in the drawing room, and nine in the study alone), she is said to have 'got a reputation for being learned'. As for her appearance, Mayor spares Mary no spinsterly signifier: she is 'dowdily dressed' with 'uninteresting hair, dragged severely back displaying a forehead lined too early'; and if possessing 'her father's beautiful eyes' – her one undowdy feature – she hides 'them with spectacles'.

As Janet Morgan notes in her introduction to the Virago Press edition of the book, Mayor herself was a clergyman's daughter who never married, a fiancé dying of cholera in India by all accounts ending any further serious thoughts about matrimony. But in all other aspects she was as different from her creation as possible: attractive, confident, and careful to make an impression. In order to emphasise the gulf between author and character even further, Morgan goes on to claim that if 'Flora had needed spectacles, she would have cast them aside'. A proposition that implies, like many we've encountered before, that the need to wear glasses is a matter of personal weakness. And, after what comes to pass in the novel (spoiler alert), that spectacles are the preserve of loser spinsters who don't care enough about their looks to win the love of a man. It also suggests a pecking order of spinsters too: those like Flora (and Davis's Charlotte Vale) who cast their glasses aside and are able to enjoy full and contented independent lives, even without men, and those like Mary, doomed to remain pitied by their relations with largely only their spectacles and a good cry for company.

A similar delineation is found in *Poor Caroline*, Winifred Holtby's pointed 1931 satire of God-bothering do-gooders then actively calling for greater censorship of Hollywood movies. Caroline Denton-Smyth, the novel's arresting central character, is an elderly spinster who establishes the Christian Cinema Company with the aim of producing more wholesome British pictures. A former suffragette and lively personality who retains 'a debonair vitality rising above her fatigue and loneliness', Caroline is marked by her eccentric dress sense, appearing often as 'vivid as a parakeet in her unsuitable green and crimson dresses' or in 'blue brocade with beads [and] chains'. She is also distinguished from the other busybodies pursuing similar types of good works – the 'middle-aged women in drab clothes' and 'earnest young women with spectacles and pimples' – by her preference for using a lorgnette hung around her neck over eyeglasses.

The character's unorthodox garb and manner were partly inspired by a lecture Holtby attended on the witch as a potential role model for free-living modern women offered by Sylvia Townsend Warner. A fellow contributor to the left-leaning feminist weekly *Tide and Time*, Warner's own great spinster novel *Lolly Willowes*, from 1926, features a maiden aunt with 'a taste for botany' who rebels against her assigned lot in life by going to the devil, quite literally. Although Lolly's eyes are said to be 'pale and blue' but not dependent on any optical aids, Warner herself was severely myopic and was never without her thick round horn-rimmed spectacles. The feeling of being naked without glasses was something she would play on in a short story published in the *New Yorker* towards the end of her life. Entitled *The Foregone Conclusion*, it opens with her ghost-writing protagonist Lucy, post-coitus, planting 'a high Spanish comb in her pubic hair' and restoring 'her horn-rimmed spectacles', and declaring to her older lover, 'There! That's as much as I shall dress!' He, in turn, tells her she looks 'very improper' and moves nearer the bed-sitting-room gas fire.*

The supposed impropriety of girls in glasses even when fully clothed is something that Warner also conveys in her memoir *Scenes of Childhood*. Recalling her confirmation in St Paul's Cathedral aged sixteen, she mentions having to do battle with her mother, Nora, about wearing her spectacles during the ceremony, Nora

---

* Rather less erotically, after holidaying on the English Riviera and finding the whole thing far too genteel for his tastes, Rudyard Kipling confessed in a letter that 'Torquay is such a place as I do desire to upset by dancing through it with nothing but my spectacles on.'

insisting they were incompatible with the traditional white dress and veil. Warner finally won the day, by arguing that she'd rather see where she was going than be thought ridiculous-looking. Entering the nave, however, Warner was relieved to see she was far from alone and that spectacle wearing was 'a handicap shared by a number of other candidates' that afternoon. But Nora, despite being short-sighted herself, would never be entirely reconciled to the fact that her only child was 'off-puttingly clever', tall and gangly with slightly frizzy hair, and needed spectacles. And cut, to her mind, such an ungainly figure. Initially raised in some luxury in India, Nora, on the other hand, had been 'an extraordinarily pretty girl' and as a young woman attending the best dances and parties that Newton Abbot in Devon had to offer the subject of considerable romantic 'fascination', not to say attention.

Warner, not unlike Mayor's Mary, was schooled at home, largely by her father George, a history master at Harrow, and, like Virginia Woolf, never went to university. Mayor and Holtby, meanwhile, attended the women's college Somerville at Oxford University, where Holtby became a close friend of Vera Brittain. Another Somerville old girl and, incidentally, also a rector's daughter was the crime writer and translator of Dante's *The Divine Comedy* Dorothy L. Sayers, whose 1935 novel *Gaudy Night* offers a fictional portrait of the college with its full complement of spectacle-wearing academic spinsters in situ.

*Gaudy Night* was intended to be the final outing for her aristocratic sleuth, the monocle-sporting Lord Peter Wimsey, a character Sayers first introduced in 1923 in *Whose Body?*, a mystery that begins with the discovery of a body in a bath, naked, aside, in a rather Conan Doyle-esque touch, from a pair of pince-nez.* Though Wimsey owed a good deal more to P. G. Wodehouse's 'silly-ass' Wooster than the cold fish Sherlock Holmes. Although

---

* Fellow author of detective fiction Ngaio Marsh would note the author's own preference for this, by then, slightly antiquated form of eyewear, describing the mature Sayers as 'robust, round and rubicund', a cross 'between a guardsman and a female don with a jolly face (garnished with pince-nez), short grey curls, & a gruff voice'.

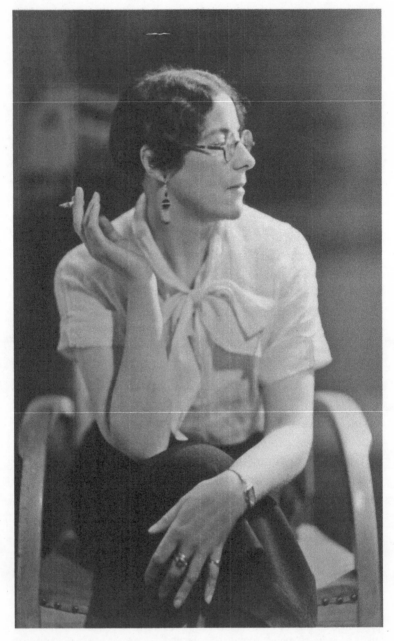

Portrait of Sylvia Townsend Warner by Harold Coster, half-plate film negative, 1934.

beginning himself as something of a caricature of the upper-class enthusiast, suave but whip-smart, a private eye with an inexhaustible private income, Wimsey would inspire Margery Allingham to create her own blue-blooded investigator Albert Campion, initially as a parody. One key difference between Campion and Wimsey is that the former, first appearing in *The Crime at Black Dudley* in 1929, chooses to shield his ever-attentive 'pale-blue eyes' behind a pair of 'tortoiseshell-rimmed spectacles' rather than don the sort of 'window-pane' monocle favoured by Wimsey, his crime-solving forerunner.

Wimsey, nevertheless, spends most of *Gaudy Night* almost conspicuously out of view. Unavoidably detained abroad on top-secret government business and kept at arm's length from the investigation elsewhere, the novel belongs almost entirely to Sayers' alter ago, Harriet Vane. Since most of the action is confined to Shrewsbury, which like its model Somerville is a women-only college, its cast is predominantly female. (The novel's male porters are a cringe-making crew of forelock-tugging working-class stereotypes.)

One of the female dons who naturally comes under suspicion, since they all do in this scholastic quad variant on the classic locked-room setting, is the bespectacled Miss de Vine. As a scholar committed to the higher cause of learning who it's plain would prefer not to *see* the undergraduates, de Vine is almost never referred to without some comment on her glasses or her myopia. Variously Miss de Vine is said to have 'large grey eyes deeply set and luminous behind thick lenses', 'brilliant, short-sighted eyes', and eyes that are 'blinking behind her thick glasses' or 'behind their thick glasses, fixed on Peter with a curious, calculating look'. When Wimsey expresses a wish to 'see her without her glasses', Vane retorts, 'I doubt whether she could see very far without them.'

Other glasses wearers pop up throughout the novel. Miss Allison, the college secretary and treasurer, for instance, keeps hers on a gold chain that she likes to sway 'to and fro slowly' when thinking. The author also equips what is obviously intended to be the most blatantly 'frightful female' in the book with a heavy pair of specs. Miss Schuster-Slatt, whom Vane has the misfortune to be seated opposite at the Gaudy Night reunion dinner, is described as a 'dark, determined woman with large spectacles and rigidly groomed hair'. Prying, gauchely overfamiliar and claiming an unwarranted 'mutooal acquaintance' in 'Your marvellous Lord Peter', Schuster-Slatt is that most ghastly of barbarians crashing the citadels of polite upper-class English society, an upstart American – to make matters even worse, also a eugenicist.

## The mysterious affair of the spinster sleuth's spectacles

One person discussed in *Gaudy Night* but who does not, in the end, appear is Miss Climpson, a middle-aged spinster with iron-grey hair netted in 'a style fashionable in the reign of the late King Edward', whom Wimsey first enlisted as an investigator in *Unnatural Death* (1927). Sadly Climpson, for our purposes, is not a spectacle wearer but does don a pair of tinted glasses and 'a hat of virtuous ugliness' as a disguise in that novel.

Published some months before the first appearance of Agatha Christie's Miss Marple in the short story *The Tuesday Night Club*, Climpson could be said to be the original spinster sleuth. If Climpson, though, does not wear glasses, her near sister in crime Jane Marple has a more complicated relationship with optical aids. And one muddied by film and television adaptations where reading glasses, along with half-knitted scarves and needles, are often fished out of capacious handbags as metonymic props for the character – the Marple equivalent of the Holmesian pipe and magnifying glass. On television, Joan Hickson, Geraldine McEwan and Julia McKenzie have all, at times, peered imperiously at assorted dim policemen, puffed-up retired colonels, flighty actresses, bearded painters, snooty dowagers, young newlyweds, absent-minded professors, weedy clerks, nosey cooks and slatternly maids through or over the top of spectacles of varying styles, Hickson in half-moons most memorably.

In the books, however, glasses are less of a given. The first full Miss Marple novel, *The Murder at the Vicarage*, was published in

Collins' new Crime Club imprint in 1930, which Christie would furnish with at least two books a year for the next twenty years. The pace of this output inevitably resulted in some minor inconsistencies in the character across the twelve novels and twenty short stories she graced, some of them ocular. Especially since Christie alternated between Marple books and those featuring Hercule Poirot, the fastidious Belgian detective with whom she first made her name back in 1922, along with writing plays and other stand-alone mysteries and stories. Described as 'a white-haired old lady with a gentle, appealing manner', Marple is, according to the Rev. Leonard Clement, the narrator of that first novel and whose vicarage provides the setting for the slaughter, someone 'who always sees everything'. In this opening book-length case we, of course, only see Marple through his eyes, that device a classic Christie act of misdirection. One that initially obscures the fact that Marple *really does* have the clearest view of all since her twinkly blue eyes look 'at the case from an entirely different angle' to everyone else, our 'unworldly' ecclesiastical storyteller included. Here, however, the only glasses this 'maiden-lady' detective is credited with owning are the 'powerful' ones that she deploys for her 'habit of observing birds'. Though the vicar suspects that this hobby, like 'gardening', is merely a 'smoke screen' that allows her to keep an eye on the villagers themselves.

Christie had just turned forty when *Murder at the Vicarage* was published, and possibly did not yet need to wear glasses herself and so didn't think to equip her more elderly spinster with them either. While Christie's fictions continued to be located in a world of swish country houses, high-end resorts and quaint villages peopled by the loaded, leisured and retired that probably even by the 1930s was becoming as fantastical as *Lord of the Rings*, they did, nevertheless, move with the times. Marple, if eternally old, does age a bit here and there. She's with-it enough to be wearing plimsolls in 1964's *A Caribbean Mystery*. And in the following year, in *At Bertram's Hotel*, she is even revealed to be around seventy-three or seventy-four years of age. This 1965 offering from Christie, and the penultimate Marple novel, professedly set in a present-day

1960s London with its Post Office Tower and Carnaby Street boutiques, involves the sleuth returning to a hotel she last visited as a fourteen-year-old girl nearly sixty years earlier. All of which if 'true' – and the truth is pretty meaningless when considering a fictional character – would 'technically' have made Marple thirty-eight or thirty-nine back in 1930 and therefore roughly the same age as Christie. More importantly for our purposes, here Marple is also said to have 'remarkable eyesight for her age'. Only three years earlier, however, in *The Mirror Crack'd from Side to Side*, the rather more sickly spinster's eyes – and her glasses – were supposedly giving her trouble. Christie, taking a bit of a swipe at the optical profession, stated that 'Even her new spectacles didn't seem to do any good. And that, she reflected, was because obviously there came a time when oculists, in spite of their luxurious waiting-rooms, the up-to-date instruments, the bright lights they flashed into your eyes, and the very high fees they charged, couldn't do anything much more for you. Miss Marple reflected with some nostalgia on how good her eyesight had been a few (well, not perhaps a few) years ago.'

Perhaps those pricey oculists came to her rescue after all, and they were responsible for the massive improvement in her eyesight that followed. Or the intervening book spent solving a murder under the sun in a high-end Trinidadian hotel worked its magic in more ways than one. Who knows? The mystery of Marple and her spectacles remains a case awaiting a suitably talented amateur to solve.

## Lyin' eyes on the cheatin' side of town

P. G. Wodehouse once took contemporary novelists like H. G. Wells and Arnold Bennett to task for not having the pluck to give their leading characters spectacles in an article for *Vanity Fair*, where he served as the drama critic,* entitled 'In Defense of Astigmatism: A Brief in Favor of Specs, Pince-nez and Goggles'.

---

* His successor in that post was Dorothy Parker.

The author of the Jeeves and Wooster books drew up a list of 'rules for novelists in this respect':

(a) Spectacles: These may be worn by (1) good uncles, (2) good clergymen, (3) good lawyers, (4) all elderly men who are kind to the heroine; by (5) bad uncles, (6) blackmailers, (7) money-lenders. (b) Pince-nez: These may be worn by good college professors, bank presidents and musicians. No bad men may wear pince-nez. (c) Monocle: This may be worn by (1) good dukes, (2) all Englishmen. No bad men may wear a monocle.

The last rule perhaps strikes the contemporary observer as the most absurd, the monocle, as previously discussed, long ago passing from the eyes of good dukes, Englishmen and aristocratic detectives to cads, bounders, Mitteleuropean generals and fascist secret police officials such as Hergé's Colonel Sponsz. At the time of writing, however, these developments lay somewhat in the future. A monocle was a trademark of Wodehouse's pre-Jeeves comic creation Rupert (sometimes Ronald) Eustace Psmith, a languorous, unflappable Old Etonian with a neat line in repartee, a fondness for Sherlock Holmes, a legal training and a tendency to emerge from unlikely romantic scenarios and criminal scrapes unscathed. And one arena in which Wodehouse also believed spectacles could be an advantage to the novelist was thrillers. 'Have you ever considered', he wrote, 'the latent possibilities for dramatic situations in short sight? You know how your glasses cloud over when you come into a warm room out of the cold? Well, imagine your hero in such a position. He has been waiting outside the murderer's den preparatory to dashing in and saving the heroine. He dashes in. "Hands up, you scoundrels," he cries. And then his glasses get all misty, and there he is, temporarily blind, with a full-size desperado backing away and measuring the distance in order to hand him one with a pickaxe.'

Wodehouse, though, is also one of the first people to use in print a decidedly streetwise American slang word for spectacles. Up there with 'Butt Me' when asking for a cigarette or 'gams' for legs or 'handcuff' for an engagement ring, the word 'cheaters', as a somewhat derogatory term for eyeglasses, has passed out of use almost entirely. But in 1920, Wodehouse casually dropped it into his novel *The Little Warrior*, besting its appearance in Damon Runyon's *Guys and Dolls* by twelve years. If pretty uncommon today, the term nevertheless retains its place in Merriam-Webster's dictionary of modern American English, where it is defined as 'US slang: EYEGLASSES, SPECTACLES'. A supposed contemporary example of its usage supplied there is 'I needed my *cheaters* to read the menu.' This is not a sentence I've ever heard anyone utter in over thirty years of visiting the United States. But perhaps I am just not eating in the right places.

Still, as a piece of slang it obviously works by resting on the hoary idea that glasses are pulling a kind of optical fast one, and that the visually less-abled wearer is somehow getting away with seeing stuff they shouldn't be able to see. Cheating, no less. The name 'wind-cheater' for a type of anorak, implying an ability to outwit gales, rests on much the same principle.

Merriam-Webster relates that more standardly a cheater is someone 'who violates rules dishonestly' and/or 'is sexually unfaithful'. And while a peculiar pair of spectacles are the namesake of Robert Bloch's mordantly creepy 1947 short story *The Cheaters*, the title also alludes to the ignoble actions of many of its characters, who are variously would-be murderers, swindlers, shoplifters, double-crossers, chisellers and adulterers. Told in a sequence of first-person narratives, the story reveals the fates of four unfortunate individuals who come into possession of the aforementioned 'cheaters'. These spectacles initially fall into the hands of Joe Henshaw, the hen-pecked proprietor of a junk shop. Despite being constantly berated as 'a bum' by his wife Maggie for accumulating ever more worthless stock, Henshaw buys unseen the contents of an old condemned mansion. He is left with almost nothing salvageable other than an old pair of silver glasses with the word 'Veritas' engraved on the bridge across the nose.

Henshaw puts 'the cheaters' on and discovers that when Maggie speaks to him he can see what she's thinking, as he puts it, 'Don't ask me to explain. I saw it. Not words or anything. And I didn't hear. I saw. I knew by looking at her, what she was thinking and planning. Like what was coming next almost.'*

Maggie and his business partner Jake, he now learns via this mental eye-wigging, have been having an affair and aim to murder him that very evening, causing him to question the part his glasses might be playing in all this. 'I could see what they were up to. I could see it. Could it be – the cheaters? Yes, the cheaters. They were cheaters. Carrying on behind my back. Getting ready to finish me off.'

Needless to say, tables get turned.†

Joe's Maggie doesn't herself wear glasses. But in genre fiction in the age of the pulps and film noir, a dame in cheaters is more often dowdy *and* devious. And never more glaringly so than in Raymond Chandler's 1949 novel *The Little Sister*. The source of the book's title is a 'prissy-looking' young lady with 'that Librarian's look' in 'rimless cheaters'. Christened Orfamay Quest, which sounds like something out of Dickens or a drowned sailor from *Moby Dick*, she is, on the surface, a puritan from the plains of Kansas. A teetotaller who disapproves of tobacco and wouldn't care to employ a detective who drinks, Quest is, as her surname implies, on a mission and hires gumshoe Philip Marlowe to find her brother Orrin who has disappeared from his Bay City boarding house. The plot of this novel, even by Chandler's standards, is as tangled as linguine, and involves blackmail, extortion, filial betrayal and a reasonable number of people getting murdered,

---

* When Donald S. Sanford came in 1960 to adapt the story for television, in an episode of *Thriller*, the *Twilight Zone*-esque series introduced each week by Boris Karloff, he was unable to find a visual way of presenting this mind-reading and opted instead simply to have the characters 'hear' each other's thoughts in voiceovers.

† John Carpenter's 1988 cult film *They Live*, based on *Eight O'Clock in the Morning*, a 1963 short story by Ray Nelson, a friend and contemporary of Philip K. Dick, also rests on the conceit of some magical spectacles that reveal a harrowing hidden truth. In this instance, a drifter acquires a pair of sunglasses that show him that the ruling elite are a bunch of skull-faced aliens who manipulate the rest of society with subliminal messages urging them to consume.

like Trotsky, with ice picks, although stabbed in the neck here rather than in the back. One of whom is supposedly a 'retired optometrist' from El Centro, but let's not go there. What concerns us is Quest's spectacles, which are an essential component of her plainness. She appears to Marlowe as featureless as her native state, which, if unfair to Kansas whose plains are not quite as plain as all that, was evidently Chandler's aim.

Marlowe regards the absence of certain accoutrements of feminine grooming – accoutrements he's clearly come to believe that no self-respecting woman in California would do without – with something close to revulsion. 'I just sat there', he states, 'looking at her glasses and her smooth brown hair and the silly little hat and the fingernails with no colour and her mouth with no lipstick and the tip of the little tongue that came and went between the pale lips.' The 'rimless cheaters', in particular, seem such an offence against nature to him that he actually suggests she change them for a different style. 'Get rid of that hat,' he tells her, 'and get yourself a pair of those slinky glasses with coloured rims. You know, the ones that are all cockeyed and oriental.'

For a man chiefly interested in the sort of glasses you pour Old Forester bourbon into – and in book after book Marlowe is a fastidious, almost obsessive-compulsive, washer-upper and wiper-cleaner of spent nightcap highballs and morning chaser tumblers – this reveals a rather canny awareness of contemporary female optical fashions. The type of spectacles he is referring to are more generally known as cat's eyes and continue to be an admired style for women. With almost butterfly-wing-shaped lenses, the top upper corners of the frame ending in elongated gestural ear-like points, the cat's eye, at its most baroque, has something of the quality of a masquerade ball mask. Hence they are also known as 'harlequins'. As an unashamedly more shapely and eye-catching frame, they draw attention to their wearers' eyes, thereby making more of a feature of them, and were judged to be generally more flattering accordingly.

They first emerged in the 1930s and were the result of an innovation in spectacle design that was arguably almost as important as the arrival of side pieces two centuries earlier, since it allowed for the production of glasses that could more readily match the contours of their wearer's face. The big change, heralded by the likes of American Optical's Ful-Vue and 'Highway' 'pantoscopic' frames of 1930-1, was for the hinges for the side pieces to be fitted on the top part of the frame. This enabled a much clearer view from the sides, since the wearer's peripheral vision was no longer obstructed by the line of their glasses, and also allowed the lenses to be angled down towards the face producing a more 'figure-hugging' frame. Although the original impetus in their development was optical and about producing a neater match between the rotations of the eye and the centre of the lens, the aesthetic gains were as great. The cat's eye was emblematic of new possibilities then opening up for designers and optical manufacturers, and especially around producing frames tailor-made for women.

Colour too, as Marlowe notes, was another area where increasingly the sex of the intended wearer would be indicated via the rims. Pink once had strongly masculine connotations, and signalling youth and vigour was considered an appropriate colour to dress boys in. Blue, for its associations through religious paintings with the Virgin Mary, was for girls. If Jay Gatsby was still able to pull off a pink suit in the 1922 timeframe of Fitzgerald's novel

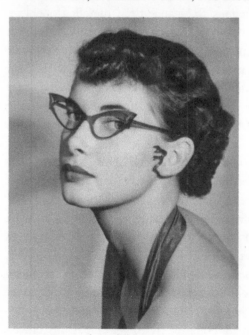

Cat's eye style of glasses, Stanley Unger for Unger & Adcock, early 1950s.

(though admittedly a book laced with homoerotic subtexts), the colour was by then already becoming more strongly slanted towards things feminine, just as blue was busily being commandeered for men only. In 1934 American Optical launched a new coloured frame aimed squarely at women under the banner 'Zyl in the Pink'. Described as 'dainty in colouring' and 'up to date with their high temples', this 'Ful-Vue' frame came in a 'pink crystal' plastic of a kind Barbie dolls would come to dream of.

In *The Little Sister*, Quest acts upon Marlowe's suggestions, acquiring a new pair of spectacles and glamming up into the bargain, her transformation setting alarm bells ringing in the detective's head: 'I looked at the drugstore and in through the plate-glass front. A girl with slanted cheaters was reading at a magazine. She looked something like Orfamay Quest. Something tightened up my throat.'

The loss of her rimless glasses can be read as a loss of innocence; the Kansan ingénue hothoused by the fetid swamp of Los Angeles proves, as it happens, to be an entirely merciless operator. But there is plenty, however, to suggest that that ruthlessness was always there and the innocent appearance was just another front. And one that served her interests well enough up until then. That costume and those 'rimless cheaters' are notably donned again later in the story, and are resumed with ease, Quest outwardly giving not the slightest hint of the dastardly deeds she has done in the intervening period.

Marlowe, though, in common with many of his gender and generation and in the profession of seeing better than everybody else, quite simply finds women without glasses better-looking. And early in the novel the detective relieves Quest of her spectacles, in what might be called the 'My God You're Beautiful' move. A move so beloved of film makers that it is still being encountered to this day, with even Juliette Binoche, as recently as 2019, suffering the indignity of having her specs pulled off her face by an amorous, younger paramour played by François Civil in *Who You Think I Am*.

In a genre where broads are as likely to get grapefruits shoved in their faces as wind up floating face-down dead in Beverly Hills swimming pools, there are probably worse things than merely being left temporarily blurry-eyed. Marlowe in Chandler's imaginings is a paragon of chivalry, and his seductions, if very pre-Me Too, are performed as graciously as the hard-boiled genre allows.

> I reached up and twitched her glasses off. She took half a step back, almost stumbled, and I reached an arm around her by pure instinct. Her eyes widened and she put her hands against my chest and pushed. I've been pushed harder by a kitten.
>
> 'Without the cheaters those eyes are really something,' I said in an awed voice.
>
> She relaxed and let her head go back and her lips open a little. 'I suppose you do this to all the clients,' she said softly. Her hands now had dropped to her sides.

As Quest surmises, the sleuth has some history in finding glasses-free girls more attractive. There is an incident, for instance, in *The High Window*, written seven years earlier, where Marlowe attempts to comfort a distraught Miss Merle Davis. Described as 'a thin fragile-looking blondish girl in shell glasses', Davis is the secretary to Marlowe's client Mrs Murdock who fails to see that her employer is setting her up to take the rap for a murder she didn't commit. With Chandler's contorted plotting this is hardly surprising. Almost no one reading this mystery, which begins amiably enough around a hunt for an errant wife and a missing rare Brasher Doubloon coin, could have seen that coming either. But her inability to see it and her poor eyesight are hardly arbitrary here. In the scene in question, Marlowe notices Davis sobbing *sans* spectacles at her office desk. He enters the room, shuts the door and puts his arms 'around her thin shoulders'. She recoils, jumping away from his arm, but when Marlowe looks at her now he sees that 'Her face was all pink and wet from tears. Without her glasses her eyes were very lovely.'

Another spectacle case closed, as it were.

*The Little Sister* was the first novel Chandler completed after working, mostly unhappily, as a scriptwriter in Hollywood. Where, nevertheless, his adaptation of James M. Cain's *Double Indemnity* for Billy Wilder and *The Blue Dahlia*, an original script for George Marshall based on a never-completed novel, both earned him Oscar nominations and reasonable sums of money.

After *The Blue Dahlia*, Chandler was eventually enticed back to Hollywood by Alfred Hitchcock to work on an adaptation of Patricia Highsmith's 1950 debut novel *Strangers on a Train*. Among Hitchcock's most stylised pictures, the final film contains one of the most arresting uses of a pair of spectacles in cinema. But Chandler and Hitchcock, which on paper could have made for one of the greatest pairings of a writer and director in Hollywood history, did not get on. Chandler was dismissed without warning after submitting two drafts. Upon acquiring a copy of the final version of the script, he dispatched an angry letter to the director, denouncing the finished article as 'a flabby mass of clichés' and complaining that his talents had been utterly squandered. Chandler had earlier moaned to his Hollywood agent Ray Stark that Hitchcock was 'always ready to sacrifice dramatic logic . . . for the sake of a camera effect', and later said he'd prefer to work with a director who realised what could be said was more important than 'shooting it upside down through a glass of champagne'.

Like many movie versions, and almost doubly so with those of Hitchcock, the film of *Strangers on a Train* diverges quite dramatically from its original fictional source material. In Highsmith's novel, Guy Haines is, for example, an architect with modernist leanings somewhat in the vein of Frank Lloyd Wright or the fictional Howard Roark in Ayn Rand's *The Fountainhead* rather than a tennis pro. Bruno Antony, who suggests the idea of an exchange of murders to avoid detection, is in the book called Charles Bruno, and so on. But of all the embellishments to the story, and by all accounts after Chandler's involvement, the one that is most conspicuous from our point of view was the decision to give the character of Miriam Joyce Haines a pair of thickly lensed spectacles.

Since Highsmith even has Bruno make a list on paper of the salient details he's gleaned from Guy about Miriam's appearance we hear quite a lot in the book about what she's supposed to look like. But there is nothing anywhere in the novel itself about her needing glasses.* By contrast the sketch provided in the film's final script offers this less than flattering summary of the character which emphasises the importance of her spectacles: 'Miriam's face is pretty because it is still young. There is a vain immaturity and shallowness about her which she will never outgrow. She is self-centred and vindictive but is confident she is irresistible to any man. She wears harlequin glasses and the myopic lenses make her eyes look as small as her calculating brain.'

Comprised almost entirely of negative aspects, with even her youthful prettiness cast as immaturity, this Miriam is an irredeemably awful – and four-eyed – piece of work, those harlequin spectacles, their name derived from the masked trickster of the Italian Commedia dell'Arte, about as firm an indicator of her devilishness as if she were reeking of sulphur, carrying a pitchfork and sporting horns. A duplicitous, scheming, money-grabbing, faithless, sexually promiscuous wife who continues to exchange flirtatious glances with Bruno right up until the moment he strangles her, Miriam is, in Laura Elliott/Kasey Rogers' consummate portrayal, a prize bitch. But she's easily one of the most arresting figures in the movie.

Miriam's glasses supply the movie with one of its most visually compelling sequences. Shot by cinematographer Robert Burks, and in a homage to the distorted perspectives of German expressionist cinema, we witness Miriam's strangulation in a reflection on the lenses of her own glasses. The spectacles, having fallen on to the grass in the struggle, act like a giant funhouse mirror, the warped figures of Bruno and Miriam flickering across them and the screen as the murder plays out to the sounds of a merry-go-round calliope. And in a further change from the book, it is these

---

* According to her biographer Andrew Wilson, Highsmith became rather miserly later in life and would make 'a special effort to drive across the border into Italy with her reading-glasses prescription because it was 20 per cent cheaper than in Switzerland'.

spectacles with their one cracked lens that the killer retrieves and subsequently presents to Guy as proof that he's kept his side of their murderous bargain.

Bruno later experiences a flashback of the murder when he meets Barbara, Anne Morton's spectacle-wearing seventeen-year-old sister who, as the script emphasises, 'superficially, in height and figure . . . resembles Miriam'. Played by Hitchcock's daughter Patricia as an eager beaver with puppy fat, Barbara has brains but is no beauty. Her spectacles, if serving to remind Bruno of Miriam, also underline how much less attractive she is than Anne, who as portrayed by Ruth Roman has the looks of the studio leading lady she was.

It's not beyond the imagination, however, to picture Roman and Patricia reprising their roles as siblings in a version of Chandler's *The Little Sister*. Patricia, you suspect, could have been rather good as the innocent-looking but villainous Orfamay Quest. While Roman, who paid her way to Hollywood by posing for crime magazine stills at $5 a pop and spent six years in bit parts before finally achieving stardom, could have empathised with the character of Leila Quest, the glamorous older sister who has remade herself as the struggling movie starlet Mavis Weld.

There's nothing to indicate that Hitchcock and co. half inched the idea from Chandler (or that it was in the author's earlier scripts either), but again it's intriguing that both the movie of *Strangers on a Train* and *The Little Sister* have duplicitous glasses wearers at the heart of their respective narratives. And that Miriam prefers the style of slanted cheaters that Marlowe recommends to Quest.

But then Hitchcock had as much form with women in glasses as Chandler. In *Hitchcock's Motifs* (2005), Michael Walker devotes an entire chapter to the use of spectacles in the director's movies, and supplies lists – similar to Wodehouse's rules for fiction – of the sorts of characters Hitchcock typically equipped with glasses. For men, these range from the 'highly intelligent, e.g. the psychoanalyst Dr Brulov in *Spellbound*' and the 'comically absent-minded, e.g. Robert's lawyer in *Young and Innocent*' to nuisances, 'e.g. Mr Fortesque in *Stage Fright*', and then a whole raft of characters that come under the general category of 'sinister'. While there are some overlaps, a further set of rules applies for women. A dame in glasses for Hitch usually signified that the character was 'intelligent/bookish but spinsterish, e.g. Pamela in *The 39 Steps*', or 'a secretary, e.g. the lawyer O'Connor's secretary in *The Wrong Man*', or 'financially grasping, e.g. Charlotte's maid Nellie in *Stage Fright*', or, and perhaps most pointedly, 'conspicuously less glamorous than the heroine, e.g. Midge in *Vertigo*' and 'Miriam . . . in *Strangers on a Train*'. For the most part, Walker argues that the women who wear glasses in Hitchcock movies 'tend to be sharp, observant and often a little threatening'. Few, if any, spectacle-wearing women get to be 'comically absent-minded' and indeed any humour has a slightly cruel streak. Hitchcock, for example, encourages viewers to consider the looking-for-love middle-aged spinster Miss Lonelyhearts in *Rear Window* all the more pitiable because she has to put on glasses to make up in the mirror.

## Beauty is in the eyewear of the beholder

A slightly similar scene was played out rather more warm-heartedly a year earlier in the romantic comedy *How to Marry a Millionaire*. Here Marilyn Monroe starred, alongside Betty Grable and Lauren Bacall, as Pola Debevoise, a comically myopic, ditsy blonde department store model cum gold digger, who out of vanity refuses to wear her glasses on dates – with the result that she's frequently unable to recognise her would-be wealthy suitors. 'Honestly, Pola, why can't you keep those cheaters on long enough to see who you are with anyway?' berates Bacall, her fellow money-mad manhunter, in a scene set in a vast mirror-decked powder-room.

This feminine sanctuary, where the three women have retreated to fix their faces and compare notes on the financial status of potential prospective husbands, is among the few places Pola is comfortable in her cat's eyeglasses. And indeed, like Miss Lonelyhearts, since she is 'blind as a bat without them' she needs to wear them to touch up her lipstick and also check her reflection in the four full-length angled mirrors that adorn the side of one wall. Having sashayed (and really no other word will do) in front of these mirrors, presenting the audience with the canyon-sized, screen-filling vista of a quartet of glasses-wearing Monroes in clingy fuchsia silk, she takes off her specs, sighs, and drops them in her purse. Striding purposely towards the exit, she misses the door completely and bangs into a section of wall to its right instead. Recovering her dignity as quickly as possible, she gropes for the handle and finally extricates herself from the room. Awaiting her outside is a one-eyed man wearing an eye-patch that she believed (until informed otherwise by Grable and Bacall) was a shiner. The remainder of the movie is chock-full of similar short-sighted misunderstandings and visual gags for the actor to fall foul of.

In her posthumously published autobiography *My Story* (most of which was ghosted by Hitchcock's script fixer Ben Hecht, though the auteur himself dismissed this particular blonde as sexually 'vulgar and obvious'), Monroe remembered an upbringing of dire impoverishment, one where her guardian, Aunt Grace, fed them for weeks on end on sacks of stale bread that cost a quarter a go and wore spectacles with one of the lenses missing because 'she couldn't afford the fifty cents to buy its replacement'. Though Grace was not a blood relation, Monroe was herself slightly near-sighted in real life. Not that she was ever seen in public with spectacles, and when presented with the scenario of *Millionaire* was extremely reluctant to don glasses on screen. The director Jean Negulesco got his way, however. And the idea of Marilyn in glasses is, in essence, treated as one long continuous joke. Pola's eventual conquest Freddie Denmark is a myope whom she meets on a plane, having accidentally boarded (for poor-eyesight-related reasons) the wrong flight. They strike up a conversation after he notices her pretending to read a book she's holding upside down. Denmark eventually convinces her that wearing glasses is fine, and dandy even, especially if you need to keep an eye out for credi-tors. That supposedly only a fellow glasses wearer seems capable of truly loving her as she is seems more of a damning indictment of the mid-century American male mindset at this juncture than anything else.*

But both the spectacle of good-looking dolls (and guys) and looking itself as a spectacular cinematic event were central to the appeal of *How to Marry a Millionaire* on its release. It was the first movie to be shot in Cinemascope, a widescreen format developed by Twentieth Century Fox to persuade once regular moviegoers to continue to patronise cinemas rather than slump in front of their television sets at home. What it promised was bigger, or perhaps more accurately broader, and better-looking movies, and Fox, opting for God over screen goddesses and the Son of Man over man chasers, chose to introduce audiences to this new format with the Biblical epic *The Robe*. Both movies, however, carried the proud rejoinder on their posters that 'You See It Without Glasses!'

That tagline was in reference to the green and red tinted specs that had to be worn to watch the 3D movies rival companies like Warner Bros and Columbia were more effusively promoting as the future of cinema. Much as with Cinemascope, the idea was to give moviegoers an experience they couldn't get elsewhere. An earlier short demonstrating the possibilities of 3D cinema from 1951, directed by Norman McLaren and widely exhibited at the time, had actually been entitled *Now is the Time (to Put On Your Glasses)* – that phrase coming to appear before all 3D features when cinemas screened them during this brief early 1950s boom time.

The eagle-eyed might also have noticed that Monroe is seen

---

* In her autobiography, Monroe confesses to having 'always been attracted to men in glasses'. And true to her word, three years after *Millionaire* she stunned certain sections of the press and her fans by romancing and then marrying Arthur Miller. A balding, bespectacled forty-something a decade older than Monroe, the author of *Death of a Salesman* and *The Crucible* was hardly most people's idea of a romantic lead. In a wedding speech congratulating the couple, the screenwriter George Axelrod quipped that he wished any children would inherit 'Arthur's looks and Marilyn's brains'. Among the general public, Miller's most identifiable feature was probably his chunky horn-rimmed spectacles. Certainly it's hard to picture him without them. So hard perhaps that in the third episode of Alex Garland's 2020 Silicon Valley sci-fi thriller *DEVS*, the tech boffin Stewart calls up a historic projection of Monroe and her third husband having sex where Miller keeps his glasses on throughout the act.

'without glasses' on the *Millionaire* movie poster. There was equally no sign of the spectacles in the image of the star, arrayed in a series of reflections of herself in that hall of powder-room mirrors, used to promote the picture. A come-hither for Cinemascope, as a lobby card it suggested that boundless opportunities to ogle her figure (and those of her female co-stars) in enhanced dimensions awaited those willing to fork out the admission fee. And they weren't far wrong. Especially as Pola, as a professional clotheshorse, spends parts of the film semi-blindly ambling across a fuller than usual screen in bathing suits and other figure-hugging garments. She might not be able to see herself for much of the movie but the viewer is treated to a damn good look at her. In the argot of dime-store novels and dirty under-the-counter books of the period, she is cheesecake in cheaters.*

That Pola, and therefore Monroe, however, ends the picture happily married and in a pair of cat's eye cheaters, and of a style swish enough, theoretically, to win the approval of Philip Marlowe, probably did provide succour to women who had no choice but to wear glasses. Unless of course they fancied spending

---

* There is, of course, an entire sub-genre of pornographic literature, and indeed out-and-out pornography, catering for those whose object of sexual fascination and indeed fetish is a well-stacked if severely dressed female librarian in spectacles. The writer and former prison librarian Avi Steinberg considered the more bookish end of the field in a 2012 article for the *Paris Review* entitled 'Checking Out'. Steinberg noted the 'conventions of the form' invariably consisted of 'the dimly lit stacks, the librarian's mask of thick glasses and hair tied into a bun, et cetera-', and listed *Bang the Librarian Hard*, *Hot Pants Librarian*, *The Librarian Gets Hot*, *The Librarian Got Hot* and *The Librarian Loves to Lick* as some of the canonical 1960s and 1970s texts cited with reverence by erotic writers at work in the form today. Helping illustrate Steinberg's piece was the cover image of what, mostly by dint of its jacket and thanks to social media, has become one of the most famous lusty lender fictions: *Nympho Librarian* by Les Tucker. A 'For Adult Readers' title published by Bee-Line in 1970, the novel came adorned with a picture of a woman, demure-looking in eyeglasses with neatly pinned-up hair yet stripped to her skimpies and straddling a topless, if still red-trouser-clad, man lying flat on his back at the foot of a bookshelf, with a large volume still clutched in his outstretched hand. Lest there be any further doubts about the likely contents of the book, enhancing this vivid tableau was a tagline below the title that ran: 'The prim miss took off more than her mask of respectability behind the stacks ... with any man who asked'.

much of their daily lives banging into powder-room walls and getting on to the wrong aeroplanes.

## Frames fashionable . . .

Writing in *Independent Woman* in 1953, the year of *Millionaire*'s release, the journalist Lenore Hailparn maintained that 'With a little care in selection, anyone can find the pair of glasses that does more for her particular facial shape and coloring; no one need assume any longer that her glasses will detract from her good looks in any way ... Who knows,' she added, presciently, 'the time may come when the woman with perfect vision who would like to alter the contours of her face slightly, may take to wearing a pair of new smart frames with just a piece of plain glass in them.'

If Dorothy Parker-esque prejudices continued, and obviously continued to be perpetrated in the culture at large, in novels and films by the likes of Chandler and Hitchcock, articles like Hailparn's and the gradual appearance of the first generation of true designer frames for women in the pages of other contemporary glossies such as *Life* and *Harper's Bazaar* in the early 1950s hinted that winds of change were definitely in the air.

To an extent their arrival at this juncture was merely a natural consequence of the emergence of a whole new range of consumer goods and domestic appliances. The Cold War would be fought with commodities as much as missiles, with the two rival political systems trying their best to outdo one another in industrial output, whizzy technological innovation and visions of material comfort. West of the Iron Curtain, gender roles still operated almost on tram lines, with decent women expected to be 'domestic, demure and dependent', in the social historian Virginia Nicholson's pithy summation. In an era when the feminine ideal, or so period advertisements would have us believe, was a wasp-waisted domestic goddess in a girdle who batch-baked wearing a frilly apron and owned pairs of gloves that matched her hats, it was probably inevitable that glasses would be turned into fashionable accessories. But also expansions in the education sector and white-collar jobs, and the larger numbers of women in employment in general, if often in more lowly secretarial and administrative positions, made girls in glasses an unremarkable sight of working life. In Britain, the establishment of the NHS in 1948 put spectacles on to the noses of anyone who needed them too. Though it also encouraged a greater uniformity in frame styles and a lower tolerance of glasses of more adventurous designs.

In America, however, where the free market reigned supreme, the notion of attaching a name from the world of high fashion to a pair of spectacles was inaugurated in 1949 when American Optical hired Claire McCardell, the American pioneer of practical, ready-to-wear women's clothes like the popover dress, to design a frame for them. Three years later they secured the services of the Italian-born Parisian couturier Elsa Schiaparelli. Arch-rival of Coco Chanel, Schiaparelli was no longer quite the fashion force to be reckoned with, having been eclipsed by Christian Dior since he unveiled his debut haute couture 'New Look' collection in 1947. But in the 1950s Schiaparelli, whose surrealistic gowns had been worn on screen by Mae West, profited from a series of lucrative licensing agreements that saw her name emblazoned on underwear and nail polish and even men's sportswear and ties. In 1951 a pair of glasses she'd created whose lenses were rimmed with blue 'eyelashes' featured in *Life* magazine, and the following year she was hired to produce a collection of ninety frames for American Optical, thereby launching the first substantial range of designer glasses in the United States. At the top of the range was a diamond-studded platinum frame, marketed as 'the Crown Jewels' and about as far away as you could get from the firm's once ubiquitous and largely unisex Windsors.

Such glasses and the ornamental frames embellished with similar precious stones produced by the London-based firm of Oliver Goldsmith were considered worthy of profiles in *Vogue*. A pair of Goldsmith's wares covered in that organ in 1954 were hailed as 'the face flattering frame'. Four years later, Tura, an American outfit established on Fifth Avenue by Monroe Levoy in 1938, launched the Turanette, a decorated cat's eye in satin shades of soft-silver, blue, pink, lime green and gold that doubled as a hair accessory. And that May's *Vogue* contained a spread with a set of models wearing an assortment of artificial-tortoiseshell frames of similarly bold designs. 'The idea', *Vogue*'s scribe explained, was 'simply to treat your spectacles as you would a diamond pin; they go with *practically* anything if they're worn with dash'. Glasses, as well as diamonds, it finally seemed, could be a girl's best friend.

# 9

# Intellectual Heavyweights

On 20 February 1960, the *New Yorker* magazine ran a kind of Whither-the-Humble-Spectacle piece on the latest trends in eyewear. Its anonymous author was convinced that they were seeing far fewer basic metal-rimmed and rimless glasses around. Pondering if such spectacles were about to join the lorgnette and the pince-nez in the boneyard of obsolete optical products, the writer sought the opinions of some local New York optometrists. This self-confessedly rather arbitrary survey seemed to confirm their thesis. Those they spoke to reported that about 60 per cent of their customers requested 'something sturdy' in the way of frames and that the darkest and heaviest styles had particular currency with actors, teenagers and longshoremen. Married men were apparently often urged by their wives to buy dark frames because of their supposed youthful-making effect. While one customer, a lawyer, was said to have confessed to feeling able to charge higher rates after adopting a pair of 'serious-looking' black spectacles. Fashion rather than money, the reporter, however, believed, was the chief motivation, observing, in a tone of superiority intended to imply that they were of a more practical cast and beyond such foolish whims, that 'people would rather wear uncomfortable glasses than be out of style'.

Seeking further answers on the fad for heavy frames the writer quizzed Mike Julian, an ad executive of a type straight out of

*Mad Men* working for the optical trade body the Better Vision Institute. 'A small stylish man in his early sixties', Julian, who it is noted wears a pair of bulky plum-coloured spectacles on the day they meet, admits to owning 'at least six' other pairs of glasses in 'various shades and weights, for various moods and occasions', including some German imports that appear to be his favourites. (That extensive wardrobe of spectacles is only to be expected from a man whose pay cheque depends on drumming up trade in frames – perhaps it was a perk of the job.) The craze for glasses with 'the biggest and blackest frames in the world for men and the fanciest frames for women', and generally referred to as 'library or intellectual specs', Julian claims was initiated in France after the Second World War, and is said to have since taken Italy, Germany and Japan by storm. In the States, however, where he estimates two-thirds of adults wear glasses and 20 million frames are sold a year to the value of $2 million wholesale, the look, to Julian's evident disappointment, appears predominantly confined to New York. Outside of the five boroughs and other enlightened East Coast enclaves and their anointed equivalents out west, he assures the writer, metal-rimmed glasses and rimless spectacles were still being worn as before. 'Go to Kansas', he exhorts, 'go to Iowa. Walk the streets of Amarillo ... You'll find plenty of rimless people out there.' Rather witheringly, he notes that for the average American wearer 'heavy frames' are thought 'too sophisticated, too intellectual'.

Pulling off a familiar *New Yorker* trick of professing to find the wearing of big-framed glasses somewhat affected while in the end celebrating the popularity of this with-it product as a symbol of the city's greater refinement in contrast to the rest of America, the piece positively enjoined the reader to get a pair straight away, lest they appear a hick. 'Rolled-gold, honestly, you poor benighted people', subscribers, even in the provinces, might be expected to reflect, rolling their eyes in dismay, before immediately testing the wire of their own spectacles, buzzing their office secretaries and demanding that they call up the optometrist and book a fresh appointment for an eye test *tout de suite*.

Glasses have, since their inception as we've seen, always been associated with the brainy and literate, if equally the sneaky and dishonest. But the widespread adoption of self-consciously 'intellectual' frames in the late 1950s and 1960s can be seen, admittedly crudely, as a barometer of the perceived importance of brainpower politically, culturally and financially in the Cold War period. A period when anxieties about the potential for nuclear annihilation mingled with optimism about scientific progress and a bright, much more futuristic future. A tomorrow when lunch might be a pill and holidays might soon be taken on Mars. And just as the technological innovations of wartime had helped birth such commercial spin-offs as aerosol spray cans, vinyl records, Minute Maid frozen orange juice and duct tape – and, as we'll come on to, plastic lenses for spectacles – so outshoots of the American Military-Industrial Complex would fund research that led to advances in global satellite communications and home computing. But building this brave new world required planners, scientists, engineers, architects, academics and economists, and a better-educated workforce. The Servicemen's Readjustment Act of 1944, better known as the GI Bill, helped with the latter by providing veterans with the funds to study and 'opening the door', as one historian put it, 'of higher education to the working class in a way never done before'.

There was also no shortage of experts whose ideas and opinions might be encountered in the burgeoning medium of print and, increasingly, on television. Here the often bespectacled public intellectual dispensing wisdom was to become as much a familiar on-screen figure as the glamorous female assistant on game shows. Dr Spock, the paediatrician whose 1946 book *Baby and Child Care* became a bible to the parents of the post-war baby boom, was just such a figure and cited in the *New Yorker*'s 1960 article, along with the trade unionist Mike Quill, as a prime example of a wearer of 'glasses with thick, dark frames'.

Interestingly, it was in this era that words like 'boffin' and 'egghead' came into widespread usage as put-downs for the brainy, the latter thanks in part to its adoption by the much-read American columnist Stewart Alsop. The term 'wonk' was also born at this time, originating in the mid- to late 1950s as a piece of Ivy League backslang – the word 'know' reversed – for an overly studious and possibly slightly effete student. Even the word 'nerd' can be dated from this period, appearing first in print in Dr Seuss' *If I Ran the Zoo* in 1950, and in that decade coming to be applied derogatorily as a synonym for 'a drip' or 'a square'.*

To wear dark, heavy spectacles was to a degree to flirt with squareness, but also to be at the cutting edge of the hip and modern. As with the earlier owlish horn-rims, it was to choose distinctiveness over discretion, to embrace the idea that a pair of glasses, something artificial and made of plastic, might be your most striking feature and a totem of your personality and character. It indicated that you were happy, possibly proud, to be thought bookish enough to sport a pair of glasses that were billed as 'library' or 'intellectual' and sought to project an aura of sophistication. Scepticism against such fanciness, as exhibited by those beyond New York's optical emporia, is baked into the word itself, since etymologically speaking it contains both the idea of wisdom ('sophist' from the Greek for 'wise man or teacher') and falsehood (the 'sophistry' and bogus arguments of that particular school of philosophers). As with food – those who profess to prefer the plain and simple over the more highfalutin – wire rims saw themselves as more virtuous, and less pretentious, because who needs that great big heavy black frame cluttering up the face? Only some stuck-up who thinks they look brighter, smarter, possibly better-read and above the common herd. Or so the argument might go.†

The idea, conveyed by the *New Yorker* piece, that heavy dark spectacles in effect went over certain people's heads arguably connects them to broader currents of mid-century modernism in art

---

* For a generation of British children, meanwhile, Brains, the wonkish scientist from the futuristic mid-1960s TV series *Thunderbirds* represented the archetype of the bespectacled boffin. Albeit in puppet form with visible strings attached.

† A more extreme example of this line of thought led to the Khmer Rouge in Cambodia during their brutal reign under the Communist dictator Pol Pot in the 1970s executing those who wore glasses on the grounds that they might be intellectuals.

and architecture. New York was just then adjusting itself to the presence of such blistering architectural exercises of up-to-dateness in concrete, steel and glass as the thirty-eight-storey Seagram Building by Mies van der Rohe (1958), the first fully modular modern office tower and the apotheosis of the Internationalist style of design; the Guggenheim Museum by Frank Lloyd Wright (1959), the high priest of American modernist architecture's final work; and the bespectacled Eero Saarinen's 'squashed-grapefruit-shaped' TWA Flight Center (1962). These were statement buildings, their shapes and presences not to everyone's tastes. There is, in any case, something quite architectural about heavy acrylic frames, and how their more strident forms play on the face, much as a new and modernistic building might stand in relationship to more familiar surroundings.

## The face of architecture

This was probably something that Le Corbusier intuited when he first adopted the hulking black spectacles that duly became his trademark back in the 1920s, the donning of these glasses specifically part of the process that saw him cultivate an entirely new persona, appearance and indeed profession. Shedding his birth name, Charles-Édouard Jeanneret-Gris, and failed ventures in watch-engraving and interior decoration like an old skin, the now promoter of machines for living re-emerged in 1921 renamed and entirely reinvented as the austere intellectual prophet of modernism and was clad accordingly ever after in a dark business suit, bowler hat, bow-tie and heavy black round spectacles. This highly contrived costume, or variants of it, was to be embraced by legions of his admirers, spurring on the whole notion of 'architect glasses' that persists still in the general collective consciousness at least.*

---

* In 1996, Mary Austin, a product development coordinator for Liz Claiborne Eyewear, maintained that for their designers 'architecture' was 'the greatest motivation for men's frames', while 'movement such as dance' inspired 'designs for women's frames'. 'They go look at buildings,' she told a reporter from *Cincinnati Magazine*, 'and shapes ... and taking walks in nature to provide different colours to use.'

The cult of Le Corbusier was to grow rapidly in the Anglo-American sphere following the translation into English in 1927 of his landmark 1923 book *Vers une architecture* (*Towards an Architecture*). Described by the critic Reyner Banham as 'one of the most influential, widely read and least understood of all the architectural writings of the twentieth century', a publication of a new transatlantic English edition by the Architectural Press in 1946 coincided with a period when Le Corbusier was himself in New York. The architect was then a member of the consulting committee overseeing the creation of the new United Nations headquarters in Manhattan.

A *corbeau* is a raven or crow in French, and many of the grand projects he envisioned looked at their best from a bird's-eye view. His 'interesting' spectacle-wearing disciples looked at the world from much the same perspective. And some of their interventions in the built environment, as often awe-inspiring as appalling, could none the less be equally short-sighted. As an early admirer of Taylorism, the American doctrine of industrial efficiency developed by Frederick Winslow Taylor that at its extreme reduced employees to almost mindless automatons performing set tasks in optimum times to maximise profits, Le Corbusier and his heirs were often guilty of failing to see humanity in all its contradictory realities.

## Hip to the horn-rims

No less uncompromising as artists who held themselves above the tastes of the general public, and just as sartorially distinctive and bespectacled as Le Corbusier, were the pianist Thelonious Monk and trumpeter Dizzy Gillespie. Along with Charlie Parker and Miles Davis, these musicians were at the forefront of bebop, the avant-garde style that broke with jazz's conventions to produce something 'smarter, harder, colder and purer', in the words of beat historian John Leland.

Draped in high seriousness with one foot in the academy and the other out on the street, bebop devotees included the emerging generation of beat writers. Gillespie named a song 'Kerouac' in 1941 after fanboy friend Jack 'that French cat' Kerouac some sixteen years before *On the Road* was published. Allen Ginsberg, known since school days as 'The Professor' because of his glasses, was another jazz-club-haunting figure on New York's bohemian scene. His poem 'Howl', subject to charges of obscenity upon its publication in 1955–6, structurally sought to imitate the short squawks and bluesy runs of bebop saxophone lines.

The French philosopher and novelist Jean-Paul Sartre, whose ideas of freedom and alienation these jazz musicians had also imbibed, was another fan. The father of existentialism visited the music joints of 52nd Street shortly after the war. He subsequently wrote that the bebop performers there 'spoke to the best part of you, the most unfeeling and most free'. Almost completely blind in his right eye since childhood and afflicted by strabismus (a squint), Sartre in his thickly lensed spectacles, with his pipe and constant stream of cigarettes on the go, and his avowal of contingent love and rejection of bourgeois marriage, represented the epitome of the continental thinker, and was something of a four-eyed style icon in his own right.

Evolving partly as an antidote to the crowd-pleasing showmanship (demeaning minstrelsy, as they saw it) that was demanded in mainstream big-band swing, bebop or bop originated in small, off-the-cuff, after-hours ensembles at clubs like Minton's Uptown Playhouse in Harlem. Heavy on improvisation, it was difficult music, and difficult to play. Audiences were expected to listen, and in studious admiration at the difficulty of it all, not to dance. This was jazz aimed at the head rather than the heart.* Miles Davis, whose own spectacle wearing would get wilder with age (on the cover of his 1974 electric-era album *Get Up With It* the trumpeter appears resplendent in a pair of hexagonally shaped wireless glasses whose lenses appear large enough to windscreen

---

* Writing in *The Jazz Scene* in 1959, Francis Newton aka the Marxist historian Eric Hobsbawm (whose own biography sixty years later by Richard Evans was illustrated with a simple cover image of a pair of heavy black horn-rims) referred disparagingly to a strain of jazz he called 'musicians' music' made by 'boppers' and 'cool' players which he pronounced 'semi-art music . . . much of it designed to be incomprehensible to the non-expert'.

a Lincoln Continental), believed he and his contemporaries were 'like scientists of sound'. Chemists, given their notorious narcotic intake, would probably be closer to the truth.

Inscrutable, cerebral, voraciously thirsty for knowledge and experience, the bop musicians cultivated tastes that ran from atonal, contemporary classical music, Afro-Cuban rhythms and wildly reworked popular standards to heroin, goatee beards, heavy rimmed specs and berets.

The sartorial flourishes, soon synonymous with bebop, were mostly down to Gillespie and Monk. The hamster-cheeked trumpeter claimed he didn't like to shave around his mouth and that a beret was the easiest hat to carry around because you could just shove it in your pocket. The heavy black horn-rimmed spectacles were simply a necessity to correct his poor eyesight. Monk was a goatee and glasses man too and had an equally natty line in headgear, adorning his own beret with a piano clip but also cutting it up over the years with an array of fur caps, porkpies, fedoras and sola topees.

His spectacles were placed front and centre on the cover of his first long-playing record in 1951. This 10-inch vinyl album was a collection of eight sides he'd cut in 1947 and only the second 'modern jazz' offering from the now legendary Blue Note records label, immodestly but not inaccurately entitled *Thelonious Monk – Genius of Modern Music*. On the sleeve, beside a shot of Monk at the piano, was an enlarged and red-tinted close-up of the jazzman's spectacle-shaded eyes. This pair of glasses were as *avant* as its wearer's music and a curious mix of rounded, weighty black horn-rim and gold wire, with a hint of welder's goggles about the combination. They were seemingly custom-made for Monk. The pianist had taken a shine to a rather pricey pair of 'heavy-framed sunglasses' in the window of a shop on Sixth Avenue and then had glasses in a similar vein run up in some cheap place in the Bronx. The same pair of spectacles, if propped up on top of his piano, can be spied on the cover of a follow-up 10-inch album for Blue Note, the rather unimaginatively entitled *Genius of Modern Music Volume 2*, which also featured some glistening vibraphone playing

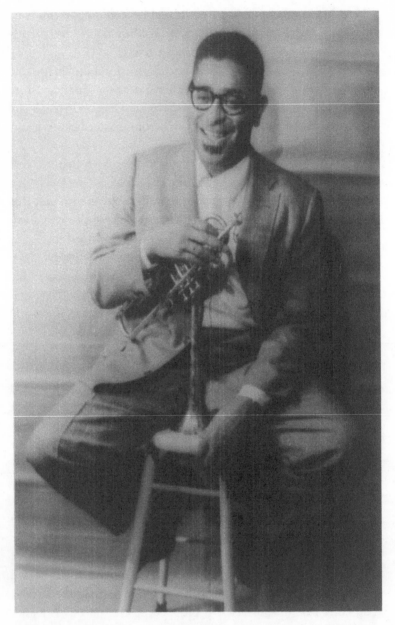

Dizzy Gillespie portrait by Carl Van Vechten.

by Milt Jackson, the horn-rimmed glasses-wearing 'Wizard of the Vibes' – as he was billed on his own 10-inch for Blue Note. And cue a photograph of Jackson on the album, dapper in a smart suit, kipper tie and spectacles, holding his mallets aloft.

The correlation between bebop and a certain type of heavy horn-rimmed glasses, more at the Gillespie and Jackson end of the spectacle design continuum than Monk's it must be said, was immediately picked up by admiring jazz wannabes. Gillespie fans in particular took to wearing berets and glasses at his gigs and in homage to their idol, and providing what later became known as the Beatniks with their style too. But the trend was well enough established by 1955 for *Downbeat*, one of the leading jazz periodicals, to carry ads for bebop glasses ('Be Smart, Wear the Original BeBop . . . with clear or tinted lenses . . . complete with leatherette case $3.95').

By then, though, bebop was positively Endsville; hard bop and cool jazz were now where it was at, its players no less eggheaded or bespectacled. In the previous November the pianist Dave Brubeck had become only the second jazz musician to grace the cover of *Time* magazine. As a financially solvent, happily married thirty-three-year-old father of four who drank only moderately and didn't touch drugs, Brubeck's jazziest feature, piano playing aside, was arguably his horn-rimmed glasses. Were it not for the musical instruments floating about his head in the cover portrait – drawn by the Russian-born illustrator Boris Artzybasheff – and the legend 'Jazzman Dave Brubeck', most news kiosk-goers could be forgiven for mistaking him for a physicist. Or Arthur Miller.

His Quartet were also early pioneers of college campus tours in America. Their 1953 album *Jazz at Oberlin* was an LP of their date at the Oberlin Conservatory of Music in Ohio on 2 March 1953. It can be seen as a progenitor of a whole sub-genre of college concert albums that would go on to spawn the Who's rocking-the-redbrick *Live at Leeds* – an exercise in maximum heaviosity alas devoid of horn-rims. Refresher courses in academic audio were to be supplied on the back of *Oberlin*'s success with Brubeck's *Jazz at the College of the Pacific* and *Jazz Goes to College* LPs following in quick succession. The cover for the *Pacific* album featured a cartoon of the group in academic gowns. Brubeck in a mortarboard looks alarmingly more like Will Hay as the beaky pince-nez-sporting schoolmaster in *Boys Will Be Boys* than any kind of jazz cat. Brubeck's subsequent fascination with time signatures, producing with the bespectacled Professor Yaffle-esque saxophonist Paul Desmond such surprisingly toe-tapping numbers as 'Blue Rondo à la Turk' in 9/8 and 'Take Five' in 5/4, saw the group move into the positively head-scratching realm of albums themed around asymmetrical mathematics metres.

In terms of glasses-wearing musical maths geeks, perhaps only Tom Lehrer enjoyed quite the same level of love among bookish college kids in that period. The Harvard-educated mathematician's self-released debut album *Songs by Tom Lehrer* was recorded in the same year as Brubeck's *Oberlin* LP. With his curly hair mercilessly tamed by brilliantine, and attired in tweed jackets, bow-ties and the ever-present horn-rims, Lehrer took to his piano as if wandering in from a seminar. Combining numbers about the Russian mathematician Nikolai Ivanovich Lobachevsky and the periodic table with withering put-downs of southern racists ('I Wanna Go Back to Dixie') and the Catholic Church ('The Vatican Rag'), and all the more devastating for being conveyed with unwavering urbanity and to the strain of tinkling ivories, his act was as if Noël Coward had majored in calculus.

When Lehrer's first album had gone through three re-pressings, he approached several major record companies to see if they might be interested in taking it on. All of them passed, seemingly. One executive at RCA, by then home to Elvis Presley, admitted that they couldn't risk adding such a controversial LP to their roster in case it led to a boycott of the cookers and fridges they also sold. Arguably no one was less rock 'n' roll than Lehrer. And as a musical genre that was a fusion of jump blues, boogie-woogie, rhythm and blues, gospel, country and western and rockabilly, and whose name alone appeared as a euphemism for sex, almost nothing appeared less rock 'n' roll than glasses. But two of arguably the most influential rock 'n' rollers were four-eyed. What's more, their spectacles were essential ingredients of their long-term appeal.

## You can't beat my glasses

Like Presley, Elias 'Bo Diddley' McDaniel was born in the state of Mississippi (and for a time earned a crust as a truck driver too).* Aged seven, however, he was sent to live with a cousin in Chicago – a path beaten from the rural Jim Crow south to the urban if still segregated north and Midwest by around 6 million other African-Americans in the Great Migration of the first half of the twentieth century. In Chicago, his adoptive mother encouraged him to play the violin. Much to her disappointment, since she nursed dreams of him becoming a concert violinist, he gave it up in favour of the guitar. 'I played the violin 'til I was fifteen,' he once recalled, 'what put the brakes on me. I looked around and didn't see too many Black violinists. That's when I grabbed the guitar, 'cause I seen plenty of Black guitarists.' He would nevertheless claim his technique with a six-string came 'from bowing the violin, that fast action'.

Unable to afford an electric model, he built his own from component parts, the unusual rectangular shape of its makeshift cigar-box body complementing the heavy rimmed spectacles he also wore and creating an image as memorable as the unique sound he forged. Drawing upon the Afro-American and Latino musical idioms from the Deep South and the electrified blues of the South Side of Chicago, his hallmark would be an infectious chugging beat, which arrived almost fully formed in 1955 on his debut and R&B chart-topping single 'Bo Diddley', the first of many self-referential numbers ('Bo's Bounce', 'Diddley Daddy', 'Bo's a Lumberjack', 'The Story of Bo Diddley', 'Bo Diddley is Loose' and 'Hey Bo Diddley' were to follow over the years).

---

* When once asked about the so-called King of Rock 'n' Roll, McDaniel would maintain: 'Elvis was fantastic but he did not start it. He was two and a half years behind me.'

Diddley would, from time to time, fight shy of being pictured in glasses on his album sleeve portraits, appearing without them but in a ten-gallon hat (itself soon another sartorial fixture), for instance, on his own country-and-western-flavoured LP *Bo Diddley is a Gunslinger* from 1960. But the musician who boasted, in song, of walking 47 miles through barbed wire and of wearing cobras as neckties looks slightly uneasy, shifty, nervy even, without them. Disarmed, you could say, despite the gun and holster on that particular cover. The specs maketh the man, and as he firmly reminded anyone who might have the impertinence to call him anything else, that was 'spelt m-a-n'.

If subsequently referring to himself as 'The Originator' for having helped invent rock 'n' roll, it can be argued that Diddley also paved the way for rap and hip hop. On tracks like 'Say Man' from 1958 he and maracas player Jerome Green traded insults over a basic Latin beat, their verbal sparring contest (a set-to-music version of a roast, or what was called 'playing the dozens' in black American communities) a clear precursor to the kind of rap battles of later MCs. A love of repetitive beats, wordplay and an immodest amount of self-referential material wasn't the only thing rappers had in common with Diddley. Darryl 'DMC' McDaniels (with an 's', and no relation) of 1980s hip hop superstars Run-DMC adopted a type of heavy-framed spectacles that could easily have been lifted from The Originator himself.

A trio from Queens, comprised of the MCs Run (Joseph Simmons), DMC (McDaniels) and the DJ Jam Master Jay (Jason Mizell), Run-DMC had been laughed off the stage for performing in chequered sports coats at an early show at Disco Fever in the Bronx, hip hop's answer to Birdland or the Five Spot. (Amusingly, Diddley and band had worn matching plaid suits as their stage wear in the 1950s.) Passing on the futuristic studded leather-and-feather duds of the likes of Afrika Bambaataa and Grandmaster Flash, who performed dressed like extras from *Mad Max*, Run-DMC reverted to wearing their 'street' clothes, soon developing a more under-stated group uniform of smart leather boxer jackets, high-end sport wear, laceless Adidas trainers, gold chains and black velour fedoras. A style that, as the music writer Alex Ogg put it, made them look 'more like an obscure Jesuit sect than hip hop outlaws'. McDaniels' Diddley-like spectacles were an essential part of the package. His preference for pairs made by the small West German firm of Cazal would see a whole new generation of New Yorkers embracing Teutonic eyewear with the same enthusiasm as *New Yorker* ad man Mike Julian back in the day.

Cazal was founded by the designer Cari Zalloni and Günther Böttcher in 1975 in Passau. This Italianate cathedral city situated at the meeting point of the Danube, Inn and Ilz is sometimes called the 'Venice of Bavaria' because of its baroque architecture and riverine location. And there would always be a touch of the rococo about Cazal glasses. Gold plating of ornamental elements such as screws and temples came as standard and contributed to their hefty $500 price tags. From the off they were intended to make an impression stylistically. Zalloni's oft-stated design credo was that 'Cazal eyewear' had to 'be recognisable from across the street'. His frames were large, technically bold, and often played with the possibilities of what a pair of glasses should look like, breaking straight lines and experimenting with polygonal shapes. In their native Germany their customer base was wealthy and conservative. The sales force was entirely male, lest women reps ruffle the feathers of opticians' wives, and they had to be smartly attired and drive the most up-to-date and perfectly policed Mercedes when visiting clients. In America, however, these remarkable glasses caught the eye of B-Boys and B-Girls who took 'Cazzies' to their hearts; DMC McDaniels' patronage of the oversized black and gold Cazal 607 style turned this particular pair of spectacles into as much of a hip-hop classic as the Roland 808 drum machine. There was even a rap act called the Cazal Boys whose 1985 single 'Snatchin' Cazals' alas highlighted a darker side to the glasses having become an essential street style accessory. Wearers were being mugged and actually murdered for their eyewear. In April 1984, the *Philadelphia Daily News* reported that in the previous few months at least ten people had been held up and robbed and three more killed over their 'Cazzies' in the 'City of Brotherly Love' alone. Benjamin Franklin must have been turning in his Christ Church grave. Cazals went on to be name checked in the lavish video that accompanied Michael Jackson's 'Bad' in 1987, the first single from his eagerly awaited follow-up album to *Thriller*.

No one, you suspect, would have been foolish enough to pinch Diddley's glasses, and perhaps especially not after he conspired to become a deputy police sheriff in New Mexico in the 1970s – a position that, just as in the old west, still came with a star-shaped badge and a gun. But the sound he created was another matter entirely. And if imitation is, as they say, the sincerest form of flattery, then one of his most sincere admirers in the fifties was the goofiest-looking rocker the world had yet seen.

Charles 'Buddy' Holly (originally Holley: a typing error on his first record contract resulted in the jettisoning of the 'e') was a tall, rail-thin, gangly, pasty-faced kid with curly hair as wiry as a Brillo pad from Lubbock in Texas. His teeth were not only as crooked as Boot Hill tombstones but also dirty brown from imbibing the region's over-fluoridated water – a condition commonly referred to there as 'West Texas mouth'. To make matters worse, in his senior year at high school in 1955 an eye test, taken at the request of a teacher, confirmed he needed glasses. A basic pair with simple plastic frames and a prescription to bring his 20/800 defect into touch was dispensed. But having already formed a country and western duo with his schoolmate Bob Montgomery – the teenagers, regularly performing locally as Buddy and Bob, were to play bottom of the bill to Elvis when the King came to Lubbock's Fair Park Coliseum for a matinée show that February – these specs were soon replaced with a slightly more fetching pair of browline or half-frame glasses.

The browline was, and indeed remains, a frame combining a thick plastic upper half and a lower metal, or lighter nylon thread, chassis. The effect is somewhat as if someone had glued Groucho Marx's bushy eyebrows on to the top of his wire rims to save him the bother of painting them on. But still it was a breakthrough when it first appeared in the late 1940s and the design has been described as one of the most 'outstanding inventions in frames for spectacles during the 20th century'. Its inventor was an Englishman, Norman William Chappell (always known as Neville Chappell), who trained as an optician in Doncaster straight from school before obtaining a position with the eminent spectacle manufacturers M. Wiseman and Co. in London. His brief at Wiseman's seemingly ranged over both technical innovation and publicity. And as the story goes, chance would have it that one day he happened to see a member of staff accidentally hack off the bottom half of a pair of acetate frames. (History fails to record if the worker was sacked for incompetence, or had their wages docked.) Chappell was apparently gripped by the possibilities of producing a frame with a lighter lower rim and a heavier plastic top half. Tinkering away on the idea, and probably ruining many a serviceable frame to achieve his ends, Chappell's design was finally advanced enough for him to file a provisional patent for what he'd call his 'Supra' frame just a month before the outbreak of the Second World War.

He looked to the United States, where he was fortunate enough to gain the ready ear and eye of Jack Rohrbach, the vice president of the Shuron Optical Company of America. Rohrbach liked what he saw. And having purchased the licence to manufacture Supra-style frames, Shuron unveiled their Ronsir Zyl line in America in 1947. Almost doing for eyewear what Dior's New Look did in the same year for dresses, the Ronsir in plastic and wire was an immediate sensation. Its stateside success encouraged Chappell to set up the Pell Optical Co. Ltd to supply glasses for the British market and he signed deals with the Zeiss company's Marwitz & Hauser wing to produce Supras in West Germany, and entered into a joint patent agreement with the French Société des Lunetiers in Paris in 1954 over their 'Nylor', an improved nylon-moulded version of the Supra.

But it was in America that the 'browline', as it was invariably known, had the most impact. By the middle 1950s browlines of varying materials, shapes, sizes and shades from Shuron, Art Craft Optical, Bausch & Lomb, Victory Optical and many other lesser-known outfits were among the most common designs of spectacles in the United States. The optician and writer Preston Fassel estimates that by 1960 'half of all eyeglass frames worn in America were browlines'. As to the root of their appeal to Americans, his conjecture is that the metal rims 'spoke to old-world conservatism' while the plastic brows, often in tortoiseshell or grained to look like wood, were 'forward thinking without being radical'.

In addition to Buddy Holly, their wearers in this heyday ranged from Kentucky Fried Chicken founder Colonel Harland Sanders and the US President Lyndon B. Johnson to the New York Giants football coach Vince Lombardi and El-Hajj Malik El-Shabazz, aka Malcolm X, the black Muslim civil rights activist. For the latter, those glasses only added to his sober dress sense, making him arguably seem even more of a threat as far as the authorities were concerned. By the end of the 1960s the style, in part because of its ubiquity among the older generation perpetuating the Vietnam war, would come to be seen as rather conservative, not to say a little reactionary – the spectacle equivalent in this new Aquarian age of messianic locks, long and flowing, of sporting a flat-top crewcut, say. And it's no accident that Michael Douglas sported both browlines and a flat top for his role as William 'D-Fens' Foster, the meek military man who loses his job and goes on a frankly racist rampage around LA in the 1993 movie *Falling Down*. Though both the hairstyle and the spectacle-type had enjoyed at least one semi-ironic revival each by then.

But back in 1955, in Lubbock on the Texan plains, a place defined more by the absence of things (hills, scenery, trees, alcoholic beverages on sale, etc.), a pair of browlines fitted up by Dr J. D. Armistead, one of the city's most trusted ophthalmologists, was about the best a young man could hope for in the circumstances.

The nineteen-year-old singer would accordingly appear in these workhorse frames in the promotional photograph that accompanied 'Blue Days, Black Nights', his debut single for Decca, released the following April. Pictured looking rather earnest, unsmiling and with a slightly worried expression playing across his face, he holds his acoustic guitar up high, fingers on frets, as if demonstrating a chord-shape to some eager play-along beginner. It was perhaps not the most auspicious start visually or musically. Although favourably reviewed by the industry paper *Billboard* which commented that 'if the public will take one more than one Presley or [Carl] Perkins, as it well may, Holly stands a strong chance', the disc, recorded in Nashville, Tennessee, with the respected country music producer Owen Bradley, only made it to number 6 in Lubbock's own chart. This against virtually zero local competition – and the record failed to catch on much elsewhere either.

A month on, however, Holly was still promoting the single with an opening slot on Faron Young's Grand Ole Opry Tour where he joined a line-up of stars that alongside Young included Carl Perkins, Ray Price, Red Sovine and Tommy Collins. Anxious about his appearance and fearful of being thought a hick, Holly had already borrowed $1000 from his brother, over half of which he used to secure a Fender Stratocaster, then the latest word in electric guitars, a top-of-the-range instrument as futuristically atomic age as a fin-winged Cadillac, but the remainder was spent on clothes: jackets and shirts in flamboyant shades of red, green and pink and pairs of shoes in red and suede. Now, and perhaps fearing his stage persona despite the posh kit and clobber would bear unfair comparison with the brooding presence of the dark-haired Perkins or the exuberance of the nudie-suit-wearing Price, Holly decided to perform without his glasses for the tour. Scarcely able to see his bandmates playing next to him let alone the audience in the stalls, it was often a disaster. One date descended into complete farce when he dropped a guitar pick and was left crawling about the stage on his hands and knees trying to retrieve it.

Conscious that this state of affairs couldn't go on but seemingly unwilling to continue as the glasses-wearing square persona he'd rejected, Holly booked an appointment with Dr Armistead the day after he got back to Lubbock from the tour. Walking into the optometrist's, he demanded to be fitted with contact lenses.

## Make contact

Rather like spectacles themselves, the contact lens was an idea that was a long time coming and its chequered development as a viable proposition was the work of many hands competing for recognition. From Leonardo da Vinci in 1508 and René Descartes in 1638 to the British physician Thomas Young and the astronomer Sir John Frederick Herschel in the early nineteenth century, the theoretical and technical groundwork for contact lenses can be traced back over several centuries. But it wasn't until 1887 that supposedly an artificial eye maker from Wiesbaden in Germany called Friedrich Anton Müller produced something nearing a prototype. A spa town on the Rhine whose thermal springs were believed to have health-giving qualities, Wiesbaden in the late nineteenth century was the summer resort of the German Kaiser Wilhelm II and a preferred place of retirement for wealthy Mitteleuropean malingerers who took the waters and sought treatment from the city's legion of doctors. One of these physicians, Dr Thomas Saemisch, approached Müller about blowing a thin glass shell to protect the eye of a patient who had lost one of their eyelids to a disease, from dry eye and inflammation of the cornea. Müller's *kontaktschalen* or contact lens seems to have been effective. The patient is reputed to have later sent a letter to Müller claiming to have worn the lens for the next twenty-one years without suffering any ill effects.

No sooner had Müller shown what could be done, however, than a bunch of German, Swiss and French eye doctors entered the fray with the ambition of creating a lens that might correct common optical conditions such as myopia. Foremost among them were Dr Adolf Gaston Fick, a German-born ophthalmologist based in Zurich, and August Müller (no relation to Friedrich), a doctoral student at Kiel University. In 1888, Fick embarked on what sounds like a series of pretty gruesome experiments involving dead rabbits' eyes and those of human cadavers. Casting impressions of these corpses' eyeballs with plaster of Paris, Fick was able to blow glass bubble lenses – scleral bowls that covered the cornea and much of the sclera (i.e. the whites of the eye) – that more accurately mapped the contours of the real animal and human eyeball. And after successively slipping lenses under the eyelids of live rabbits using a glucose unguent derived from grape juice, Fick experimented on himself with the human variety with seemingly positive results. He claimed to be able to wear his lenses for up to two hours at a time and engaged Ernst Abbe of the scientific instrument makers Carl Zeiss to help him develop some optically enhanced lenses.

August Müller, who was severely myopic and was looking for a means to free himself of glasses, was charting a similar course around the same time. Also working with casts of dead men's eyes, in 1889 he and the Berlin optician Otto Himmler successfully created blown and then ground contact lenses with optical powers. The only problem was they were excruciatingly painful to wear and could only be tolerated for about half an hour at the most, and even then only after the eye had been anaesthetised with cocaine. Nevertheless, some of Müller's researches would prove invaluable to later contact lens makers. And as largely the go-to-guys for Fick and many other early experimenters, the firm of Zeiss, after many further trials and errors, were to finesse a corrective contact lens that they began manufacturing commercially shortly before the outbreak of the First World War. By 1918 they were already looking to celluloid as a potentially thinner, lighter and more flexible alternative to glass. But it would not be until the 1930s that the first plastic contact lenses were created when, almost simultaneously, the Hungarian Istavan Gyorffy started tinkering about with a new form of sheet plastic (polymethyl methacrylate or PMMA, marketed in Germany under the brand name Plexiglas as a substitute for windows) and the American William Feinbloom contrived a lens in a combination of glass and bakelite. It was also in this decade that another Hungarian, Josef Dallos, who was Jewish and had been forced to flee to London from his native Budapest in 1938, greatly improved methods of tailoring contact lenses to the wearers' eyes by making use of a soft moulding substance called Negocoll that came from dentistry.

A couple of years after the Second World War, and again independently but concurrently, both the German inventor Heinrich

Wöhlk and the American optometrist Kevin Tuohy were to fashion smaller and lighter lenses that just fitted over the cornea and did away with the sclera-covering outer rim. Infamously, Tuohy came up with the idea by accident when part of one of his plastic lenses broke off. Sticking it in his eye anyway, he discovered that he could see just as well without the additional portion. These dinkier cornea lenses, by allowing more oxygen to get to the eye, were more comfortable to wear and therefore could be worn for longer, often up to ten or twelve hours a day. They could also be fitted without the long and painful process of making a mould of the eye.

In America, following their arrival on the market, contacts were to grow in popularity throughout the 1950s. *Business Week* in 1958 reported that while only around 50,000 people had worn contact lenses in 1945 – and most of those for serious eye conditions such as keratoconus (a thinning of the cornea) – there were now anything between 2 and 3 million wearers in the United States. The paper maintained that 'two out of every 76 people who required optical aids used contacts'. Most users, it revealed, were women and the ratio was about 'three women to two men', although the number of men opting for them was 'increasing', and '80 percent of the users of contacts' in its survey claimed they 'wore them for appearance sake'.

Even if contacts were lighter, thinner and smaller than they'd ever been before – and the lightest and thinnest lens to date, the Microlens, the result of a very Cold War collaboration between a trio of British, West German and American oculists, Frank Dickinson, Wilhelm Sohnges and Jack Neill, was launched in 1953 – Buddy Holly was still looking at sticking a pair of hard impermeable discs of PMMA in his eyes. Gas-permeable lenses and hydrogel soft lenses, the latter the inspired creation of the Czech scientists Otto Wichterle and Drahoslav Lim in the early 1960s and made using a rotating drum powered by a child's bicycle, were not to go on sale until the 1970s.

*Business Week* would cite the figure of $150 to $300 for a pair. Holly paid Armistead $125 for his contact lenses. And although prices might have increased in the intervening three years, it's possible that the singer's lenses were not of the finest quality. Though with his rather expensive tastes when it came to clothes and guitars, it is difficult to see Holly settling for second best. Perhaps the very latest micro lenses had yet to reach west Texas. But whatever the case, he found them agonising to wear and could scarcely keep them in for more than ten minutes, making them virtually useless for public appearances and stage work. Holly despondently put his browlines back on and headed out on the road again.

## Off your rocker

The inadequacy of those contact lenses inadvertently changed the course of rock 'n' roll. For a year later Holly was still wearing his glasses when he and his new backing band the Crickets hit the top of the charts on both sides of the Atlantic with their single 'That'll Be the Day', the song's title (and chorus refrain) picked up from a line of dialogue drawled by John Wayne in *The Searchers*. And it was a grinning, happy-go-lucky-looking Holly in said spectacles, with a Fender Stratocaster guitar held at the butt almost like a parade-ground rifle, who a few months later took his place beside the rest of the group on the full-colour cover photograph for their debut LP, *The 'Chirping' Crickets*.

The Buddy Holly who found fame in 1957 presented teenage record buyers, and especially the weedier, paler, more sun-starved and less corn-fed variety to be found on these rain-lashed shores, with a uniquely endearing idol. Where Elvis, Little Richard, Jerry Lee Lewis and even Bo Diddley were sexual and slightly dangerous, Holly was boy-next-door homely for all he sang of lovin' and turtle dovin'. The spectacles conveyed the idea of diligently completed homework, good high school grades and chaste prom dates – girls in vast petticoated skirts driven home on time, their lipstick intact, and the buttons on their angora cardigans and straps of their bullet-bras unmolested.

Where Elvis, like Frank Sinatra, was an interpreter of other people's songs – one of the best when on form and presented with the right material, if also alas at the mercy of it when not ('Muss i denn' anyone?) – Holly wrote many of his own numbers, stealing what he needed from elsewhere of course, along with collaborating with Crickets drummer Jerry Allison and producer Norman Petty. Telegraphed subtly to those who picked up the signals – and Holly's Stratocaster cut through the airwaves like Morse code – was the notion that songs could be written by the musicians themselves as a unit and didn't have to be bought by the yard from tune merchants on Tin Pan Alley or Denmark Street. And that in order to cut it as a rock 'n' roller, looking like Elvis might not be quite so essential after all. Here was a guy who sang with an odd hiccupy inflection, throwing in a-heys and a-hey-a-heys here and there as if yodelling or gargling with water, and wore glasses. What might previously have been considered shortcomings turned out to be strengths. And when it came to his glasses, Holly, on the good counsel of the Everly Brothers, would up the ante and acquire a pair of heavy black horn-rimmed frames of a type that, as a Google search will confirm, remains to this day synonymous with the singer.

Professional performers since childhood, the Kentucky-born Don and Phil Everly took Holly under their wing after first touring with him in 1957. In New York they introduced him to their preferred outfitters, Phil's, a menswear shop on Third Avenue that specialised in Ivy League threads. Holly was an immediate convert and soon he and the rest of the Crickets were sporting collegiate duds. With his curls tamed by Jake Goss of Lubbock's Shag 'n' Shear shop and having spent $300 getting his teeth capped, practically all that remained of pre-hits Holly was his old browline glasses. These, Don and Phil suggested, really had to go. They argued that the singer should get a pair that made, as Phil subsequently told Holly's biographer Philip Norman, 'a real upfront statement', one that proudly said 'OK, I wear glasses, and here they are.' Which is precisely what he did with the heavy black frames seemingly purchased somewhere in New York – the Big Apple proving once again to be the home of big glasses.

It was this more suavely bespectacled Holly that toured the UK.

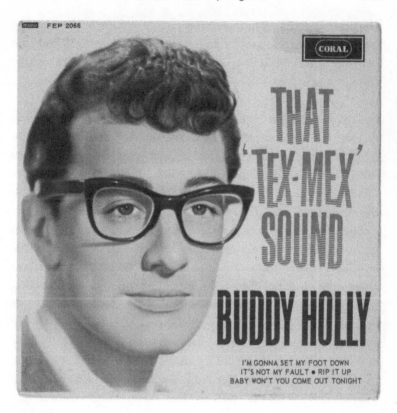

Buddy Holly, That 'Tex-Mex Sound'.

This Holly that romanced and married María Elena Santiago, a cute Puerto Rican girl who worked as a receptionist at his music publishers in Manhattan's Brill Building. This Holly that broke with Norman Petty and embarked on a new life and musical direction in New York, one that saw him recording with spine-tingling pizzicato string arrangements that plucked at the heart on songs like 'Raining in My Heart' and 'It Doesn't Matter Anymore'. And it was this Holly, tired and weary and only part of the way through a twenty-plus-date winter tour of iced-up Midwestern towns, who on the dismally chilly evening of 3 February 1959, after a gig at the Surf Ballroom in Clear Lake, Iowa, clambered aboard a four-seater Beechcraft Bonanza bound for Fargo, North

Dakota. That tiny plane, carrying Holly, Ritchie Valens and the Big Bopper, was barely 5 miles into its flight when it crashed into a cornfield, killing all three musicians and the pilot outright. Holly was just twenty-two.

In a grisly epilogue to the tragedy, the spectacles he was wearing that day – 'the day the music died' as Don McLean hailed it in the lyrics of 'American Pie' – came to light some twenty-one years later. On 27 February 1980, Jerry Allen, the local district county sheriff, came across an envelope in the Cerro Gordo courthouse that contained four dice, a watch that had belonged to the Big Bopper, the parts of another watch, and Holly's glasses, their lenses smashed but the frames apparently intact. The discovery made headlines around the world, and there was an unseemly scrabble among the more fanatical and morbid Holly fans to acquire these holy relics of rock 'n' roll's fallen saint. A desperate Walt Guyer of Mill Creek, Delaware, reportedly sent a cheque to Allen for $502.37, a sum that comprised his entire life savings, in the hope of seeing off other bidders. This tasteless circus was only brought to an end that October after Holly's widow, María Elena, filed a petition calling for the court to hand the spectacles over to her. Her wish was finally granted following a hearing with the District Judge, B. C. Sullivan, on 20 March 1981.

But the half-life of those horn-rims was to be a good deal more positive. In Holly's wake, four-eyes would be good enough for aspiring English rock 'n' rollers such as Hank Marvin of the Shadows. Elton John, in his autobiography *Me*, would in effect blame Buddy Holly for his spectacles. Recalling his time at Pinner County Grammar in the late 1950s when he was 'expressly forbidden from wearing anything' with any 'connection to rock and roll', he writes that 'The closest I got to sartorial rebellion was my prescription glasses, or rather, how much I wore my prescription glasses. They were only supposed to be used for looking at the blackboard. Labouring under the demented misapprehension that they made me look like Buddy Holly, I wore them all the time, completely ruining my eyesight. Then I had to wear them all the time.'

As an adjunct to this, John claimed that following this, he also gave up masturbation because he feared going blind. 'While plenty of musicians will tell you that Buddy Holly had a massive impact on their lives, I'm probably the only musician that can say he inadvertently stopped me wanking,' he maintains. But the sexual revolutions of the 1960s were to sweep even spectacles along with them, glasses finding wearers among cinema's ace faces and young meteors.

# 10

# I Spy with My Little Eyeglasses

Few, it's fair to say, would ever have described the horn-rimmed glasses-wearing guitarist Hank Marvin as possessing matinée idol looks. But in the early 1960s the Shadows with Cliff Richard became bona fide movie stars in England's answer to Elvis's big-screen musical outings: *The Young Ones*, *Summer Holiday* and *Wonderful Life*. Two of these were directed by the Canadian Sidney Furie, for whom the Shadows would supply songs for the soundtrack of his likeable 1962 teenage social-issue picture cum courtroom drama *The Boys*. But it wasn't really until the arrival of Furie's *The Ipcress File* in 1965 that Anglo-American movie audiences can be said to have been truly presented with an all-out spectacle-wearing male action movie lead. And a south London one at that too.

There had, of course, been romantic men (and women) in spectacles before then. Gregory Peck, as the noble lawyer Atticus Finch, in owlish horn-rims in the adaptation of *To Kill a Mockingbird*, for example. And on the continent, the Italian heart-throb Marcello Mastroianni, for whom the phrase 'suave' could have been invented, had worn glasses in Federico Fellini's 1963 film *8½*. A movie about movie making, Mastroianni starred as Guido Anselmi, a Fellini-esque film director dogged by creative doubts who spends most of his time ducking out of sight of his increasingly anxious cast and crew. Accordingly, for much of the

picture the actor's eyes are protectively framed by distancing pairs
of large black horn-rimmed eyeglasses and dark-tinted sunglasses,
which he peers over and pulls off and on as the situation dictates.
The actor is effortlessly debonair and chic while doing so, his spectacles as immaculately stylish as his black suit, soft collared white
shirts, skinny ties, maestro cape and broad-brimmed hat. The
contemporary designs of his eyewear were variously (if not conclusively) attributed to such luxury Italian brands of the period as
Terri Brogan, Polo and Persol. The latter's sunglasses Mastroianni
had helped put on the map by wearing them in *La Dolce Vita*, the
film that made him an international star in 1960. Nevertheless,
possibly the most stylish pair of spectacles in *8½* are the narrow
rectangular black horn-rims worn by Anouk Aimée, who plays
Mastroianni's on-screen wife.

As a spy movie, *The Ipcress File* is also about looking, or perhaps more precisely surveillance (along with kidnapping and
brainwashing), and a picture that plays equally with inventive
cinematic framing devices. Events are observed over other people's
shoulders and conversations heard through half-closed doors. As
Michael Caine, who played its central protagonist Harry Palmer,
once astutely commented, it was 'filmed ... as if someone else
was watching it'. And Palmer, like Anselmi, observes the world
through a pair of heavy-rimmed spectacles. Though in this
instance Caine's Palmer is, as he says, never without his glasses,
'except in bed'* – a confession that prompts their come-hither
removal by Sue Lloyd, playing the intelligence office vamp Jean
Courtney. It's a scene that neatly, and quite brilliantly, reverses the
typical cinematic stereotype of the male lead moving in for the
romantic kill after first depriving his passive female love interest
of *her* glasses.

Palmer is, in fact, first glimpsed in bed and without his glasses
in the title sequence of the movie – itself preceded by a rapid

---

* The claim is palpably false in any case. Earlier in the film Palmer is seen to
remove his glasses and tuck them into his jacket pocket before fighting a sinister
bald-headed man on the steps of the Royal Albert Hall.

plot-setting prologue involving the disappearance on a train of an absent-minded scientist called Dr Radcliffe* and the murder of his assistant, whose body, eyes left wide open, is seen unceremoniously dumped on a mail truck on the station platform. Woken by the bell of a wind-up alarm clock, Palmer switches a bedside lamp on and gingerly stretches a hand out over the sheets on the right-hand side of the bed, which has evidently recently been occupied but now lies empty. Surprised to discover no one there, he sits bolt upright. His blue eyes, which match the colour of his pyjamas, scan the room. In one of the film's many visual sleights of hand, the perspective now switches to Palmer's point of view, and we are briefly presented with a blurry myopic impression of his surroundings. He fishes for his glasses, a pair of brown plastic horn-rims which sit temples in the air, lenses down, on a bedside table, and puts them on. Looking out again, we are presented with an in-focus tracking shot of the interior of a one-room apartment. Beyond the bedroom there's a lounge area with a sofa and armchair and a table where a bottle of liquor, almost empty, and two large brandy-style glasses with dregs in them sit. After that, taking up much of the rest of the place is a contemporary open-plan kitchen, well equipped, with stacks of copper pans, teak units and an *à la mode* breakfast bar with two stools.

It is into this space that Palmer, still wearing just his specs and pyjamas, heads to prepare coffee. And 'prepare' is the word, for in his hands it is revealed to be a laborious, almost anally retentive, business. Not for Palmer the mere ladling of brickdust-brown instant Nescafé into a mug with a shot of hot water and away to face the day, oh no. He must grind his own beans using a special gadget, a piece of equipment that he operates, eyes half shut, in a state of ecstatic reverie, the grinder whirring in sync with John Barry's jangling cymbal-driven theme music. In between washing and dressing and tidying up the flat, the coffee making proceeds in a series of similarly fastidious actions, with fresh water boiled,

---

* We know he's a scientist because he reads a copy of the *New Scientist* and we know he's absent-minded because he leaves his camera behind in the car.

precise quantities (two scoops) of coffee and water measured out, and just the right sort of spoon and the dinkiest of cups and saucers and the shiniest of chrome and glass cafetières arrayed. Nothing is left to chance. Even a bean that accidentally strays on to the counter is retrieved and put in its proper place.

By the time Palmer, who has yet to utter a word, finally sits down to drink his coffee and study the racing page in the paper, an indelible picture of the character as something of a connoisseur has already been nailed home. After all, hardly anyone in Britain took this much trouble over their coffee back in 1965. With the retrieval too of both a woman's bracelet and a gun from the tangled sheets of his bed a few seconds later, it is also made abundantly clear that his glasses have done him no obvious harm in terms of getting to sleep with women who can afford to leave their jewellery behind after the act. Or gaining employment as a secret agent.

The movie was loosely based on Len Deighton's debut novel, a snappily written espionage thriller with a touch of Raymond Chandler about its hardboiled prose and the tortuousness of its plotting. Most of which Furie dispensed with entirely for the movie. (Which isn't to say that the film version is exactly easy to follow in places.) But published in 1962, the same year as the Cuban Missile Crisis and the release of *Dr No*, the first of the James Bond movies, it was an instant bestseller. With the Cold War getting ever frostier and spy pictures doing good business at the box office, the rights for Deighton's book and its projected sequels were immediately snapped up by Harry Saltzman, the Canadian co-producer of *Dr No* and the 007 franchise. As the author recalled in an introduction to a new edition in 2009, Saltzman 'had decided that *The Ipcress File* and its unnamed hero could provide a counter-weight to the Bond series'. Prior to Bond, Saltzman had brought gritty, socially realistic kitchen sink drama to the big screen, backing adaptations of John Osborne's controversial (for its day) Angry Young Man play *Look Back in Anger* and Alan Sillitoe's Nottingham-set novel *Saturday Night and Sunday Morning*. And in contrast to Fleming's upper-crust Bond, Deighton's protagonist/narrator was determinedly working-class; his lack of deference

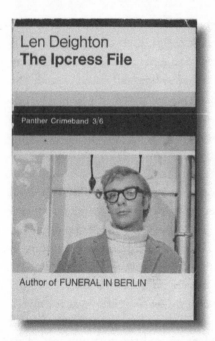

Len Deighton
**The Ipcress File**

Panther Crimeband 3/6

Author of FUNERAL IN BERLIN

*The Ipcress File.*

too was of the zeitgeist, chiming as it did with the mood afoot following the Profumo scandal.

In the novel itself, the London-born Deighton even chose to make his bolshie unnamed hero a northerner. An autodidact from Burnley in Lancashire, he reads the *New Statesman* and has a superior appreciation of the finer foods of life compared to his supposed betters. With his mohair cardigans and a thorough working knowledge of Soho's continental delicatessens, bistros and espresso bars, he's a bit of a proto-mod or modernist. Someone able to spot a Charlie Parker rip-off in a Sammy Davis Jr number, if nevertheless retaining a soft spot for brass band music. Caine's Palmer, meanwhile, and perhaps to further emphasise his speccy brainy side, listens to Mozart – at least when he's entertaining, and therefore trying to impress, classy birds (to use a derogatory phrase of the period) from the office at home.

There is, however, only a single blink-and-you'll-miss-it mention of him wearing glasses in the book, and this occurs curiously after he's purposely damaged someone else's bins. Deighton's main man is on a first-class flight to Rome when he finds himself seated next to a man in spectacles. Overweight and overbearing, and the eater of a packed lunch of sausage sandwiches who has the poor taste to attempt to order a port and lemon from the stewardess, Fatso (as our hero dubs him) is the plane passenger from hell. He's also almost too suspiciously awful to be true and so our spy conspires to 'accidentally' break his glasses and swipes his wallet to discover more about him. Surreptitiously inspecting the contents of the latter, he finds, among other things salient to the story, three photographs of 'passport style – full face, profile and three-quarter positions of a dark-haired, round-faced character; deep sunk eyes with bags under horn-rimmed glasses, chin jutting and cleft ... even though the photograph was in black and white. I'd seen the face before; most mornings I shave it.'

That's it. His horn-rims go unremarked from here on in. And elsewhere in the novel, if desisting from actively damaging any more pairs, he shows no great affinity with other spectacle wearers either. Referring only dismissively to Colonel Ross's military-issue wire frames, he expresses extreme irritation, in particular, at another operative's use of his glasses as a kind of prop: 'He had a pair of heavy black spectacles of the sort with straight side bars. These latter facilitated his pulling his glasses half off his face just before telling or showing you something, then snapping them back on his nose to lend emphasis to what he was saying.'

Ironically, the decision to equip Caine with glasses for the part in the film came from Saltzman and stemmed from a similar irritation for the way glasses were often used far too ostentatiously in movies by non-spectacle-wearing actors.

Caine was short-sighted in real life and always wore his glasses off-screen, and it was at a dinner at the producer's Buckinghamshire house that the actor maintained that Saltzman first proposed the idea. They'd been discussing how they might create a more believable thinking man's Bond when Caine noticed that the producer had been staring at his glasses for some time. Saltzman, as the actor recalled in his autobiography *What's It All About?*, then raised the possibility of making them a potential feature of the character. 'I always hate it in films', he informed Caine, 'when actors who do not normally wear glasses are made to wear them and don't know how to handle them. You know exactly what to do with them, so why don't we have Harry Palmer wear some in the film? It will also help to make the guy look more ordinary.'

It was over another meal, this one cooked by Deighton at his home, that the on-screen Palmer gained his culinary dimension.

Before breaking into fiction, Deighton, who'd studied at St Martin's and the Royal College of Art, worked as an illustrator, graphic artist and the art director at a London ad agency. But his mother had been a professional cook. Inheriting her interest in food, he became an accomplished amateur chef. Combining his skills with pen and pan, he began in the early 1960s to produce an acclaimed weekly cookery comic strip for the *Observer* newspaper, these strips forming the basis for his *Action Cook Book* published in the year *The Ipcress File* came out.

Caine's Palmer, it was duly decided, would not only enjoy good food but inherit his creator's skills with an egg whisk, seducing the love interest Courtney with a home-cooked meal. This again was intended to distinguish Palmer from Bond. 007, it was reasoned, could only be imagined wining and dining his dates in restaurants with wine lists as long as your arm and seemed otherwise wholly dependent on hotel room service for victuals for sustenance and seduction. Bond, it could be added, orders drinks but is never seen mixing them. And Furie consciously intended Palmer's prissy coffee making to be both the equivalent of Bond's shaken-not-stirred martini and something of an antidote to it. For he not only prepares it himself, but as a stimulant rather than an intoxicant – this drink sharpens rather than dulls his mind.*

Deighton would come to tutor Caine in the art of cracking eggs on set, and cut-outs of his cookery strips, pinned up here and there, were to form part of the interior decor of Palmer's kitchen in the movie. Concerns were apparently raised by some film company executives that a cooking Caine would be thought gay. To assuage their fears Furie, who only the previous year had made the homoerotic British biker feature *The Leather Boys*, promised to 'butch up' any scenes where food was involved, with Palmer, for example, shot engaging in a kind of shopping trolley duel

---

* A perusal of the *Action Cook Book* entry on coffee confirms Deighton's own disdain for the likes of Nescafé as a beverage at least. 'Instant coffee,' he wrote, 'although not worth drinking, should be kept in the flavouring cupboard. Use it when making coffee-flavoured sauce, cake, mousse, caramel, frosting or cream.'

with his superior Colonel Ross in order to show that he was a real man and not some effete foodie. Oddly enough, considering how unorthodox it was at the time, no one seems to have objected to Caine wearing glasses.

The part, though, gave Caine the freedom to wear his glasses in public, and in future film work, without damaging his ability to be seen as a likely leading man. Just as his working-class London accent, which in previous eras might have precluded him from being considered for certain roles, was no longer an impediment, neither was being a speccy.

# 11

# Working Glass Heroes

Just a few months after *The Ipcress File*'s release, the July 1965 edition of *Vogue* profiled Len Deighton and John le Carré in a feature that considered the emergence of less fantastical secret agents entitled 'The Men Who Throw Cold Water on Hot Spies'.* The issue also carried adverts for the Marcia range of decorative browline-style frames ('Exquisite in their own right, Marcia Frames perfectly complement your good taste in jewellery ... available in combinations of sable on smoke, onyx on silver, smoke on silver and azure on silver'). And, most pertinently, that month the magazine's regular 'Beauty Bulletin' column was devoted entirely to spectacles.

Subtitled 'How Not to Miss a Thing ... The Techniques for Doing It Dashingly', the piece made a case (yet again) for viewing spectacles not simply as visual aids but as fashionable accessories. Alluding to its readers' easy familiarity with acquiring stately piles, its writer maintained that 'Unlike the perfect country house and the lifetime love, spectacles are hardly meant to be

---

* Pre-dating the publication of *The Ipcress File* by a year, the former MI5 agent John le Carré's debut novel *Call for the Dead* had also featured a spectacle-wearing spy in the form of George Smiley. A character whose 'only fidget', according to le Carré, 'was to polish his glasses on the silk lining of his tie and when he did this his eyes had a soaked, naked look which was embarrassing to those who caught him at it'.

forever. And it strikes us that where spectacles do a poor job of everything except the improvement of vision, it's because they've been chosen with some vague hope for eternity – like copper pipes or herringbone-brick terrace.' Warming to their theme, they continued:

There has never been a piece of fashion that could offer a life-time guarantee as such – and the important thing to keep in mind about spectacles now is this: they're part of fashion: they're no longer glass crutches. Spectacles have become fashion to the extent that women with no eyesight problems are writing their own prescriptions ('20/20 but plenty of frame'). Spectacles have become fashion to the extent that what's great today will almost certainly be classic a year from today.

Spelling out the advantage of wearing spectacles, the writer considered the 'woman whose face' was 'not bony in a strong way'; such a person might, they argued, be 'short of the sort of feature that reaches out and grabs people and sticks in the memory for keeps'. But with 'the addition of noticeable spectacles, most soft-featured women', they believed, acquired 'a bonier, more racé look instantly'. Spectacles, they argued, could also 'provide a sneaky way to hide tired lines, re-contour a face, divert attention from the undereye department, or slink around wrinkles – and be amusing about it meanwhile'. As one unnamed female interviewee had apparently quipped, 'Why go to a plastic surgeon when tortoise is quicker?'

Giving it plenty of frame across the spread were a series of pictures of models in glasses, shot by Bert Stern. One of the last people to photograph Marilyn Monroe – his now immortal ethereal images of the star posing in the nude, her modesty protected by swathes of gauzy scarves, were taken only six weeks before her death – Stern had a good track record with eyewear. In 1962 he'd been hired to produce the movie poster still for Stanley Kubrick's adaptation of Vladimir Nabokov's controversial novel *Lolita*. The photographer was fortunate to stop off at a branch of Woolworths en route to the shoot with the film's fourteen-year-old lead Sue Lyon. On a rack in the store he came across a cheap pair of red plastic heart-shaped sunglasses that he instantly bought and took to the session. His sexually provocative colour photograph of the young actor (though still two years older than the character in the book), posed wearing these sunglasses, scarlet-lipped and licking a pinky-red lollipop, became the definitive image of the movie – even though the film itself was shot in black and white and Lyon wore a completely different pair of sunglasses.

Stern's spectacle shoot for *Vogue* was considerably less sleazy but was evidently still intended to convey the idea that a girl in glasses might welcome passes from eligible gentlemen at least. The central image to the spread was a full-page colour photograph of a model with centre-parted blonde, chin-length hair wearing a dark-pink Emilio Pucci shirt fastened at the midriff. She meets the viewer's gaze, her lips, cupcake frosting pink, in a pout, and her eyes, hooded with pale eyeshadow, peering out above a pair of plastic half-moon 'sky blue spectacles'. These spectacles are said to 'offer instant accommodation for the far sighted'. Superimposed above her is a pair of big round plastic tortoiseshell frames described as 'owl eyes that miss nothing' with 'straight skinny side-pieces' whose great virtue, it is stated, is that 'they mess up the hair not at all'.*

While the model's sky-blue numbers were at the more playful, op art end of the style, half-moon spectacles were then already enjoying a wider revival among spectacle wearers, though by and large in more muted shades of clear or black plastic. The American Optical Company credited Fred Astaire as a possible trailblazer for

---

* And continuing on the topic of spectacles and hairstyles, elsewhere in the piece the Hollywood socialite Lady Nancy 'Slim' Keith was credited with making it acceptable to put one's horn-rims to use as temporary hairbands in polite company. One of the few photographs of Diana Vreeland with spectacles from this period, and a casual family portrait of her with her son Frederick and grandson Alexander, perhaps telling, shows the *Vogue* editor rocking these glasses in a top-of-the-head look.

their renaissance: the all-singing, all-dancing Hollywood star had been pictured wearing some on television. A Milwaukee optician interviewed by *Time* the previous year, however, had maintained that television itself was responsible for the fashion since 'the half spec' enabled people who only needed 'glasses for reading to go through the evening paper and watch TV at the same time without taking their glasses off'. This sounds reasonable enough. But as Richard Corson astutely points out in his near contemporary book *Fashions in Eyeglasses*, it could also be argued that people 'might not have been so quick to adopt them . . . had they not seen them on TV (or on Fred Astaire)'.

In any case, their reappearance in the mid-1960s, which in retrospect seems more like a fault line in the decade between its mod and hippy phases, was on a par with a more widespread raiding of granny's attic for inspiration. Reacting against the progress-can't-be-stopped tide of the shrink-wrapped and the off-the-rack, discerning tastemakers were increasingly to be found trawling the likes of the Portobello Road market for antiques, and adopting old policemen's capes and red guardsman's jackets as the height of King's Road dandy fashion.

*Vogue*'s survey reveals that optical design was similarly engaged in a process of thumbing its own back pages, if often with equal gleeful irreverence. Another Stern picture, and a parallel image to the main photograph, shows a helmet-haired Kacia Newman reading a book while modelling a pair of upside-down half-moon plastic specs. Specifically for the near-sighted, their topsy-turvy far-out design is every bit as kinky as one of Mrs Peel's catsuits in *The Avengers*, *Vogue*'s reporter saluting 'immense square-eyed frames and great oval owl eyes' and 'horizontal ovals' and 'hexagonals' as 'the hottest things on the market today'.

Perhaps the oddest old-school optical aid the piece championed was a new line in 'sight stick wands' for women who wished to be more discreet about their need for glasses. Essentially a monocle-on-a-cane lorgnette, here was a full-on *incroyables* throwback, a device that could possibly have still been made-to-order by the veteran umbrella makers James Smith & Sons. Something John

Steed, Mrs Peel's bowler-hatted and vintage Bentley-driving partner, might conceivably have used as a weapon instead of a sword
stick in an episode of the series.

The revival of such an instrument along with a shift to oval,
round and hexagonal frame shapes was indicative of what
Corson at the time saw as a shift towards ever more 'aggressively old-fashioned spectacles'. Citing an article from the *New
York Times* in November 1965 on the 'trend to elderly eyewear',
he identified a coffee-shop boutique called Serendipity as one
potential source of the fad. About 'a dozen years ago', or so the
*New York Times* claimed, the coffee shop had acquired, for a
pittance, the entire stock of an elderly optometrist who'd gone
bust. It began selling on this arcane range of glasses, 'slowly and
quietly to visionary customers', until 'three years ago' when the
'traffic in Benjamin Franklin spectacles and the round, steel-
rimmed style admired by Soviet politicians started booming'.
Writing in 1966, Corson reported that these 'granny glasses'
were 'flooding the market'. A year later that flood was arguably
to turn into a tsunami as John Lennon adopted the style as his
own. After all, the Beatles, by his own estimation, were at this
point 'more popular than Jesus'.

## Living is easy with eyes closed

In the field of 1960s pop Lennon was, if anything, something of
a late adopter of this type of frame. John Sebastian of the chirpy
American folk rock band the Lovin' Spoonful had been wearing
his little round wire glasses when the group's debut single 'Do You
Believe in Magic' smashed into the American *Billboard* top ten
back in July 1965. For the group's third album, *Hums of the Lovin'
Spoonful* released in November 1966, Sebastian also wrote '4-Eyes',
a kind of anthem for spectacled youth. The song, whose chorus is
voiced from the angle of a school-yard bully who taunts a myope
after pinching their glasses, exposes the prejudices glasses wearers
suffer from childhood by reeling off the common insults thrown
their way. From being thought icky by girls and considered a queer

by boys in the playground to looking too severe in tortoiseshells upon graduation, it's perhaps both an exorcism of some personal demons by Sebastian and a spirited exercise in table-turning reclamation. Think a 'Short People' for spectacle wearers and you'll get the idea.

But for Lennon the round-rimmed glasses would help him regain some of his independence after three insane years of Beatlemania, a change of look that reflected a shift in his own perspective about the need to escape his allotted role as a loveable, if irascible, mop top in the toppermost of the poppermost group in the world. Appallingly short-sighted (and with the added issue of an astigmatism) since childhood, Lennon had been fitted with glasses aged seven. Embarrassed by their thick lenses, and believing, as he later confessed, that 'glasses were cissy', he avoided wearing them whenever possible – a habit that continued into adulthood and for the first half of the Beatles' career, even after he'd acquired a spiffy enough pair of black horn-rims.*

Unlike his marriage to Cynthia, no attempt was ever made to keep Lennon's spectacle wearing a secret from the fans. In an early interview with *New Musical Express* in 1963, readers were informed that Lennon appeared glasses-less in public as he didn't 'want the group to be accused of any imitation' of the Shadows. But perhaps fear of being mistaken for their Hamburg circuit

---

* Another sixties pop star and firmly established spectacle-dodger since childhood was Bob Dylan, who in the mid-1960s and having 'gone electric' preferred to shield his eyes with a pair of Ray-Ban Wayfarer sunglasses (rumoured to be fitted with prescription lenses 'as thick as Coke-bottles') than ever be seen in spectacles. Though he did briefly flirt with an old-time wire-framed pair during the years of his marriage to Sara Lownds and retreat to Woodstock in upstate New York towards the decade's end. Dylanologist and biographer Daniel Mark Epstein has gone so far as to suggest that the singer's myopia might have had an 'aggrandizing' effect on his hearing, and his extraordinary facility with music. 'Where others', he writes, 'heard a phrase he heard a paragraph; where some heard a theme he heard a fugue.' Since he could 'not read the blackboard', Dylan, he maintains, 'became an audiodidact, one who learns mainly through his ears rather than his eyes, from the sound of voices rather than words on a page'.

and Cavern Club rivals Freddie and the Dreamers also played its part. Riding on the coat-tails of the early sixties Merseybeat boom and enjoying chart hits on both sides of the Atlantic, this Manchester group were fronted by Freddie Garrity, a diminutive former milkman who wore large horn-rims and skipped clownishly about the stage like a demented marionette. As endearing as this undoubtedly was to a certain section of the record-buying public, and especially in America, it can't exactly be said to have made wearing glasses in pop appear any cooler. If anything, it perhaps only perpetuated the idea that it would always be a bit comic – that joke best left to funny-looking limeys with eyesight as poor as their teeth, Garrity far closer to Peter Sellers than Elvis Presley. If alas probably closer still to Peter Glaze, the buffoonish glasses-wearing host of BBC TV kids' variety quiz show *Crackerjack!* Lennon himself, if revering Buddy Holly and the Goons and admiring Hank Marvin, though much less vocally so after the Beatles' own success, plainly appears to have subscribed in part to this view.

Michael Braun, who trailed the group in 1963-4 during their first year of fame, quizzed Lennon about why the musician kept 'ostentatiously removing the glasses' he 'constantly' wore off-stage, and was told: 'Mustn't spoil the image.' Braun would subsequently record that not even a petition signed by 200 French female Beatles fans and specially delivered to the group at their hotel in Paris calling for 'John Lennon to wear his glasses on stage' at that evening's show at the Olympia Theatre could convince him to perform with them on.

Like Holly, Lennon experimented with contact lenses but with no more success, tending, by all accounts, to drop and lose them on the dressing-room floor which resulted in him having to go on without them. When they'd started out, gigging in tiny venues and clubs, there had possibly been some distinct advantages to not being able to see. The sight of rows of bevvied-up Birkenhead Teddy Boys yelling obscenities at you inches away from your face could be more than a little distracting. In variety, Harry Secombe of the Goons, the BBC radio comedy show whose anarchic humour fired Lennon's imagination as a schoolboy, had, for instance, left his glasses off to keep the audience out of view and conquer crippling stage fright. As the Beatle confessed to his friend and biographer Ray Connolly, though, the experience of playing to vast crowds you couldn't see was rather more unsettling. 'Can you imagine', he told Connolly, 'what it's like hearing all that noise and playing and singing and not seeing a bloody thing? It's frightening.'*

But exhausted by the rigmarole of performing in cavernous American sporting arenas – some, this time round, picketed by the Ku Klux Klan in response to reports of Lennon's comments about the group and Jesus, and undertaken amid death threats – the Beatles retired from touring following a grisly final date on 29 August 1966 at the Candlestick Park baseball stadium in San Francisco.

Relieved of live duties and looking for new directions, that September, only a month after the release of the group's ground-breaking LP *Revolver*, Lennon accepted the offer of a non-musical acting bit part in Richard Lester's satirical movie *How I Won the War*. Based on a novel by Patrick Ryan and with a script by the playwright Charles Wood, who'd collaborated with Lester on the Beatles' second movie *Help!*, the film was a wearingly zany send-up of militarism and cinema's own perpetuation of the heroic myths of the Second World War. It starred Michael Crawford as Lieutenant Earnest Goodbody, an

---

* The choice to wear glasses or not was largely Lennon's own. But this was not a luxury usually afforded to female singers and musicians in an industry where sexism was rife. The Greek singer Nana Mouskouri, who in 1963 represented Luxembourg at the Eurovision Song Contest, had to fight to keep her glasses on and was sacked by one Athens nightclub for not looking elegant enough when she refused to remove her spectacles. Self-conscious about her appearance, and believing that her eyes were too wide-set, Mouskouri felt the black square-framed glasses she favoured not only masked this defect but also shielded her from the audience. Wearing them gave her the confidence she needed to sing on stage, and they came to define her public image. One American newspaper, the *Gazetteer*, in 1965 patronisingly described her as looking like 'a pretty PhD candidate about to do a thesis on Greek ethnographic song'.

overeager upper-class twit charged with leading an absurdist mission to build a cricket pitch between enemy lines in Tunisia. Lennon played Musketeer Gripweed, a working-class Scouse grunt with a ready line in snarky off-hand gags who is said to have once supported Oswald Mosley. For the eight or so minutes Lennon is on screen he acquits himself well enough. But the movie, sold heavily (or oversold) on the basis of his participation, was neither a commercial nor a critical success. It remains, at best, a period curio.

To play the part, however, Lennon submitted to a haircut and also donned a pair of round wire Windsor-type spectacles with brown plastic-coated tortoiseshell rims and hook-ended side pieces. After six weeks' shooting in Almería in Spain, the Beatle, having found the lengthy process of film making tedious, returned to London armed with a new song and still wearing Gripweed's round metal Windsors. Or ones much like them without the plastic detailing, anyway. The song was 'Strawberry Fields Forever' and had been written in the downtime off-set at a Spanish mansion whose wrought-iron gates reminded him of the entrance to an old boyhood haunt, the Strawberry Field (no 's') Salvation Army children's home and gardens at Woolton. The spectacles were to receive their first major public airing (months ahead of the film) when Lennon made a guest appearance on the Boxing Day edition of Peter Cook and Dudley Moore's BBC TV satirical series *Not Only But Also*. A year earlier Lennon had performed on the show extracts from *In His Own Write*, a bestselling book of his comic stories, drawings and nonsense verse. This time he put in a turn in a sketch as a doorman in top hat and tails stationed outside 'London's most fashionable lavatory spot'. 'Follow your nose, sir,' the freshly bespectacled Beatle advises after ushering Cook, playing a pipe-smoking visiting American TV reporter whom Lennon has just relieved of a £5 entrance fee, down the steps of a public convenience.

Around this time Penguin published a paperback collected edition of Lennon's writings and drawings. Entitled *The Penguin John Lennon*, its first impression featured a cover designed by art director Alan Aldridge with portraits of the Beatle by the legendary sixties London snapper Brian Duffy. On the front a spectacle-free Lennon, a little chubby about the face (as he was on the album sleeves of *Rubber Soul* and *Revolver*), was shown wearing a Superman shirt and striking a comic-book hero pose. Aldridge, perhaps conscious of copyright, reworked the Superman logo so that Lennon's own initials were emblazoned across his chest. On the back of the jacket, however, was another Duffy image. Here a beaming Lennon was shown wearing two pairs of round wire spectacles across his face, their lenses filled in with cartoon drawings of eyes, as if the musician had the benefit of sixth sight – insect vision, kaleidoscope eyes, rather than Superman's usual X-ray powers. But the truth, perhaps accidentally intuited in these knockabout snaps, was that Lennon with his new glasses would achieve a kind of reversal of Clark Kent and Superman. He was stronger with spectacles on.*

The glasses arrived at the moment when the Beatles, retreating into the studio like artists rather than entertainers with fickle concert-goers to please, were becoming ever more serious, and seriously experimental, about their output. As they set about making pop music at album length, on long-playing vinyl that came sleeved in covers designed by the contemporary artists Peter Blake, Jann Haworth and Richard Hamilton, Lennon's spectacles underwired the enterprise. 'All You Need is Love', 'Give Peace a Chance' and the proselytising of macrobiotic diets and anti-Vietnam bed-ins would all be much easier to accept from a man in goggles similar to those worn by Mahatma Gandhi. If unfortunately, alas, also Heinrich Himmler. And, less publicly, Adolf Hitler, whose admittedly rather more rimless style of reading spectacles with hook sides by Optiker Ruhnke were among the posthumous effects recovered from the Führerbunker in Berlin in 1945. Hitler, who refused to be photographed in glasses, believing that any hint of defective sight would undermine his authority, was

---

* A similar photograph by Bob Gruen, with Lennon wearing multiple pairs of glasses, was used on the sleeve of his 1974 solo album *Walls and Bridges*.

one of the figures Lennon, 'just to be a naughty boy', put forward for inclusion on the cover of *Sgt Pepper.*\*

But rather like another much-loved beetle, the 'People's Car' by Volkswagen (acclaimed by Hitler as 'The Strength Through Joy Car'), these glasses were taken up in earnest as badges of youthful anti-authoritarianism. In her poem 'New York Visit 1969', published in the *New York* magazine on 7 April that year, Judith Viorst provided a succinct survey of Manhattan's late-sixties counter-cultural demi-monde. A city where almost everyone seemed to be 'a drop-out with principles ... a vegetarian with insights ... or a black revolutionary with charisma', and she, as 'a nice Jewish girl from New Jersey' attempting to have a 'wicked' time in Greenwich Village, feared not being able to quite 'pass' in 'last year's pants length'. As she wrote, in the final stanza:

> *Everyone in New York*
> *Had ... An unconventional sex life,*
> *John Lennon glasses*

In the next line of the poem she adds that everyone also appeared to have 'A secret place to buy 1934 fur coats', which again underlines the degree to which vintage wear, the trend the spectacles themselves formed part of, was then *à la mode*.

## From the cradle to the grave

Until he formally changed it by deed poll to 'Ono' in a ceremony conducted at the Apple building on Savile Row on 22 April 1969, Lennon's middle name was Winston, after Churchill. Exorcising this permanent reminder of his status as a war baby was conceived as something of an anti-imperialist act on a par with his subsequent returning that November of his MBE in protest against Britain's

---

\* Gandhi was another person excised from the finished album's photo montage, after Sir Joseph Lockwood, chairman of EMI, raised concerns about it being considered sacrilegious in India and jeopardising sales there.

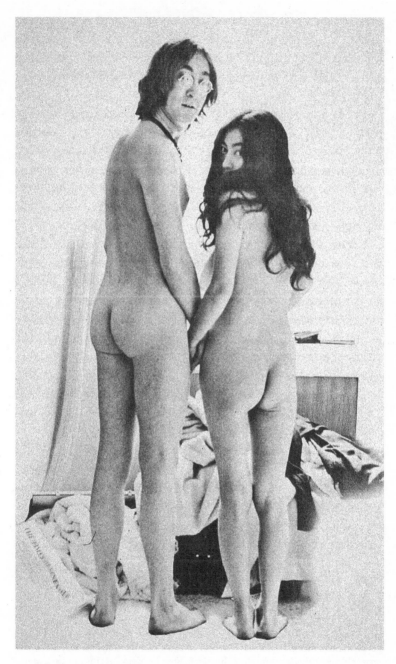

John Lennon and Yoko Ono.

involvement in Biafra, though he'd later come to use the pseudonym Dr Winston O'Boogie when moonlighting on records by
the likes of Elton John, whose own eyewear in the 1970s was to
add a whole new meaning to the word 'spectacle' when it came
to glasses.*

But Lennon's chosen frames were arguably also war babies. The
plain gold-filled round-rimmed pantoscopic style with a centre
joint, pad bridge and curl sides he acquired in 1966 were at the time
readily available in Britain on the NHS at a cost of ten shillings
and eleven pence (just £9.62 in today's money according to the
National Archive's Currency Converter). Though in 2005 one of
Lennon's own pairs sold at auction in London for £55,000.

Richard Corson writing in 1966, the same year that Lennon
first took up with his wire frames, noted the conservative tastes
of spectacle wearers in Britain. In the States just two years earlier
an industry body called the Fashion Eyewear Group of America
had been formed specifically to promote groovy new homegrown
glasses. And while a trade organisation called the Optical Council
had been attempting to do much the same thing in Britain since
the early 1950s, Corson observed, slightly wryly, that 'Many
Englishwomen seemed impervious to lizard and woodgrain and
Op' designs and 'still wore pink translucent plastic frames prescribed by the National Health'.

During a British parliamentary committee session in 1991, the
Labour MP David Hinchliffe, recalling his own Lennon-like aver-
sion to wearing glasses as a child, maintained that 'In the 1950s and
1960s, NHS spectacles would not have been worn by anyone who
was concerned about his or her appearance.' But the reality was
that an overwhelming majority of never-had-it-so-good Britons

---

* At the height of his mid-1970s fame, when he was dazzling US stadium
audiences with costumes adorned with plumes of marabou feathers, John, as
he writes in his autobiography, 'had a pair of glasses made in the shape of the
word ELTON, with lights all over them'. If visually stunning, they impaired his
performance, as 'the combined weight of the glasses and the battery pack that
powered the lights ... squashed' his nostrils and caused his singing to sound as
if he was holding his nose.

were content to lump it with NHS glasses, which were from the outset and by government diktat intended to 'be of good quality but not luxurious standard of appearance', and which, while they might grumble, suited their needs admirably enough, and at little (or to begin with no) cost. Price largely trumped fashion in an era that, despite the emergence of more rampant consumerism, continued to be coloured more by experiences of war than Warhol. While perhaps only Henry Ford offered models in as limited a range of designs and colours, the NHS scheme, launched in 1948, lasted into the 1980s.

Personally, having caught really only the final decade of NHS glasses, and after the passing of nearly forty years, it's the cloth-covered metal clip-shut cases that now linger most vividly in my mind, especially as my own current spectacles are hardly a million miles off the NHS frames I was first presented with as a child. About the size and shape of a Cornish pasty and as hard as an armadillo's shell, these carapaces appear, in my memory, almost congenitally conjoined with soft plastic zip-up pencil cases on the top edge of graffiti-scarred wooden school desks. The pencil cases usually contained a compass that many clearly put to ill use gouging names and obscenities into desk lids. Nothing so seditious or vandalistic was possible with the contents of a glasses case. Or certainly not those, like mine, with concave lenses for short sight. Whatever we'd read in William Golding's *Lord of the Flies* about how the overweight myope Piggy's spectacles were used to create fires for these boys left stranded on their desert island was nonsense, as a bright sunny afternoon of dull double maths spent trying, nonchalantly, to kindle the contents of a wastepaper basket with my specs more than confirmed. Divergent lenses are useless as burning glasses. The focal point is all wrong; pyromania requires the eyewear of the hypermetropic. And that novel was an O-level set text back then too. But those glasses cases required handling with care. The spectacles sat inside them almost like an oyster that needed to be shucked out of its shell. As tautly sprung as a mouse-trap, opening the case alone presented a challenge. The loss of a finger appeared a serious possibility if the thing sprang shut unexpectedly halfway through. The noise the case made when it accidentally snapped to, a violent clack somewhere between a music-room woodblock and a cap gun, could send a hushed exam room into paper-scattering shock.

Such cases, and especially by the late 1970s and early 1980s, seemed almost excessively sturdy, something akin to a sit-up-and-beg bike when there were far sleeker drop-handled racing models out there. In this, though, they stood against brushed black plastic alternatives and ever-rising disposability. The protection they offered to glasses was almost noble in its old-fashioned commitment to keeping them from harm. But the spring-lidded spectacle case *was* old-fashioned, of pensionable age no less by then. A child of the Edwardian era, its design was patented in 1908, the year that saw the publication of Kenneth Grahame's *The Wind in the Willows*. Its inventor was Francis James Willmott of Willmotts Ltd. A manufacturer of cases for jewellery and spectacles based in Evesham, Worcestershire, the company had originally been established in Birmingham's jewellery quarter in the 1880s and were to open a showroom for their wares in Clerkenwell near Hatton Garden before the outbreak of the First World War. In 1908 Willmotts had only recently merged with Smythe & Co., another case maker from Birmingham. Smythe's owner E. L. Payton shared Mr Toad's love of automobiles and held an interest in the Austin Motor Company, whose works were outside the city in the then still largely rural Longbridge. If spectacle cases and cars seem an unlikely convergence of business interests, both Willmotts' spring-lidded line and the bodywork on Austin's motors were made from rolled sheet steel.

The spring-lidded spectacle case had by the 1920s become a staple across the industry, with Dale Cases of Bethnal Green and Lessar Brothers of Birmingham, among many others, including American Optical in the States, producing their own variants. The East End firm of M. Wiseman & Co.'s model, fitted with hinges that it was claimed were 'perfectly constructed to avoid creaking', was marketed as the 'Summit' in 1933. But unbeknown to them the peak for the spring-lidded case still lay some years off, and its greatest boon was the creation of the NHS. And Wiseman's, like Willmotts, having turned their machines over to war work for the duration of the conflict, were to be major beneficiaries of contracts for the new health service.

By the time it was up and running, Willmotts' own spring-lid case was pushing forty but stood on the brink of becoming ubiquitous. For each pair of NHS spectacles was to be supplied with a free metal case. If adding to the per unit cost, it probably saved the government money in the long run by helping to prevent damage to the frames and lenses. On the back of supplying the NHS, Willmotts became the largest manufacturers of spectacle cases in Europe and by the 1970s were churning out between 100,000 and 150,000 of them a week.

If Willmotts set the standard for NHS cases, then M. Wiseman & Co. arguably had the most influence on the styles of glasses supplied. It would become one of the biggest manufacturers of spectacles for the service, providing, at its height, 1.5 million people with government-subsidised glasses a year.

The company was founded in 1898, when Max Wiseman,* aged just nineteen, and following his involvement with importing frames from the DuPaul Young Optical Company, another American spectacle maker from Southbridge, Massachusetts, and the Bay State Optical Co. in nearby Attleboro, had become 'inspired and tremendously enthusiastic at the possibilities of gold-filled being the future of spectacles'. As he was to recall in *The Optician* in 1941, 'at that time steel and solid gold were the principal materials for spectacle frames', but the products from American and later German manufacturers, in lighter and more durable rolled gold, were far superior and soon eclipsed those in blue steel or too-easily-tarnished gold plate. While establishing a lens-making plant in Perivale in 1926, Wiseman continued to source frames from Germany until 1932. That year, and following

---

\* Wiseman was originally Weissman and anglicised his name shortly after the outbreak of the First World War on 23 October 1914, publicly announcing the change by deed poll with a notice in that week's issue of *The London Gazette*.

Britain's departure from the Gold Standard, those imports were banned, resulting in Wiseman taking the dramatic step of acquiring the entire contents of a spectacle-making plant in Rathenau. The machinery along with ten technicians willing – even eager, with the political clouds in their native land darkening – to relocate were transported wholesale to the Algha Factory, a former print works in Hackney Wick – an industrial district in the East End of London that had been the birthplace of Parkesine, an early form of plastic. With the outbreak of war, many of Wiseman's German spectacle makers were interned in Scotland as enemy aliens, but the machinery (much of which is still in use today) and some of those technicians supported the war effort by producing lenses for gas masks and other protective eyewear.

Prior to the establishment of the NHS, Wiseman's made a range of glasses that were available to those who paid into the National Health Insurance (NHI) Scheme, either as private individuals or through the membership of a friendly society or union. Many of these ophthalmic benefit frames (OBAC), including the round wire Windsor panto, formed the basis of the first National Health glasses. In 1949 Wiseman's offered eighteen options in nickel, gold-filled and cellulose acetate on the NHS, ten of which until 1951 were completely free, the remainder requiring small additional fees.

The NHS range would ebb and flow before settling down in the late 1950s to about ten basic workhorse frames in nickel, rolled gold and plastic, roughly half of those variants of the panto Windsor with either high or centre bridges and coated and uncoated rims. A further token of individuality could be obtained by choosing either curl- or hockey-ended sides (because of their resemblance to that game's stick). And there were a few choices in colours for the plastic models and finishes too.

The 'pink translucent plastic' frames mentioned by Corson were, with complete insensitivity to other skin shades, officially billed as 'flesh-coloured'. While Corson might have sneered at them, glasses in this colour had originated in the luxury end of the market. In the 1930s, (Philip) Oliver Goldsmith, a former salesman for the optical outfit Raphael's who'd struck out on his own as a spectacle maker with premises on Poland Street in Soho, had developed the first 'flesh-coloured' frame after experimenting with a plastic called Erinoid. Goldsmith called the frame 'Dawn', a play on the female name and the first light of day, since he believed it represented a new era in spectacles for women. Oliver Goldsmith as a brand would become noted for its attention-grabbing eyewear, especially after his son Charles (later also to call himself Oliver) took over the business in the 1950s, and when some of its ornate jewel-studded cat's eyes reached chandelier-like glitziness. This particular style, however, was sold on its apparent 'unobtrusive-ness'. The frame, being supposedly closer in colour to the wearer's face, was rendered less visible, somewhat like a chameleon blending in with the surroundings. Or so the idea went. That idea would continue when the pink acetate frames were offered on the NHS, where they were most commonly prescribed to women and young girls;* the kids' range mostly consisted of mini-me adult frames with curl sides to stop them falling off when children pelted across muddy fields during games.

For those who did yearn for something just a tad more distinctive and were willing to pay a little bit extra, by the 1950s there were also what the optical historian Joanne Gooding terms 'NHS hybrids'. These were frames that had to be purchased privately from the optician but were of a suitable shape that they could then be glazed with regulation NHS lenses. Here too, though, the man (and woman) from the ministry had a say in what qualified as a compatible frame. Only styles meeting the strictures of the patterns set down in the Ministry of Health's guidelines were acceptable. Two-tone coloured frames, like the Supra for example, were not welcome on the NHS.

However, in 1960, Vertex Optical Ltd of Rochdale, one of the manufacturers of the most ubiquitous of all NHS frames, the mighty cellulose acetate number 524 – the squarish frame, most

---

* Though perversely so too were ones in an ice-blue plastic that only a Smurf would have found 'unobtrusive'.

commonly in black or brown, that when anyone refers to 'NHS glasses' is usually the one they are thinking of – unveiled its Pussy Cat NHS hybrid range.

Advertised as 'The Style Setter for 1960' and 'The frame with the upswept look' and available in 'Four Unique and Exclusive Colourglow shades: peach, lilac, blue and red', it was a cat's eye type of feminine frame that many in the ministry considered too fashionable by half.

In its aftermath a Standing Ophthalmic Advisory Committee was awarded the remit to adjudicate on future contentious frames. The issue would come to a head three years later when Michael Birch (Designs) Ltd was refused a licence to offer their bi-coloured plastic cat's eye Candida frame as an NHS hybrid, a decision finally overturned on appeal. But government officials, concerned that more fashionable frames would increase take-up among those who could afford private frames and add to the cost to the exchequer, remained committed to insisting on the 'elimination of styling aspects' in NHS frames.

And in 1964, when a spectacle-less Lennon and the Beatles were taking America by storm, the General Optical Council, the official government body with which all opticians wishing to practise had to register, restated its draconian restrictions on promotion in the industry. Under its 'Rules on Publicity' – The General Optical Council (Rules on Publicity) Order of Council (SI No. 167, 1964) – advertising was to remain restricted to trade periodicals, with only public announcements like the change in the name of a firm allowed in newspapers; any publicity material had to be 'dignified and restrained', optical goods were 'not to be displayed with any goods except accessories, sunglasses or optical instruments' and no statements of prices were to be displayed in windows or on the outside of premises, and even premises signs 'had to be "appropriate" to the practice of business'.

In 1970, twenty-two years after their initiation, and with some of the basic frames remaining virtually unchanged, *The Optician* warned that NHS glasses were becoming widely regarded as 'functional but second best'. Six years later Barbara Castle, when she was the Minister for Health in Harold Wilson's second Labour government, told the same paper that she believed the range had become so out of date it was like forcing people to wear 'a badge of poverty across their faces'.

But again, that the round panto frame in particular stood slightly outside of fashion was in its favour in the late 1960s. While Lennon did not exactly give up all his earthly goods upon donning his glasses, a certain sackcloth-and-ashes renunciation of the trappings of the material world was a component of the flower power counter-culture that the Beatles embraced. A culture surprisingly well stocked with counters selling beads, ethnic clothing and copies of the *I Ching*, and dealers offering supposedly mind-expanding substances for sterling pounds, shillings and pence (LSD, in old lolly).* The austerity of the NHS panto Windsor fitted too with the dressed-down-in-workwear-denim egalitarian side of the hippy dream. They could be worn by either gender while eating mung beans and brown rice off a handmade-looking pine table from Habitat, or while attending a demonstration.†

However, just as Val Doonican's ability to knock *Sgt Pepper* off the top of the album charts and the arrival of Richard Nixon in the White House in 1968 were ominous signs that Haight-Ashbury was not everyone's idea of heaven on earth, equally the decision of the French fashion house Christian Dior to put its name to a range of spectacles by Tura of Fifth Avenue that year hinted that

---

* One of the new trends advertised in *The Optician* in 1966 was for slightly back-to-the-land frames themselves fashioned in woods such as teak, rosewood and charcoal.

† In Uli Edel's 2008 film about West Germany's Red Army Faction *The Baader Meinhof Complex*, the glasses worn by Martina Gedeck playing the journalist-turned-terrorist Ulrike Meinhof follow her political radicalisation, her square metal browline-esque spectacles giving way to round wire numbers as she takes up arms in the struggle. Bruno Ganz, meanwhile, who'd already appeared as Hitler in tortoiseshell-coated wire rims in *Downfall*, was cast as Horst Herold, the chief of the Federal West German police who led the hunt for the gang. Ganz wore, as his real-life counterpart did, glasses with rectangular plastic brown frames, a pair of specs that in the context of the movie unequivocally positioned him on the side of 'The Man' – if a thinking man, at least, in the actor's sympathetic portrayal.

consumerism, even with students rioting on the streets of Paris, was in more robust health. Its founder's New Look, with its surfeit of skirt fabric, had in 1947 thumbed its nose at clothing shortages and pieties about austerity. And the House of Dior, despite the industrial unrest of the decade to follow, appears to have similarly grasped the zeitgeist better than those storming the barricades over changes to the curriculum.

While students in London were protesting against the Vietnam war outside the American Embassy in Grosvenor Square and occupying the Hornsey Art College, the Optical Council had been busily dispatching a fleet of mobile caravans kitted out with displays of promotional material to visit sixty-six sites in the capital and across the provinces as part of a campaign backed by 'educational' cinema adverts to make the British public become more 'eyecare and eye-fashion conscious'.

Arguably, the 1960s were to conclude with the dawning of the new age of designer spectacles rather than Aquarius. And wooden glasses, to paraphrase a subsequent lyric by a Reagan-supporting Neil Young, were to prove just a hippy dream.*

By the time the Berlin Wall had fallen in 1989, NHS glasses were already no more. And the Algha Works were turning out gold-filled panto glasses under the upmarket brand of Savile Row, a name derived from the plush West End street some distance from Hackney Wick famed for bespoke tailors rather than civically inclined manufacturing, if also briefly home to the Beatles' Apple Corps HQ, and on whose rooftop the group made their final public performance.

In 1990, over twenty years on from that epochal event and a decade after Lennon's murder at the hands of a crazed fan, the late Beatle's estate signed a contract with the Eagle Eyewear Company

---

* In much the same vein as 'the hippy wigs', Danny the Drug Dealer in *Withnail and I*, Bruce Robinson's cinematic ode to the late 1960s, complains are on sale in Woolworths, the London optical firm of Alexander Jerome launched a somewhat blatant counter-cultural cash-in line of glasses. Its 'Hippy Range' boasted '6 metal styles for the eyewear of today' in a variety of round, oval, octagonal and square frames.

of Whitehouse, New Jersey, to produce and distribute a range of glasses frames in his honour. Manufactured for Eagle in Italy by Demenego, the John Lennon Collection was to contain four styles modelled after those he'd worn in the 1960s and 1970s, including the squarer P3-esque plastic variety he'd adopted in the final years of his life, a pair of which he'd been wearing when he was shot outside his home in the Dakota Building in New York.*

Each style was marketed with Lennon-themed names, 'Revolution', 'Imagine (or The Dreamer)', 'The Walrus' and 'Double Fantasy', and every pair bore the words 'John Lennon' prominently emblazoned on the side pieces and came with a leather case embossed with his signature – an endorsement from beyond the grave that it remains difficult (however difficult and unconscionable Lennon might often have been) to quite imagine (no pun intended) the musician himself making. There was also a card inlay that featured a cartoon self-portrait, a sketch by Lennon depicting himself as little more than a mop of hair and a pair of round glasses. Which perhaps most seductively of all offered an image of the prematurely deceased musician at ease and immortal in their eyewear.

---

* His widow Yoko Ono was criticised for using a photograph of those glasses, their lenses splattered in blood, on the cover of her solo record *Season of Glass*, less an album than a concept piece about grief, and one that is as poignant, poetic and haunting as it is harrowing and discomforting, released just six months after Lennon's death.

# 12

## Spectacles Take Off . . .

To consider the extraordinary ubiquity of the aviator style of spectacles in the 1970s and 1980s, it perhaps helps to think a little about aeroplanes. For on 9 February 1969, crowds gathered at Paine Field in Everett, Washington, a former US Army Air Force base used during the Korean War, to witness the launch flight of the largest transport plane in the world. With a tail taller than a six-storey building, the Boeing 747 jumbo jet was a double-decker aircraft with a fuselage as humpbacked as a whale and four fuel-guzzling engines. Over 230 feet in length, and with seats for 400 passengers and a cruising speed of some 600mph, the 737, if briefly stalled by the oil crisis in 1973, put ever more affordable air travel within reach of millions. Entering service in 1970, the plane nicknamed the Queen of the Skies would become one of the most successful classes of commercial aircraft ever built. Initially, it tempted passengers with its promise of more spacious leg room and onboard facilities such as piano bars and lounges. These amenities were soon removed to make way for more revenue-generating seats. But the aircraft and air travel itself continued to be viewed as prestigious even though they were becoming increasingly common. By 1972 over half of Americans had flown and the number of air passengers had quadrupled since 1955. In Britain too, where only 3 per cent of the population had holidayed abroad in 1952, improvements in aviation and the arrival of cheaper package deals from companies such as the Travel Club of Upminster, Horizon, Gaytours, Intasun and Universal Sky Tours meant that some 5 million Britons, roughly 10 per cent of the population, were heading overseas by the end of the 1960s. And the US airline Pan Am would deploy its first 737s on the New York to London transatlantic route in 1970, making the jet as familiar a sight in the skies over Britain as the migrant swallow.

In popular culture, disaster movies like *Airport*, the second highest-grossing movie (after *Love Story*) in America in 1970 and based on a best-selling door-stopper by the monumentally successful schlockmeister Arthur Hailey, reflected the measure of the fascination and fear jet air travel inspired. Flying might be safer than driving, or so the statistics constantly maintained. But since the stakes were infinitely higher and the consequences that much more dire, the enterprise would always be tinged with a hint of danger. Which only added to its continuing glamour.

In an age when security remained, by today's standards, astonishingly lax, the phenomenon of 'skyjacking' became close to an epidemic between 1968 and 1972 when dozen of planes, such as Western Airlines Flight 701, were commandeered by hijackers professing political aims and diverted to the likes of Havana or Algeria. This added a further frisson to the experience, as well as providing material that was grist to the mill of the *Airport* franchise. The plot of the third outing of the series, *Airport '77*, concerned the targeting by art thieves of a private 747, its well-stocked piano lounge teeming with the rich, famous and sinister (Christopher Lee), owned by a wealthy collector played by James Stewart in his final film role. Captaining the jet, and the voice of reason at the heart of this cinematic catastrophe (in all senses), was Jack Lemmon, the actor appearing with a giant slug of a moustache across his top lip and in an almost permanently crisp blue short-sleeved shirt with epaulettes, courtesy of legendary costume designer Edith Head.

And the social cachet that the flyers of planes enjoyed above other professions in this era was to result in many elements of their get-up, from 'pilot' shirts (as sported by the Roxy Music singer

Bryan Ferry) to moustaches (ditto) and aviator-style sunglasses (also ditto), crossing over into contemporary seventies fashion. And if beginning as sunglasses, aviator-type frames also made the transition to spectacles and as load-carriers for clear corrective lenses in the early 1970s, becoming in the judgement of the American optician and industry commentator Preston Fassel 'as optically emblematic of that decade as zyls [i.e. black plastic horn-rims] in the 60s'.*

Fassel, writing for *20/20* magazine in 2013, saw this development less in terms of the expansion of jet-propelled flight and more as a somewhat embarrassing symptom of the collective nervous breakdown in response to the chaos of everyday American life. Reeling from the dramatic social changes of the 1960s and still dealing with the ongoing horror of the Vietnam war, Watergate, conflicts in the Middle East and with sky-rocketing gas prices on the horizon, 'Americans', he argued, 'almost as if to overcome the struggles going on around them . . . turned to big things. Big pants with big legs. Big jackets with big lapels. Big turtlenecks with big . . . turtlenecks. Big patterns. Big hair. Big squash necklaces. Big shoes. Big glasses.'†

The aviator, to his mind, was 'the perfect icing on the 70s gonzo cake'. Though he doesn't mention it, the freewheeling non-fiction writer Hunter S. Thompson, exemplar of New Journalism and the so-called 'gonzo' style of immersive writing, was another devotee of the style. As a spectacle frame, aviators were, he maintained, 'massive enough to swallow up the wearer's face, while lacking the aesthetic boldness of plastics that made oversize lenses look halfway decent' prior to that.

---

* Michael Caine, ever a barometer of spectacle trends, would convert to aviators in the 1970s, portraying Mickey King, a wealthy hack writer, in a pair of large plastic models in Mike Hodges' comedy-crime movie *Pulp* (1972). And by the time the Shadows reunited in 1977, even Hank Marvin would have abandoned his horn-rims for a pair of aviator-style spectacles. Cliff Richard, having since found God, did the same.

† Shirts with pointed 1970s collars were, by the 1980s and in my part of the world, disparaged as 'Gatwicks', in honour of the airport.

While there is some truth to this, the 2020 television mini-series *Mrs America*, while chronicling the failure to secure the anti-discriminatory Equal Rights Amendment (ERA) in the 1970s, served as a reminder that the feminist writer and activist Gloria Steinem was one of the foremost wearers of gold aviator spectacles of that era (though, admittedly, often with a slight hint of tinting about the lenses). And aviator spectacles, if worn by a member of the Women's Liberation Movement, could be both radical and chic.

As its name suggests, the aviator had its origins in aviation and by some accounts its design was shaped by the input of the American army flying ace Lt John Macready. As the flight instructor of the US Army Pilot School in Brooks Field, Texas, during the First World War, Macready had written the manual that gave a generation of American flyers their wings. After the war he headed up the army's first test flight programme at McCook Field, near Dayton, Ohio. In 1922 Macready set a world altitude record of 40,800 feet and in the following year, with Lt Oakley Kelly, he made the first non-stop transnational flight across America in a single-engine Fokker T-2 monoplane. This east-to-west-coast odyssey from Long Island, New York, to San Diego, California, took them nearly twenty-seven hours to complete. He's also credited with making the first ever crop-dusting flight and participated in the first aerial survey of the United States in 1924.

One of the problems Macready and his cohorts immediately encountered when they started to fly higher and higher into the sky – in planes with open cockpits built largely out of steel tubing, wire and plywood – were the freezing conditions. At heights of over 30,000 feet temperatures could drop as low as minus 80°F. To guard against such conditions, the pilots wore padded leather flying suits and fur-lined helmets and goggles. But the goggles, if helping to stop the pilots' eyes from frosting up, were still not sufficiently tinted to offer much protection against the bright glare of the sun in the upper atmosphere. According to his daughter, Sally Macready Wallace, the pilot then began working with Bausch & Lomb to produce a pair that would guard against the dazzle of the stratosphere.

Macready seemingly got his goggles, and ones with a heat-absorbing dark green-grey tint. But a more commercial outcome of this collaboration was that in 1937 Bausch & Lomb also launched a line of sporting sunglasses aimed at golfers and fishermen. These tinted shades offered those seeking to drive Byron Nelson off the fairways or hoping to chase blue marlin with Hemingway in Key West 'real scientific glare protection'. With teardrop-shaped tinted lenses and a metal wire frame 'as delicate as a biplane's strut', in science writer and historian Pagan Kennedy's arrestingly poetic phrasing, these glasses were aimed at the pro-am sports market and sold for several dollars when cheap sunglasses could be had for a few cents. More contentious remains the apparent similarity of these glasses to a range of frames the British firm of Max Wiseman & Co. had already been manufacturing for about two years, following their own work on protective goggles for the Royal Air Force. However, come the Second World War, both companies would supply their respective forces with optical kit and Macready was recalled to active duty, serving with the 12th Air Force in North Africa. Bausch & Lomb was to provide the US Air Force with glare-beating spectacles, and gun sights and equipment for aerial photography and mapping, as well as binoculars, sextants and rangefinders for the navy.

But it was arguably Douglas MacArthur, the overbearing American army general who commanded the Allied forces in the southwest Pacific, who became most famously associated with Bausch & Lomb sunglasses during the conflict and far beyond. Along with a heavily braided cap and a peculiar habit of snacking on lettuce heads, the sunglasses were as much a part of MacArthur's contrived public persona as the corncob pipe that appeared to have taken root in his mouth. One of the most enduring images of President Trump's avowed favourite general is a black and white photograph of MacArthur landing with his troops at Leyte in the Philippines in 1944. Having made good on his promise to return to the Filipino people after his withdrawal from the islands following their capture by the Japanese after the Battle of Bataan two years earlier, MacArthur wades purposefully ashore knee-deep in water. Eyes shaded by aviator sunglasses, the general looks every inch the vainglorious martinet, convinced of his own invincibility. The shades and the corncob pipe would accompany him to Korea in the early 1950s, where his gung-ho arrogance over pursuing an all-out war against Chinese-backed forces in the north would lead to him being removed from command by President Truman.

The story of young people repurposing military gear to their own ends is pretty much the whole story of post-war fashion and runs from ban-the-bombers at Aldermaston donning naval duffel coats and mods sporting American army parkas to hippies in military greatcoats and combat jackets. Not to mention the adoption of P3 spectacles, Lennon's wartime-issue granny glasses, and aviator frames on civvy street.

But in some respects the ex-military spectacles Gloria Steinem selected were all the more subversive for the subtlety with which they indicated her personal politics – and that the personal *was* political was the rally cry of the movement. Like high boots, originally the preserve of chevaliers, here was another item of masculine military attire being co-opted by a woman. And in her appearance, Steinem confounded prejudices about what a women's 'libber' was supposed to look like. In essence, Steinem looked more like Daphne from *Scooby-Doo, Where Are You!*, say, than the frumpy, bookish Velma. While it's an urban myth that the characters from this punctuation-defying cartoon TV series were modelled after typical attendees of the Five College Consortium, Velma, the tomboyish smart-cookie in heavy zyl spectacles, is usually taken to represent Smith College, the exclusive women's liberal arts college in Northampton, Massachusetts, that Steinem herself attended.

In her memoir-cum-feminist self-help manual *Revolution from Within: A Book of Self-Esteem*, Steinem recalls being prescribed spectacles in sixth grade and that as a student at Smith College in the late 1950s she was a plump 'mousy girl with harlequin glasses and a pony tail'. Born and raised in Toledo, Ohio, just over two hours' drive from Dayton and Macready's airfields, Steinem admits to consciously distancing herself from her family and her

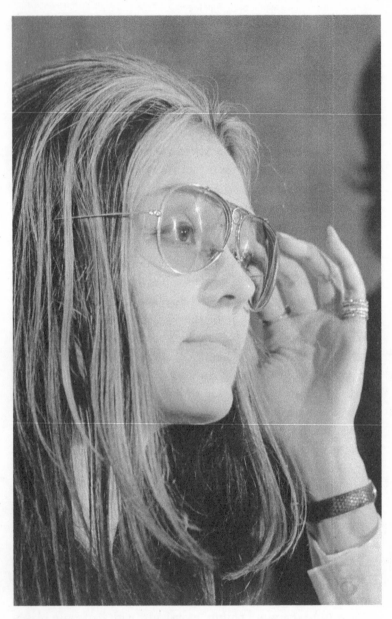

Gloria Steinem at a news conference.

Midwestern background when she arrived in New York. After a two-year fellowship in India, she was trying to make a living as a freelance writer. Taking inspiration from Audrey Hepburn's portrayal of Holly Golightly in *Breakfast at Tiffany's* because she identified 'with the poor prematurely responsible childhood [the character] had escaped by walking down a dirt road a little farther every day', Steinem chose to restyle herself after the actor in that movie. As she writes: 'I laced my dark hair with obvious blonde streaks, just as she had done ... I also copied her huge sunglasses in order to hide the fleshiness left over from a chubby childhood that overhung my eyelids and displaced my contact lenses so often that I gave up wearing them.'

Reflecting on this forty years later, Steinem believed she'd merely swapped one socially sanctioned female image, '1950s "collegiate"', for another, '1960s "rebellious"', without really thinking about who she was. Feminism came to her rescue, though, and she embraced 'a simple, comfortable, jeans-sweater-and-boots uniform' that lasted her for a decade. If simple, it was also all the more effective for the retention of a pair of oversized glasses. The aviators, along with the mane of leonine hair, she retrospectively claims were emblematic of a lack of self-esteem about her appearance, something instilled in her since childhood, that she wore to hide behind, just as she'd become stoop-shouldered as a teenager trying to disguise her height. But armour, in concealing a weakness, also confers strength, and the spectacles surely helped empower her to do battle with the patriarchy. They were not a pair of glasses that could easily pigeonhole her as a Velma-esque bluestocking. They therefore only added to the disarming quality of her appearance, even if the media was often more interested in her appearance than her ideas. The 11 August 1972 issue of *Life* magazine, with a cover story illustrated with a photograph of a Braniff Airways 727 jet considering the 'Perilous War on the Skyjacker', ran a two-page spread headed 'Gloria in Excelsis: It's the Steinem Look'. This was a photo feature with headshots of fifteen women, all sporting Steinem-style specs and hair, and readers were invited to guess which one was the activist herself.

After an operation on her eyelids more than thirty years ago, Steinem abandoned her aviator glasses for sleep-in soft contact lenses. Writing in 1992, she maintained that letters 'asking: Whatever happened to your big glasses?' continued to pour in. By then, however, aviators had already completed their journey from the spectacle of the thoughtful radical to the frame of conservative reactionaries. Computer nerds. Radio One DJs. Horror writers. And out-and-out creepy loner weirdos. A brief roll call of those who tarnished their public image would have to include President George H. W. Bush, Bill Gates, Mike Reid, Simon Bates, Stephen King, Shaun Hutson, the Unabomber Ted Kaczynski and the serial killers Dennis Nilsen and Jeffrey Dahmer. It's Preston Fassel's hunch that it was the publication, following his eventual arrest, of police mugshots of Dahmer with a wispy blonde moustache and in gold clear-lensed aviator glasses that sounded the death knell for the style in the States. A killer blow they have never quite recovered from. And that no amount of knowing irony seemed entirely capable of fully overturning either, as proven by Jon Heder's turn as the eponymous aviator-sporting geek in *Napoleon Dynamite*, an all-quirk-no-soul indie comedy whose bad-is-cool aesthetic reflected the post-millennial penchant for trucker caps and Pabst Blue Ribbon beer. The *Vogue* fashion photographer Terry Richardson, once known as much for his clone moustache and plastic-framed aviators as more recently for a litany of outstanding accusations of sexual assault against young female models, hardly helped the matter. Perhaps only Rose Byrne, starring as Steinem in *Mrs America* and in what she has aptly described as the writer's 'superhero' spectacles, can redeem them, by once more putting them back on the faces of young women seeking to make society change for the better.

## Power dressing

In 1973, a year after the Equal Rights Amendment calling for an end to all forms of sexual discrimination had been approved by the Senate, Karen Nussbaum and Ellen Cassedy, two young clerk-typists at Harvard University, founded an organisation to fight for better pay and conditions for women office workers. While a third of all working women in America held clerical positions in the 1970s, their jobs were often menial or held little scope for advancement. Sexism was rampant and systemic in male-dominated offices and corporations. Formed initially with just eight other women secretaries from the Boston area, 9 to 5 soon grew into a national association for working women. In 1979, the year Margaret Thatcher became Britain's first female Prime Minister, its cause received a boost when the actor and political campaigner Jane Fonda undertook a whirlwind tour of six cities in America – New York, Boston, Baltimore, Pittsburgh, Dayton and Cincinnati – to urge female workers to organise and fight for their rights. Through Nussbaum, she met a group of forty secretaries who told her about the indignities they'd suffered at work and also shared their dreams about getting even with their misogynist bosses. Inspired by their stories, Fonda decided that her next movie would be 'a feminist revenge fantasy' screwball comedy with three female leads, and she hired the screenwriter Patricia Resnick to work undercover as a secretary at an insurance office to garner more material. Entitled *9 to 5* (or *Nine to Five*) in tribute to Nussbaum, the film's jaunty theme was to be written and performed by country music star Dolly Parton – who also made her acting debut in the movie as Doralee Rhodes, a buxom secretary perpetually sexually harassed by her chauvinist pig of a boss.

Fonda, meanwhile, played Judy Bernly, a housewife forced to seek clerical work after being abandoned by a husband who'd run off with his much younger secretary. Keen to make a good impression, Bernly arrives for her first day at the office done up like a corporate Holly Hobbie, in a ludicrous hat with a bow, her hair fussily overdone and wearing a frilly blouse that could have been pilfered from Mrs Thatcher's wardrobe – Laura Ashley meets Laura Ingalls Wilder, say. Topping the whole thing off are a pair of giant clear plastic glasses with a gold chain attached, a pair of spectacles that the film critic Christopher Lewis, in discussing the movie's supposedly 'aggressively 80s aesthetic', recently described as the 'visual equivalent of the synthesizer from Dancing in the Dark'.*

For while trousers and lapels would get narrower and hair for both men and women shorter as the 1970s slipped into the 1980s and Thatcher and Ronald Reagan set about gutting welfare pro- grammes and marketising a society the former maintained didn't exist, spectacles, like shoulder-pads, were to get even bigger. While the 1980s is often called the 'designer decade', the seed beds of a highly brand-conscious consumer culture were already germinating in the late 1970s.

In 1978, the Federal Trade Commission had abolished all remaining restrictions on advertising the prices of eyewear in America. And with Christopher Reeve, in a substantial pair of brown plastic tortoiseshell specs, about to bring Clark Kent to the big screen in Richard Donner's *Superman* movie (and Clark gets a decent chunk of the picture: Kal-El's Superman cape and tights aren't donned until a full fifty minutes into the film), the trade journal *Retail Week* confidently offered the prediction that the coming year would see 'most of the major market department stores' using 'larger amounts of designer eyewear', and that 'plas- tic frames' would 'sell slightly better than metals' though 'metal frames' would remain 'stronger in men's than women's'. As if illustrating the point, the following summer, and with the second season of TV soap *Dallas* airing, Texas State Optical ran a state- wide advertising campaign to promote its new range of designer eyewear, urging would-be purchasers to 'Try on a Fabergé, Dior, Givenchy, de la Renta'. Its print ads in local glossies featured a photograph of a blonde with flyaway Farrah Fawcett hair, her mouth – lips glossed bright red and teeth pearly white – open in a

---

* In the 1982 movie *Tootsie*, Dustin Hoffman, playing Michael Dorsey, a strug- gling actor who dresses in drag to gain a lead part in the medical soap *Southwest General*, wore remarkably similar spectacles (and frou frou blouses) as his female alter ego Dorothy Michaels. According to *Totally Awesome Movies of the 80s!* the glasses, at first opposed by the film's cinematographer Owen Roizman, were found in screen tests to have 'further feminized' Dorothy by making Hoffman's prominent nose 'less noticeable' and 'creating a more noticeable gender separa- tion between the Dorothy/Michael characters'.

blow-up sex doll pout, and cheeks blushed pink. Her blue, equally immaculately made-up eyes are behind a pair of large rounded plastic light-tortoiseshell glasses with side pieces that fixed to the lower part of the rim, giving them an oddly upside-down cast. 'The difference', a tagline maintains, 'between just wearing glasses and a Fabergé from TSO.' 'Convenient credit', the ad also claimed, was 'available', implying that the designer look could be acquired by Texans not possessing the Ewings' ready wealth.

In Britain such mainstream press ads remained prohibited. But in January 1979, and partially in response to developments in America, a report compiled by Roy Hattersley, the Secretary of State for Prices and Consumer Protection in the Labour government, was published that argued the ban on displaying prices and advertising should be lifted:

We consider it important that competition should be permitted to play its part in encouraging efficiency and cost saving. If this distinction is accepted then the restrictions on price display and advertising appear in a less favourable light. Far from protecting the consumer, they may bolster high cost production methods and high retail margins in the supply of spectacles and their component parts. If in addition it is the case that prices at the prescription house level are fixed by reference to generally accepted price lists, such improvements in production methods as are introduced are likely to result in higher profits to the more efficient producers but no savings to consumers.

As with the Labour government's proposals for the sale of council homes, the report's more pro-market recommendations would be adopted wholesale and carried further by Margaret Thatcher's incoming Conservative administration. In their second term, the Conservatives would sign the death warrant on the NHS frame range by introducing a means-tested voucher scheme for those who qualified for free spectacles and relaxing the rules on advertising and pricing, a move akin to the 'Big Bang' in the City, that opened up the industry to free competition.

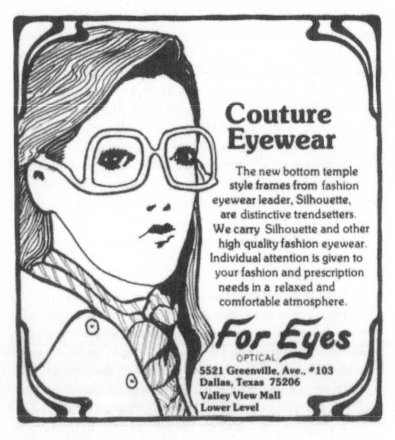

Couture Eyewear US advert, 1977.

Perhaps rather portentously, the number one record at the time of the election of Britain's first female Prime Minister in May 1979 was 'Bright Eyes', the mawkish ballad about life ebbing away from a dying rabbit written by Mike Batt for the animated movie *Watership Down* and sung by Art Garfunkel. And certainly spectacles were to become both more colourful and much more of a commercial commodity during her tenure. The optical chain Specsavers, established in the Channel Island tax haven of Guernsey by Doug and Mary Perkins, two enterprising optometrists who'd previously owned a network of opticians in the West Country, was among the first new names on the high street to seize upon the opportunities offered by deregulation in the 1980s.

One of 1979's other big hits was 'Video Killed the Radio Star', a magnificent sci-fi-infused synth-pop number inspired by a J. G. Ballard short story that offered an airplay-friendly vision of a not-too-distant future where machines wrote symphonies and radio DJs had been supplanted by video cassette recorders and TV screens. Performed by the Buggles, a studio group comprised of producer-musician Trevor Horn and keyboardist Geoffrey Downes and conceived as a kind of 'robot Beatles', the song was promoted, aptly, with a whizzy video. Garnished with what then passed for state-of-the-art solarising colour effects, and with a few allusions to Fritz Lang's *Metropolis* (cue a woman in a glittery leo-tard and fright wig in a glass tube), the video found the pair and a few cohorts cavorting about in matching silvery leather jackets and skinny ties amid racks of synthesisers, flickering TV screens and piles of old radio sets. Horn, singing into an antiquated 1950s chromium microphone, had on a pair of outsized white plastic glasses, spectacles that rendered the Buggle almost bug-eyed. These glasses would become as much Horn's trademark in the 1980s as the bombast of his production work on records by Yes, ABC and Frankie Goes to Hollywood. Artists who were after a big, 'epic' sound that appeared to match the vaulting Greed is Good ambitions of the era beat a path to the guy in the big glasses. However, as he revealed to the *Guardian* in 2018, the inspiration for the glasses came from fellow skinny-tie-wearing New Waver Elvis Costello. 'I came out of the opticians', Horn recalled, 'with these big specs and said to Geoff, "I'm a Buggle now."'

## Glass scratched

The Buggles' debut album, released in the opening month of the new decade, was entitled *The Age of Plastic*, and lenses in spectacles would more often be made from that material rather than glass from this point on. The knock-on from this was there was greater scope for experimentation with the shape and size of the frames themselves as bigger glasses were no longer so heavy for the wearer. *Industrial Design Magazine* in 1980, in an article on eyewear headed 'Go for the Distinctive', noted that 'Plastic was lighter and allowed more flattering lenses which intrigued some designers'. Those at the fashion houses of Christian Dior and Givenchy were two such cited in the piece.

The story of a workable plastic spectacle lens really goes back to the 1940s when the Columbia Southern Chemical Company in Barbeton, Ohio, a subsidiary of the Pittsburgh Plate Glass Company (PPG), developed a new clear plastic resin, allyl diglycol carbonate. This fresh compound combined well with cloth and paper to produce sturdy laminated 're-inforced' materials and was eventually trademarked as CR-39 after its batch number (i.e. Columbia resin batch number 39). When America entered the war, a use was eventually found for the substance in fashioning lightweight fuel tanks for B-17 bombers, and also as a replacement for glass in the inspection tubes on the plane's fuel lines, which were vulnerable to shattering in combat and spraying the cockpit with gasoline. With the onset of peace and the cancelling of many military contracts, PPG were left with a railroad car tank full of 38,000lb of surplus allyl diglycol carbonate. Unsure what sort of shelf life this stuff might have or if the resin could self-harden over time, leaving them with a worthless hulk of tank-shaped plastic, the company began desperately scouting about for a civilian buyer for this military dead stock. Somehow or other the news reached the ears of Robert Klark Graham.

A eugenicist who with the ambition of breeding a race of quite specifically white super beings would, in the late 1970s, go on to establish the Genius Sperm Bank (officially the Repository for Germinal Choice) housed in an underground bunker in the backyard of his ranch in San Diego, Graham is one of optometry's most odious characters. It is then all the more depressing that he should amass a considerable fortune — one that bankrolled his racist breeding schemes — from a product formerly used in the fight against Nazism. But Graham, alas, is the man who not only saw the potential in CR-39 but who was also instrumental in it becoming the main substance for plastic lenses.

A one-time employee of Bausch & Lomb, in 1945 Graham was working with evidently something of a roving brief in the sales department of the Univis Lens Company of Dayton, Ohio, which also owned The Unbreakable Lens Company of America (TULCA), an optical outfit based in Los Angeles that had been beavering away on producing viable plastic lenses in Plexiglas since before the war. Graham duly acquired a few gallons of the spare CR-39 for the boffins at TULCA, and buoyed by the initial reports came back for the rest. When its parent company closed the plastic lens unit down amid concerns about the cost and the threat of copyright infringement claims over existing patents in the UK, he left, taking all but one of the research team with him, and formed his own company in Pasadena. By 1947, Graham's Armorlite Co. was ready to start production of their own CR-39 lenses, and after its six-year global monopoly expired, Essilor in France and SOLA in Australia, and on home turf American Optical and even Univis itself, all began making optical lenses from the resin.

However, a huge problem with using CR-39 for spectacle lenses was that in comparison with glass, it scratched far too easily. Armorlite's own scientists explored some 2000 different abrasive-resistant coatings alone. And while some improvements were made to make the lenses less prone to damage, and shrinkage, none of them seemed to cure the problem satisfactorily.

It wasn't until the 1970s when the Minnesota Mining and Manufacturing Co. (3M) – whose products included magnetic audio tape, the non-stick pan coating Teflon and the Scotchgard water repeller – got involved that a solution was found. 3M seemingly discovered that the answer lay less in the protective coating per se (though it wasn't negligible) than in the environment in which it was applied. Dust and all other impurities had to be completely eliminated before any protective coating worth the name could be added to optical lenses. After spending two solid years refining their coating process, 25,000 pairs of hard resin lenses with the new 3M treatment were released into a test market in five American states in 1978. The trial was so successful that in 1979 3M acquired Armorlite outright and they began churning out lenses with the new scratch coating under the trade name RLX Plus, which although sounding like an errant droid from *Star Wars* would transform the use of plastic in spectacles. By 1983, over 50 per cent of the US market had already gone over to plastic lenses.

During the same period both hard gas-permeable and 'extended wear' soft contact lenses (Bausch & Lomb's 'SofLens' was the first on the market) for the near-sighted received approval from the US Food and Drug Administration. The pop artist Andy Warhol, who on moving to New York in the 1950s and attempting to make it as a commercial artist in advertising had purchased children's spectacles to save on the expense, was a convert to the latter. Although in 1981 he confessed to finding it 'so scary to wake up in the night and be able to see'.

Following the election in 1980 of the former actor Ronald Reagan, the US also had their first contact-lens-wearing President. Reagan had started out in radio as a sports announcer on an Iowa station where his myopia, diagnosed at thirteen and with an acuity of 20/200 corrected by thickly lensed spectacles, represented no obstacle. But on moving into acting and relocating to Hollywood, 'Dutch' was quickly advised to leave his glasses off, and earned himself a contract at Warner Brothers after completing a screen test without them in 1937. Ironically, he'd go on to play a radio announcer (without spectacles) in his first movie role in *Love is on the Air* (1937). His short-sightedness kept him from active combat when he tried to enlist in 1942, and resulted in Reagan spending most of the war producing training films for the US army in Burbank, California. He would, nevertheless, while appearing as an informant for the FBI, testify before Joseph McCarthy's communist witch-hunting House Un-American Activities Committee in Congress in horn-rims in 1946. By the time he entered politics in the mid-1960s, he relied upon a pair of hard plastic Tuohy corneal contacts fitted by the Hollywood optometrist Estelle Herron. When delivering political speeches, however, he would remove the lens from his right eye. Much like wearing a monocle, this enabled him to gauge the audience's reactions at a distance with his left eye and still see his notes at close range with the other. It seems that the President, who was left-handed but had been forced to write with his right at school, was more adept at removing his right lens than his left. For in 1987, and after appearing with a visibly puffy left eye when delivering a speech on budget reform, the White House physician Dr John Hutton was forced to issue a statement reassuring the public that Reagan had merely bruised his lower eyelid while taking out a contact lens.

Reagan has been described as 'the First Reality TV Star President': as the host of *General Electric Television Theater* on CBS in the 1950s and early 1960s the actor had opened up his brand-new 'all-electric' hilltop home in the Pacific Palisades to the show's viewers. And in the opinion of the film critic David Thomson, as President, Reagan still 'played the role of a possible friend' and was 'the first man in the office entirely comfortable' with the medium of television.

Other new arrivals in 1981 included IBM's PC, their first personal computer, and the twenty-four-hour music video channel MTV, the station launching, with a wink and a nudge, with a screening of 'Video Killed the Radio Star'. MTV's entrance, in the view of *Wired* magazine's 2012 survey of 'The Decades that Shaped the Future', signalled 'the dawning of a new era in which visuals would rival audio when it came to cultural impact'. Reagan, whose hearing was almost as bad as his eyesight following an on-set accident with a pistol in the late 1930s and who began wearing a hearing aid in 1983, was a president fully in tune with that shift.

The proliferation of new technological devices, at work and in the home, from personal computers and VCRs to video games, along with the expansion of cable television in the States, was to dramatically increase the amount of time people spent gazing at screens. And with people leading longer and healthier lives too, spectacles would accordingly become a much more necessary evil for those who might previously have tried to do without them. Perhaps catching wind of the direction of travel, the sunglasses maker Foster Grant was to dip a toe into the optical market with their

'Spare Pair' range of off-the-shelf reading glasses in 1980, the line soon becoming the second most popular in the field in America.

In 1980 the then comparatively little-known Italian fashion designer Giorgio Armani designed the costumes for Richard Gere in *American Gigolo*. Gere starred as Julian Kaye, a money-grabbing, shallow, narcissistic male escort in Los Angeles. He is first seen on screen at his tailor's and next needs to do a line of coke in order to slip into his loose-fitting but immaculately cut Armani two-piece suit. The movie consequently induced Armani mania in America and set the sartorial template for boxy power dressing by every wolf on Wall Street for the remainder of the decade. The following year, on the back of the film's success, Armani launched a ready-to-wear casual range for men, his 'designer' jeans becoming one of the most sought-after garments on the planet. A fragrance was to come in 1982, and Armani also began selling underwear and gradually moving into accessories.

It was then that Leonardo Del Vecchio, the founder and chairman of the Italian optical company Luxottica, approached Armani about the potential for licensing a line of eyewear. An Armani suit, Vecchio reasoned, might be beyond the means of most people but a pair of spectacles bearing the designer's name could be an option for the aspirational and one that wouldn't trash the brand either. A deal was eventually signed in the late 1980s, just as Michael Douglas was strutting his stuff in striped shirts and braces as the unscrupulous financier Gordon Gekko in Oliver Stone's *Wall Street*. The encyclopaedia-sized cell phone that Gekko uses at one point to call his protégé Bud Fox (Charlie Sheen, cast, perhaps less believably now, as the trader who finally gains a moral conscience) from a beach to go off on a Roy Batty-esque reverie about the sunrise and making himself rich is as 'aggressively 80s' as Jane Fonda's glasses. Which are themselves matched for eighties-ness in the movie by the window-pane-sized plastic numbers James Spader wears while uttering such immortal lines as 'What's in it for *moi*?'

Fonda, in any case, would come to be less well remembered for those *9 to 5* spectacles than her workout books and videos, the first of which were released in 1982. That initial tape was to become the *Thriller* of home videos, shifting 17 million copies worldwide, and remains the biggest-selling video cassette of all time. The critic Richard Schickel argued that in presenting 'fit, buff women as feminist exemplars', Fonda's foray into video exercise manuals was 'perfectly timed' for the 1980s, and that the actor offered 'a tamed, earned liberationist feminism, without the threatening hysteria of the movement's earlier days. It accomplished', he added, rather uncharitably, if not entirely inaccurately, 'a political goal. But better still, it made her a bunch of money, and redeem[ed] her in the eyes of most Americans, as success stories always do.' The association of wealth with health and fitness was to merge with bottom-up 'fresh' street wear and sportiness in spectacles, from hip hop artists like Run-DMC's adoption of German 'Cazzies' teamed with laceless Adidas sneakers and chunky jewellery (see Chapter 9) to the desirability of Ralph Lauren's waspish country club Polo-branded glasses, only gaining in fashionability.

## Breaking out of the frame

Keith Haring, whose dynamic works with motifs in bright pri-mary colours of jiving babies and barking dogs would be exhibited alongside the work of other New York graffiti artists like Jean-Michel Basquiat, Fab 5 Freddy and Kenny Scharf at the Fun Gallery in the East Village, drew a kind of ironic self-portrait of a skeleton figure in silver glasses as one of his earliest subway pieces. Gay, slight of build and bespectacled, Haring was to die tragically young at thirty-one of AIDS-related complications, lending the tag a bitter poignancy. Immersed in the melting pot of New York's downtown art and music scene, when rents remained low and crime high, Haring was a regular at venues such as the Mudd Club and Paradise Garage, and would supply images of anthropomor-phic beat boxes and body-popping figures for record sleeves for the likes of the NYC Peech Boys, Emanon, Grace Jones, Malcolm McLaren, Sylvester and Run-DMC. Haring's own glasses, mean-while, were frequently restyled by Scharf, the artist with whom he briefly shared an apartment in Times Square. 'Kenny', Haring once related, 'was constantly painting everything in the house . . . from telephones to the television to everything else. My glasses were lying there and he said, "Let me paint your glasses." Starting from then on I'd go onto this ongoing thing of every two weeks having a different paint job done on my glasses.'

Those lacking an in-house designer were in any case soon able to buy multicoloured, striped and patterned frames from firms such as Anglo-American Optical or Brulimar, whose 'Zoe' women's frame came in a splatter paint finish with shades of Jackson Pollock. One of Tura's none-more 1980s campaigns headed 'Finding complements is easy!' featured an assortment of go-getting people in glasses from a tennis player in a headband with a racket to a businesswoman in a chalk-stripe double-breasted power suit and pearls to a Don Johnson lookalike in a cream jacket over a T-shirt, and boasted that they had 'the widest selection of eyewear colours', and advised potential purchasers to 'Enjoy matching your eyewear style to your lifestyles' (plural, notably).

Haring would produce designs for the Swiss company Swatch, whose range of brightly coloured plastic watches was launched in 1983 in response to the cheap digital models produced by Japanese companies such as Casio. Backed by the tagline 'The New Wave in Swiss Watches', Swatch watches were promoted with a television commercial on heavy rotation that depicted sporting types pumping iron, doing aerobics Fonda-style, wind-surfing, swimming and skiing, all soundtracked by a World Supreme Team-style turntable-scratching and a hip-hop beat. And a similar mix-and-match aesthetic was prevalent in spectacles with 'fun' fashion sporty frames in colours as varied and lurid as jellybeans.

What in a sense had begun as a glorious liberation from the constraints of supposedly dreary old brown, black and metal glasses frames perhaps too easily tipped over into zany for the sake of it – like the comedy socks and cartoon character ties that had possibly at first looked amusing in branches of new eighties accessories outlets such as Tie Rack and the Sock Shop but which quickly became the attire of dull accountants trying to prove they had a personality or sense of humour. So too the

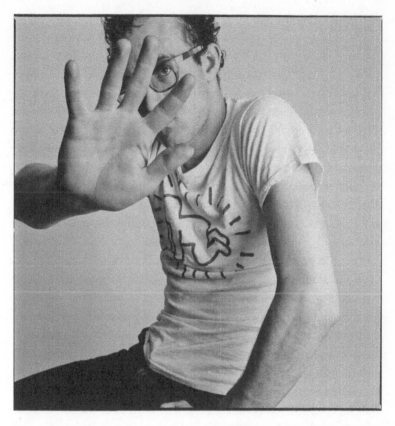

Getty Artist Keith Haring is photographed for the *Soho News* in May 1981, in New York.

oversized coloured plastic spectacle gradually came to be seen as outré and 'wacky'. Rather more good-for-a-laugh sitcom star Su Pollard than informed Channel 4 wine critic Jancis Robinson; too much jolly chubby actor and game show fixture Christopher Biggins and not quite enough acerbic restaurant and architectural reviewer Jonathan Meades. Blame the hyperactive breakfast TV presenter Timmy Mallett, if you like.*

---

* Though Biggins would later appear in drag as a wire spectacles-wearing Queen Victoria in Meades' 2001 television essay 'Victoria Died in 1901 and is Still Alive Today'.

## Glasses to kill for

Among the litany of brand names referenced in Bret Easton
Ellis's 1991 satirical novel *American Psycho*, cancelled by its original publishers Simon & Schuster after being denounced prior to
publication by *Time* magazine as a 'childish horror fantasy about a
Wall Street yuppie whose tastes run from nouvelle cuisine to the
most appalling acts of torture, murder, and dismemberment ever
described', was the designer eyewear maker Oliver Peoples.

Ellis, responding to his critics in the *New York Times* in March
1991, had explained that he 'was writing about a society in which
the surface became the only thing. Everything was surface – food,
clothes – that's what defined people.' The 1980s, he maintained,
had been 'a perverse decade', and Patrick Bateman, his twenty-six-
year-old shallow, amoral, murderous, label-obsessed investment
banker protagonist was a representative of that fact, merely exaggerated for comic effect. Bateman is prissily exacting about every
conceivable product he consumes, from facial scrubs by Caswell-
Massey and linen suits by Valentino Couture to the 1980s-only
albums of Genesis and Phil Collins ('all the albums before *Duke*
seemed too artsy, too intellectual') and Huey Lewis and the News
that he listens to on compact disc, naturally. And like those real-
life serial killers Dennis Nilsen and Jeffrey Dahmer (apprehended
just a few months after *American Psycho* was finally published),
Bateman wears glasses. Though of a very particular kind, under-
standably. Not for him the metal aviator spectacles of loners, losers
and weirdos. For sunglasses he takes a Ray-Ban Wayfarer, perhaps
just to be safe.

He doesn't wear glasses because he needs them either, since
his are fitted with 'non-prescription lenses'. But they are another
carefully selected facet of his look and intended, like everything
else that he owns, eats, drinks, dresses and washes in, to convey
his wealth, status and superior discernment. The glasses he actively
chooses to wear are 'Oliver Peoples redwood-framed glasses',
a style and brand also worn by some of his hyper-competitive
peers, with, and unashamedly without, prescription lenses. In a

bar, banker drinking buddy Taylor Preston 'takes off his glasses (Oliver Peoples, of course) and yawns, wiping them clean with an Armani handkerchief'. Elsewhere, when attending a work meeting, his friend Craig McDermott 'walks in . . . carrying a copy of this week's *New York* magazine and this morning's *Financial Times* wearing new non-prescription Oliver Peoples redwood-framed glasses'. And one day, while out shopping in a Paul Smith clothing store, Bateman is depressed to notice that two other Wall Street guys he runs into, Charles Hamilton and his closeted gay colleague Luis Carruthers, both have exactly the same slick-backed hairstyle and Oliver Peoples spectacles as himself. He is reassured, fortunately, to remember that unlike theirs, his glasses 'at least, are non-prescription'.

At the time of *American Psycho*'s publication, Oliver Peoples had only been in business for just over four years and the company had made its impression by consciously reacting against 1980s glasses design. As one of its current creative directors Giampiero Tagliaferri told *20/20* magazine in 2017, on the occasion of the firm's thirtieth birthday, 'When Oliver Peoples was founded in 1987, the brand challenged the ostentatious eyewear trends of the era with its decidedly classic aesthetic.' Nevertheless, their backward-looking vibe did chime with the era's burgeoning yearning for timeless staples of the past. A yearning that had already produced the revival of the fly-button Levi 501 jeans, boxer short briefs and, in some of the preppier New York social circles, wing shirts with detachable collars, if Whit Stillman's *Metropolitan* was to be believed.

As its co-founder, the optician Larry Leight would reflect in 2011 that he was after an 'American intellectual' look: 'A look; a style of eyewear that doesn't really exist any more, but we focused on an intellectual, unisex, smart and simple-looking frame. Like Manolo Blahnik does heeled shoes or Levi's does jeans, we created something that will be forever known as a retro, intellectual category of eyewear.'

## Eyeing the future

On 13 March 1991, the *Seattle Times* was one of a number of US papers to carry a widely syndicated story about a survey conducted by the optical retailers LensCrafters. Established in 1983 by Dean Butler, a former marketeer at Procter & Gamble who'd worked on campaigns for Cheer laundry detergent and Folger's instant coffee, LensCrafters had prospered, despite much scoffing from more established players, by offering a while-you-wait glasses-in-an-hour service and a thirty-day money back guarantee on all pairs sold. Expanding expeditiously in the 1980s and early 1990s – in 1986 alone it was estimated to be opening almost two new stores a week – within months of the *Seattle Times* piece LensCrafters would outpace its nearest rival Pearle to become the largest optical retailer in America. Butler, having sold up in 1987, was to repeat his winning if high-street-diversity-eroding formula on the other side of the Atlantic by going on to set up the Vision Express chain in the United Kingdom.

What the paper reported, however, was the findings of a poll of people working in recruitment undertaken by LensCrafters about different styles of spectacle frames. Personnel directors had, it was claimed, been presented with a photograph of the same man either 'wearing dark-coloured plastic frames' or 'lighter wire-frame glasses' and were asked to surmise their profession and evaluate their income. Those shown the picture of the man in the dark plastic specs thought he was a school teacher and probably earning only about $30,000 a year. On the other hand, those presented with the wire-framed wearer pronounced him a stockbroker and awarded him an annual salary of $200,000. If illustrating just how financially undervalued education had already become by the early 1990s, the message readers were encouraged to take home from this rather unscientific-sounding piece of market research was that they could look up to $170,000 richer by changing to a wire-framed pair of glasses. And although it was never stated, dangling in the air was that faintest of hints that LensCrafters might just be able to help with that.

The wire frames are rimless with oval-ish lenses and of a similar kind to ones that Frederic Grethel, vice president of sales and
marketing for Essilor's Logo Paris range – then promoting itself as
'eyewear for the man at the top' and 'The Professional's Brand' –
termed 'power eyewear'. This resurgence in smaller and narrower
frames was both an inevitable stylistic reaction against the fashions
of the previous period – the spectacle version, say, of Ikea's urging
of a chucking out of Laura Ashley-esque chintz in favour of nine-
ties flatpack Nordic simplicity – and also technologically driven by
the appearance of dynamic new materials. In particular titanium,
and also 'hyperindex' lenses, which were 45 per cent thinner and
lighter than conventional plastic lenses and 50 per cent thinner and
80 per cent lighter than glass lenses.

A naturally occurring element, titanium ore had first been discovered in the black sands of the beach at Manaccan in Cornwall
by the tubercular clergyman and amateur chemist William Gregor
back in 1791. A process for extracting a pure form on an industrial
scale wouldn't be arrived at until the 1930s, and it was not until
the 1950s and 1960s that it was put to use in aviation, shipping and
Cold War aerospace and hailed as a miracle metal. Lightweight,
amazingly strong and highly resistant to corrosion, it was soon
deployed for sheet roofing and shock- and shatter-proof sports
equipment such as tennis rackets and lacrosse sticks, and for reinforced attaché and flight cases. The first commercial use of it for
eyeglasses was in Japan in 1981 but it wasn't until the late 1980s that
European and American manufacturers got in on the act.

Lindberg Optical from Denmark, a country where minimalism is close to a national state of being – the company ascribed to
a design philosophy it termed 'reductionism' – introduced their
barely-there, rimless AIR Titanium frames in 1988.

Less austerely beautiful but just as ground-breaking, that same
year Marchon of Melville, New York, which manufactured
glasses under licence for Calvin Klein, launched its 'Auto-flex'
eyewear range made with Flexon. This was a newly patented
titanium composite material with a 'metal memory'. Its roots lay
in research by NASA in the 1960s into an alloy for a missile heat

shield that was found to return to its original form despite having been pummelled with a hammer. Publicised as 'smart' eyeglasses, imbuing them with intelligence and a touch of class, these remarkably springy 'Flexon frames would snap back into shape even if twisted like a pretzel'. Or so it was claimed back then. The firm is rather more circumspect now, its website currently warning that although 'Flexon frames are durable, they are not indestructible. Flexon frames should not be twisted more than 90° and Flexon temples should not be twisted more than once around the finger.' Still, the bendy-ish frame was here to stay. And titanium, perhaps by the nature of its very newness, its malleability and the historic connections to aerospace, would encourage frames of a more futuristic bent, just as the clock was starting to tick down to the millennium.*

But as with titanium as a material for spectacle frames, further innovations in the use of computers in designing and selling eyewear would come from Japan, though the Japanese eyewear retailer Paris-Miki was to choose Paris and its outlet in the Louvre as the place to trial its computerised Mikissimes Design System in 1994. This in-store tool was really the first of its kind to offer customers an interactive experience in selecting and styling their eyewear. Developed over five years, it eliminated the need for customers to keep physically trying on spectacles to find a pair to suit them. Instead of yanking frame after frame off the racks, or wading through countless drawers, the optician would simply take a digital picture of the customer's face. The Mikissimes Design System would then analyse this image for distinctive facial characteristics. Having already been fed a set of adjectives about the sort of styles the customer liked ('formal', 'traditional', 'sporty', 'elegant' etc.) the system would then recommend certain rim sizes and shapes, and present the potential purchaser with a series of digital images

---

* A Flexon print and television advertising campaign due to air in the autumn of 2001 and carrying the lines 'Just Amazing' and 'If only all metal were Flexon' and featuring a structure similar to the Empire State Building in New York bending out of the path of the low-flying jet had to be pulled following the 9/11 attacks on the World Trade Center.

with the specs superimposed over the photograph of their face. Once a suitable style had been found, the customer could, with the aid of the optician, further customise their frame, adjusting the size and shape of the rims and the bridge, hinges and sides until they reached a look that satisfied their fashion sense and met their optical needs. To begin with, customers were presented with a final photo-quality print-out of themselves wearing the frames and could leave the shop in an hour with their own custom-made frame. Over time, however, and as customers grew ever more accustomed to seeing digital images of themselves on screens, such print-outs became largely superfluous.

## Yesterday, today and tomorrow

The internet, in presaging the virtual over the actual and the digital over the physical, would leave few areas of life unchanged, and augmented reality beyond anything that had previously been visualised. But it's fascinating to reflect on how much of internet activity from the outset has been devoted to retrieving and archiving aspects of the past. From early cult film fan chatrooms to YouTube, and from forums like Friends Reunited to social media giants like Facebook, the latter dissolving the difference between acquaintances largely forgotten and fellows only recently met on a timeline with no regard for chronology, yesteryear has often never seemed more present than online. 'Vintage', a term originally applied only to cars and wine, had been in circulation in fashion circles since at least the early 1970s. But the arrival in 1995 of 'AuctionWeb', a site founded by Pierre Omidyar out of a spare bedroom in his Silicon Valley town house and inaugurated with the sale for $14.83 of a broken laser presentation pointer, was to help lend 'vintage' and its near sibling 'retro' an even greater financial resonance. On eBay (as it was soon renamed), the defunct, the obsolete, the abandoned and the completely busted might still be desirable to someone out there. And as Omidyar's opening trade had shown, sellers found they were able to offload almost any old rubbish and earn a far from negligible sum. The clearing out of cupboards and the disposal of recently obsolete pairs of glasses, or those left over from childhood or once owned by distant and deceased relatives, was to put thousands, millions even, of old spectacles on to the market.

Simultaneously designers, artists, film makers and musicians, later helped by the ease of being able to look up old stuff online, began to make more deliberate use of the recent past – at first, perhaps, with some degree of eyebrow-raising post-modern irony, but gradually in deadly post-everything earnest. When Kurt Cobain of Nirvana appeared with his long bleach-blonde hair chopped off and in a pair of heavy horn-rimmed glasses in the video for 'In Bloom', a promo that parodied a spot on a black and white TV show like Ed Sullivan's, he was intentionally and ironically mocking the idea that he was grunge rock's pin-up. Hair-metal rivals Guns & Roses didn't do glasses. Nor did they wear dresses or old men's woolly cardigans. Heroin and loud guitars were about all they had in common.

But progressively, and especially after the millennium, any sort of line between what was deliberately chosen to make some sort of arch or kitsch point and what might simply be considered retroliciously, geekily chic à la Wes Anderson's cinematic output or Jarvis Cocker's wardrobe disappeared. Those wishing to wear once-dormant mom and pop frames like the harlequin or the browline could just as easily pick up period models online or from specialist dealers in deadstock as buy a new repro pair or a modern style that tipped its hat to a so-called 'heritage' line.

The Algha Works' Savile Row brand were able to offer rolled-gold panto round-rimmed frames, once available on the NHS and worn by John Lennon, that were 'not like the originals' but were '*the* same original frames', handmade in exactly the same way, in the same factory, and using the same materials and almost all of the same tools and machinery as before.

Published in 2002, when printed books about how to use the internet were still considered a money-spinner, *Virtual Vintage: The Insider's Guide to Buying and Selling Fashion Online* contains a section on eyewear that provides both a snapshot of the wares then turning up on eBay but also illustrates the degree to which consumer tastes were already being driven by label recognition and celebrity endorsement. 'Whether you are looking', the guide's authors gushed, 'for the signature Lafont titanium eyeglasses worn by TV reporter Ashleigh Banfield or a pair of vintage Bausch & Lomb Ray-Ban Wayfarers, there are plenty online through which to browse ... We've seen vintage Versace, Christian Lacroix, Gianfranco Ferré, Oakley, and Giorgio Armani in these auctions.' Since Armani didn't branch out into eyewear until the end of the 1980s, this also indicates the shrinking timescale with which items could be classified as 'vintage'.

The actor and heiress Gloria Vanderbilt is generally held to have got the celebrity glasses ball rolling when in 1976, the same year her designer jeans first went on sale, an eyewear line in her name appeared, with the Italian star Sophia Loren following soon afterwards in 1980. Some rather glittery Gloria Vanderbilt Collection specs would serve as a punchline in 'The Glasses', an episode of cult 1990s sitcom *Seinfeld*, when George, a short, bald and neurotic wire-rimmed spectacle wearer, accidentally buys a pair to replace his own, which have been stolen at a health club, only to discover to his embarrassment that they are 'lady's glasses'.

By then, however, George could equally have mistakenly purchased 'lady glasses' endorsed by the likes of the supermodel Christie Brinkley. Brinkley's glasses, made for her by Nouveau Eyewear Inc., were sold on the basis of 'offering all-American beauty with a simple approach to style'. Come the twenty-first century and with magazines such as *Hello!* and *OK!* catering to the public's seemingly insatiable demand for ever more mundane details about celebrities' lives, 'signature' spectacles would become a ubiquitous part of the optical market. The range of celebrities willing to put their name to pairs of glasses today runs the whole gamut from the former Spice Girl Victoria Beckham to the snooker star Dennis Taylor.

Taylor's original giant upside-down frames with their plate-window-sized lenses had been created specially for him by the trained spectacle maker turned TV snooker commentator and billiards enthusiast Jack Karnehm. If looking more than slightly ridiculous, these spectacles, the elevator shoes of eyewear, enhanced Taylor's peripheral vision and almost certainly helped him win the world championship in 1985. The trademarked 'Dennis Taylor "Pro-Snooker" glasses', modelled after his tournament-winning pairs and sold by the Brulimar Optical Group in 2016, would come in a green-baize-coloured case featuring his autograph. This was also etched on to the side pieces of the frame in the unlikely event that anyone mistook them for a style of snooker spectacle worn by Ray Reardon, or Hurricane Higgins, say.

In the United States, Zyloware Eyewear, the company responsible to this day for Gloria Vanderbilt glasses, produces spectacle lines for a whole roster of celebrity clients including the musician and *American Idol* judge Randy Jackson, the Cuban-American TV presenter Daisy Fuentes and the former professional basketball player Shaquille O'Neal. None of whom might be described as A-listers. A more recent entrant into the field, though, was the one-time Disney teen idol, actress and singer Hilary Duff. Her 2018 'Muse x' spectacle collection with GlassesUSA was marketed in the language of motivational coaching and sold as empowering aids to female self-esteem. As an accompanying press pack puff put it, 'Every part of the line from the small personal messages to fans to the packaging help in conveying the message of being confident in yourself. Duff said in a statement, "When you are comfortable in your own skin and proud of who you are, you can focus on what's important in your life."' We might well wonder just how at ease anyone who *needed* a pair of Hilary Duff specs to feel confident about themselves really *was*, but that's consumer capitalism for you.

Duff's spectacles were pitched at the more affordable end of the market. But questions over the value for money of some designer glasses have been parried away by claims about the potential therapeutic benefits of choosing a labelled pair over a less prestigious kind. In 2007, Pierre Fay, the vice president of Luxottica, declared that 'Brands can be key to patient satisfaction and patient compliance in wearing their eyewear prescription.' As Mandy Rice-Davies once put it, well he would say that wouldn't he? At the time of writing, among the names Luxottica owns or licenses are Armani, Brooks Brothers, Burberry, Chanel, Coach, DKNY, Dolce & Gabbana, Michael Kors, Oakley, Oliver Peoples, Persol, Polo Ralph Lauren, Ray-Ban, Tiffany, Valentino, Vogue and Versace.

The Italian company also holds the American LensCrafters optical chain and its one-time rival Pearle Vision, along with Sears Optical, John Lewis Optical, David Clulow and Sunglass Hut.

In 2018 it consolidated its hold on the global market by merging with the French lens manufacturing giant Essilor to form the mammoth combined entity EssilorLuxottica. Perhaps not since the earliest days of their invention more than seven centuries ago have Italian and French spectacle makers wielded so much power. Although much of the making now, of course, is outsourced to China, a country where some 90 per cent of teenagers and young adults are estimated to be short-sighted. While the wearing of glasses has perhaps never been less stigmatised or as fashionable, they are also more necessary than ever. With ever greater parts of our lives, and from infancy, now spent indoors looking at screens, the world is facing up to a potential epidemic of poorer and poorer sight. But technology, if a factor in causing this situation, could also offer a solution.

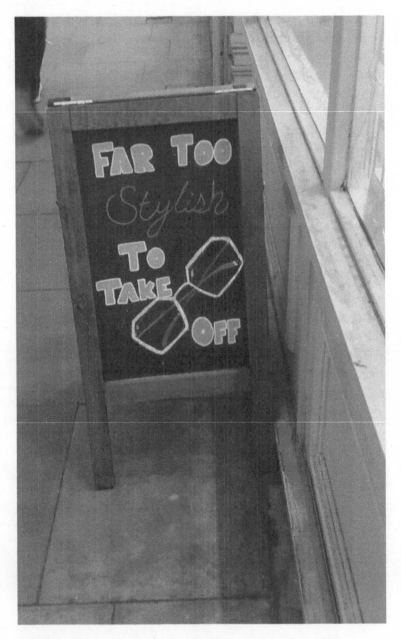

Optician's board on Stoke Newington Church Street, London, 2020.

# 13

# 20/20 in the Twenty-first Century

'The coloured part of the eye, that's basically a water washer with poster paints on. The black bit for the pupil is photographic paper.' John Dixon Salt, a retired ophthalmic optician and collector of antique ophthalmic equipment, has just pulled out a glass-covered tray full of artificial eyes. Presented in rows, and glistening slightly under the electric lights, they appear disturbingly like engagement rings in a jeweller's shop, and shimmer like a passing shoal of fish. The Ancient Greeks, we now know, not only painted but also attached marble sculpted eyes to the bows of their ships to ward against evil and guide them safely to their destinations. We are, as it happens, by the sea. Though in Worthing, my home town, far from the Aegean on the rather chillier shores of the Sussex coast. I learn that these eyes are most likely as old as I am, and rather special, since they were hand-made in acrylic by Dixon Salt and his late father William in the 1970s. They offer, though, a glimpse even further back in time. For by then it was already highly unusual for a high-street optician to make their own artificial eyes. But as Dixon Salt stated, his father was 'effectively a Victorian gentleman' who'd always made them and brought his son up to do the same, and using a truly ingenious array of common household products to craft replacements that might pass for the real thing. 'The veins', he told me, gesturing with pride at one eerily convincing rheumy

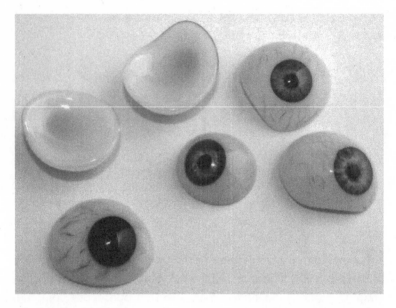

Handmade artificial eyes.

pale-blue eye, 'are either felt-tip pen, or bits of a silk ribbon, the silk embedded in.'

Unlike traditional artificial eyes, those glass baubles constantly mistaken for marbles or dropped in pint pots in silent comedy skits, the Dixon Salt eyes are hemispherical discs, i.e. about a quarter slice of a globe in shape and thickness. The mock eye part, he explained, was fitted on the front of a perspex knuckle that slotted into the eye socket. The muscles in the socket could then fasten on to the knuckle, with the result that the fake eye, if positioned correctly, could move in tandem with the patient's remaining healthy eye, making it less easy to detect. Getting the whites to match, however, was, he added, a real challenge. 'The older you are, the yellower the eyes are, and you don't want one eye yellow and the other Dulux white.' A solution to the problem, he told me, was found by chance one day when a bit of tobacco from his father's pipe accidentally fell into the mixture and 'produced a lovely nicotine yellow that was just perfect'. A Senior Service cigarette was kept on hand thereafter apparently.

Slim, his evidently once dark hair threaded with silver but still thick and full, Dixon Salt is a youthful sixty-something who wears glasses for reading and close work. But only sparingly so during the afternoon we spent together. When we met at his home, a charming 1930s semi straight out of Metroland, in November 2019, he'd only recently closed the family practice his father had first established in this resort and retirement town back in 1956 (a canny move, given the rising number of elderly residents, many of them needing spectacles, which would reach 31 per cent by 1961 and 34 per cent a decade later).

Dixon Salt's own retirement, though, has allowed him to further indulge his somewhat busman's holiday-like interest in ophthalmic antiques, an enthusiasm that sees him not only acquiring rare frames and optical equipment but also mastering the techniques of making and repairing older forms of spectacles using traditional tools and materials. A bone frame was a project currently in the works, he informed me. And he even confessed to experimenting with spectacle making by candlelight to get a better sense of the conditions in which his optical forebears had had to operate. But his whole collection is displayed in a dedicated workshop at the back of the house, a man cave and *wunderkammer* of optical delights that his children, when young, christened 'Dad's sulking room'. A sign that they gave him with this splendid rejoinder and a picture of a dinosaur printed on it still hangs on the door.

In the cabinets of brown wood and glass that line each wall and in various drawers and trays in desks and chests are examples of almost every type of spectacle and optical instrument conceivable, from rivet spectacles in leather, silver and pearl locket lorgnettes, cane spyglasses and blue-steel railway glasses to carved spectacle cases, charts for testing colour blindness and a set of gruesomely diseased fake eyes used to train students to recognise common ailments. A full set of NHS frames in their original perspex display case prompts reminiscences about the mad rush for eye tests in the months before fees were introduced in the late 1980s. 'We had patients', he recalled, 'we hadn't seen in fifteen years suddenly turning up, it was madness. And once the deadline had passed we hardly saw a soul for the next eighteen months.' Dixon Salt remained within the NHS, and still believes wholeheartedly in the service, but feels that in terms of spectacle design it did rather 'hold us back'. 'We didn't have a lot of colour for a long time,' he comments drily as we both peer at the brown, black and 'flesh-coloured' pink 524 NHS frames, lodged in a block of clear plastic like prehistoric insects in amber. And perhaps no less representative of a lost world. In identifying antique spectacles, he told me, it's often subtle differences in the design or materials that offer a clue to their country of origin. Historically Americans, for instance, preferred squarer and more rectangular frames with straighter bridges, while English frames were rounder with arched bridges. Where information on auction sites such as eBay can sometimes be a bit sketchy, such details have helped him spot a few misdescribed or undervalued gems over the years and avoid some obvious duds and fakes.

Of all the things he showed me that afternoon, though, the artificial eyes had it.

I'd earlier asked Dixon Salt about the state of the nation's eye-sight and if he thought things were better or worse now than they were twenty or thirty years ago. He replied unequivocally that from a medical point of view things were 'fantastically better'. 'Oh my God, just look at the surgical treatments, the medication, the anti-inflammatories, the anti-autoimmune drugs. They are superb. We are capable of saving sight left, right and centre now.' He and his father's eyes, if as lovingly conceived and executed and as much works of art as optical aids, were somewhat brutal reminders of a time, just within my own lifetime, when life prospects were decidedly grimmer. Offering a brief summary of why such lines thankfully became less necessary, Dixon Salt reeled off, on his fingers, the reasons: antibiotics, deindustrialisation, improvements to health and safety regulations at work and, perhaps most impor-tant of all, the absence of any further world wars. Armed combat along with insanitary living and working conditions and a lack of access to affordable medical care were, he argued, some of the major causes of eye loss in the first half of the twentieth century.

And these really were the bad old days, their after-effects lingering on for decades. He himself remembered encountering appalling eye conditions in local hospitals as a young graduate in the late 1970s that have now all but vanished, largely thanks to modern pre-emptive treatments.

But he nevertheless did fear that some of the practical knowledge about how lenses were cut, edged and produced and spectacles manufactured and repaired – part and parcel of somewhere like his father's practice – are in danger of being lost.

His own collection is predominantly British, and its frames and ephemera, if deliberately erring on the more antiquated side, still summon up some ghosts of spectacle makers and opticians only comparatively recently passed, such as Hadley of Surbiton and Dollond & Aitchison. Worthing itself was home to the Marylebone Optical Works, Dollond & Aitchison's specialist plastic lens making plant, located barely a mile from Dixon Salt's house and closer still to my childhood home where my parents continue to live. During a miserabilist adolescence blighted by acne, myopia and the music of the Smiths, I cycled past it most days. It closed sometime in the mid-nineties, hanging on longer than hundreds of other British lens and frame makers who fell when optical manufacturing started to move overseas in the 1980s.

Back then, though, I was in the minority. Today, one in five teenagers in the UK are myopic. And the condition now affects twice as many ten- to sixteen-year-olds than when I was born, nearly fifty years ago. While a third of the UK population is currently estimated to be short-sighted, in southeast Asia the figure reaches 70 per cent, and a 2012 study of South Korea found that a staggering 96.5 per cent of nineteen-year-old men there were myopic. If the surge continues to rise at this rate, half the world's population is expected to be myopic by 2050.

In a piece for the spring 2019 issue of *Acuity*, the house organ of the College of Optometrists, Madeleine Bailey ran through some of the potential factors behind this sudden increase in short-sightedness. Reading them, and reflecting on my own early teenage years spent skulking in my bedroom, the curtains drawn

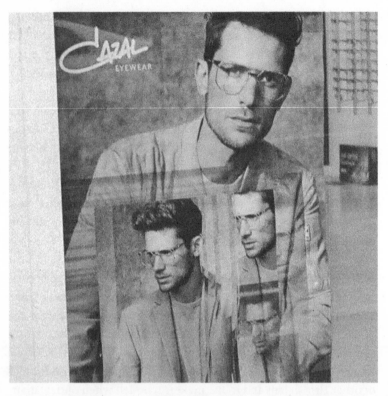

Cazals window display, opticians Kingsland Road, Dalston, London, 2020.

on sunny days, thumbing *Absolute Beginners* and *The Outsider* and poring over issues of *Sounds* and the *NME* while listening to *Power, Corruption & Lies*, *Fried* and *Brilliant Trees*, I felt more than a pang of regret about what I might inadvertently have done to my eyes.

As Bailey writes, while there is 'a clear genetic component to myopia', a 'possible culprit' for 'the rapid change over the past few decades' has been that 'our lives are increasingly lived indoors'. She cited recent research in Australia and Asia that had shown 'that time spent outdoors' helped 'to protect against the development of myopia'. Though it didn't 'prevent existing myopia getting worse'. Bailey conceded that 'No one knows exactly why' or 'which aspect of spending time indoors' might be 'the key factor in myopia'. But one theory is that 'light stimulates the release of dopamine in the retina' and prevents the overgrowth of the eye that leads to myopia. Alternatively, less exposure to sunlight and correspondingly lower levels of vitamin D 'may have a similar effect on eye growth'.

If the causes continue to be a bit of a mystery, Bailey reports that the optical profession believes it has a duty to engage with much more active interventions to halt its spread among the young in order to avert a potential global catastrophe in eye health. Aside from the need to wear glasses to see distant (or not so distant) objects, myopes are also at greater risk from suffering from glaucoma in later life, a disease that remains one of the leading causes of irreversible blindness in the world. At a minimum, children, and especially those with short-sighted parents, it is argued, must be made to pursue more of 'an active lifestyle . . . spending time outdoors'. Which is easier said than done, even without a lockdown. As the shy, bookish offspring of an actually rather sporty myope, the last place I ever really wanted to be was outside and exercising when I could be inside and reading. And we didn't even have the internet. The smart money inevitably is on 'the science' providing a more lasting solution. Trials in Hong Kong and elsewhere using soft multifocal contact lenses have produced some positive results in slowing myopic progression in children aged between eight and thirteen. While in southeast Asia, eyedrops with a low-strength dosage of the alkaloid atropine, more commonly used to treat low heart rates and reduce saliva during surgery and as an anti-cholinergic, appear to have had a similarly retardant effect, forestalling the advance of myopia in children for at least as long as the treatment continues. At the time of writing, concerns remain about potential side-effects, including the possibility of premature presbyopia and cataracts, and its use is at present unlicensed in the UK. Though a study, known as CHAMP or the Childhood Atropine for Myopia Progression, is currently being undertaken by the University of Ulster.

Daniel Hardiman-McCartney is not only a clinical adviser to the College of Optometrists but also a Liveryman of the Worshipful Company of Spectacle Makers. Though perhaps unusually in his own private practice in the horsey Suffolk market town of Newmarket, he doesn't sell spectacles. With a goatee beard, spiky black hair and in dark brown horn-rims and a denim shirt, he could pass for a prosperous former grunge musician rather than a medical professional. But in person, and later over email, he provides plenty of food for thought on where optometry and glasses could well be heading.

Adding to my sense that the odds were always stacked against me, he tells me that eldest siblings have a greater likelihood of being myopic, though he confesses that 'with myopia we still do not fully understand it'. But Hardiman-McCartney is extremely positive about the potential for reducing its 'progression by around 50% with both contact lenses or eye drops'. If a cure is 'unlikely to become available within the next ten years', it is, he thinks, 'a plausible idea and perhaps will become a reality' within his lifetime.

'With presbyopia,' he adds, 'several companies are working on implantable lenses, which can adjust between distance and near mimicking the focusing of the natural eye. These lenses would be implanted during the widely performed cataract operation. I would guess they may become publicly available within the next decade. This could result in a generation of over seventy-year-olds who do not need glasses, for distance or reading.' As it stands already, he calculates that 'roughly a hundred thousand refractive surgical procedures are undertaken every year in the UK. That may be with laser surgery or lens implants. Results are generally good, reducing the need for spectacles once taken.'

The idea of making incisions into the cornea to flatten the eye and reduce myopia, known as 'radial keratotomy' (RK), was first suggested in the 1880s by Dutch ophthalmologist Leendert Jan Lans, after his experiments on rabbits. The procedure wasn't attempted on humans until the late 1930s, and in Japan by Tsutomu Sato. The technique was subsequently improved upon by both the Spanish ophthalmologist Professor José Ignacio Barraquer and the Soviet eye surgeon Svyatoslav Fyodorov, the latter acquiring his knowledge of the procedure after visiting Japan shortly after Sato's death in 1960. But the operation was not performed in the United States until 1978. It was only with the arrival of precision-cutting excimer lasers – developed by IBM for Ronald Reagan's cherished Star Wars weapons programme and first demonstrated in the field of optometry and on the corneas of monkeys and rabbits by Stephen Trokel in 1983 – that an accurate enough tool for the procedure really presented itself. In 1995, approval was granted for doctors to perform the first type of laser eye surgery, photorefractive keratectomy (or PRK), on patients. Since its introduction four years later, what's known as laser-assisted in-situ keratomileusis (or LASIK), pioneered by the Greek ophthalmologist Ioannis Pallikaris, has become the more commonly recommended form of corrective surgery. This involves cutting a flap in the cornea and then altering its underlying tissue with a laser, either flattening the cornea to cure myopia or steepening it for hypermetropia and righting its shape to correct an astigmatism. Once the cornea has been amended the flap is put back into place, almost as if nothing has happened.

Like botox and other formerly clinical cosmetic treatments, laser eye surgery is now readily available on the high street. The chain Optical Express, which bills itself as the 'UK's number one laser eye surgery provider' and offers it at many of its hundred-plus outlets, describes it as 'a simple procedure that takes anything from a matter of seconds to just a few minutes, depending upon the level of correction that's required'. Yet such surgery is not suitable for all patients, nor is it without risk. A survey by the consumer magazine *Which?* in November 2019 of 958 people who'd had laser eye surgery found 'that 11% said their vision was worse than expected after surgery'. They also reported that '15% of all respondents who had the surgery in the past five years said that they weren't well informed that this deterioration in eyesight could happen'.

Hardiman-McCartney thinks that 'it is the role of practitioners to ensure people are aware of the risks of surgical intervention'. As he says, the oft-quoted 'risk of one in a thousand may seem very low, but that may mean a hundred people each year having worse vision than they intended with a surgical method of correction'. Looking to the future, however, he still believes that 'it remains within the realms of the plausible that in fifty years the majority of people in wealthy countries will not need to wear glasses or contact lenses. Myopia will be reduced, perhaps cured, presbyopia will be corrected surgically, and refractive surgery will be the preferred correction.' Among the other even more imminent innovations that Hardiman-McCartney mentions are 'smart' contact lenses capable of measuring eye pressure to diagnose glaucoma and others that can test levels of blood sugar for diabetes, which are already in development.

Turning the clock back to his own initiation into the industry, he recalls that when he started out almost 'the only appointment that was offered was a sight test or contact lens fitting' whereas now optometrists offer a 'menu of services' and 'are increasingly involved with providing appointments relating to ocular health'. Certainly this is true of my own experience of being tested for glaucoma, something that I can't honestly recall featuring much in earlier decades. But again that might just be more my age (and ageing) than the age itself.

Like all retailers, opticians have had to adapt to online competition. But Hardiman-McCartney is certain that sight tests will soon 'take place from the comfort of your home on an app, perhaps combined with a saliva genetics test. AI systems will monitor the results and refer those at risk of needing spectacles or eye care to health professionals.' For optometrists and ophthalmologists, he maintains, 'those professions will become more targeted, focusing on those who require eye care or have complex prescriptions rather than for routine screening and prescribing spectacles. With an ageing population', he adds, dryly, 'there will be plenty of work.'

While medical advances could eventually make spectacles obsolete, he's convinced many people will still choose to wear glasses 'for fashion and to consume information'. He reminds me that initially much of the press around Google Glass, the Silicon Valley giant's disastrous 2012 foray into smart eyewear, was positive. It was briefly the wannabe wearable gadget drooled over by tech execs and fashionistas alike. Beyoncé, Bill Murray and, er, Prince Charles were all photographed wearing it. *Time* magazine named it one of the 'Best Inventions of the Year'. It was treated to a twelve-page spread in the September 2013 issue of *Vogue*. Entitled 'The Final Frontier', in reference to *Star Trek*, it was illustrated with a series of photographs by Steven Klein that looked like stills from a science fiction movie, an aesthetic emphasised by an opening line that claimed: 'Beyond the blue horizon lies a futuristic vision of fashion – a beautiful minimalism tailored for the brave and the bold.' Striking a suitably dystopian note, one picture, framed by a model with oil-sleek shiny black hair caught adjusting her Google Glass with a gloved hand, and in a Stella McCartney amethyst felted-boucle coat priced at $3855, was captioned, 'Cloaked against the autumn chill in monochrome coats or suits, the trio wanders Ransom Canyon like future humans returned to the abandoned earth . . . ' As it turned out, of course, Google Glass's prospects as a fashion accessory were as bleak. Roasted in the tech press over the inadequacy of many of its much-trumpeted features and vilified more generally over concerns around filming and privacy with wearers mocked as snooping 'Glass-holes', it was quietly withdrawn in 2015. With far less fanfare but much better results, however, and largely unbeknown to the general public, the company continued to tinker with a version for the workplace. And after trials at GE, Boeing, DHL and Volkswagen, its Glass Enterprise Edition, or Glass EE, was released in 2017 without any fashion shows or sky-diving teams to promote it. It continues to prosper in factory and in hospital settings. In medical wards, the ability to call up medical records digitally and photograph and film a patient's symptoms and share them with colleagues has helped speed up the diagnostic process with many positive outcomes. It has been estimated that by 2025, 'nearly 14.4 million US workers' could well be wearing smart glasses. If suffering a similar series of setbacks to Google, the photo-video-messaging site Snapchat is also presently on to its third generation of camera-spectacles for consumers.

Hardiman-McCartney argues that because of the long periods we spend looking at our phones and screens, smart eyewear is 'sensible on several levels', and once issues over trust have been overcome, 'displays in spectacles or contact lenses' could 'become as common as headphones'.

Tech inevitably will also alter how the spectacles are made and purchased. 3D printers could allow customers to design their own bespoke frames. Virtual try-ons, first pioneered in-store by Paris-Miki back in the 1990s, are already a common feature of many online optical websites, including those like Cubitts, who represent the emergence of what might be termed 'artisanal opticians'.

On departing the College of Optometrists, my head full of our conversation about a potential spectacle-less future, I amble up from Charing Cross into Covent Garden, an area described as 'a great resort of gallants' by Samuel Pepys when he visited it to watch a Punch and Judy puppet show on 9 May 1662, just a month after first complaining of problems with his eyes. The diarist might have been surprised to find vendors of glasses more numerous than gallants in the district these days. A stroll around the main plaza and surrounding side streets, and amid the bars, restaurants, theatres, clothing shops, buskers and living statues, reveals opticians and optical stores of various shapes and sizes, from behemoths like Boots the Chemist and mid-sized chains such as David Clulow (operated by Luxottica) and Ace & Tate to smaller vendors such as Tom Davies 'Bespoke Opticians', Ollie Quinn and Moscot, and quirkier boutiques such as Spex in the City, Bailey Nelson and Cubitts.

Named in honour of the Georgian master builders Thomas, William and Lewis Cubitt, responsible for many of the stuccoed terraces, crescents and squares of Belgravia, Pimlico, Clapham and Millbank, along with Kemp Town in Brighton and Osborne on the Isle of Wight, Cubitts have a young, fogeyish penchant for history. Its Covent Garden outlet, until recently a branch of the stationers Scribbler, and in contrast to the sterile Apple computer silver and white of other optical outlets, is done out with lots of darkwood timber. This is a self-proclaimed reference to the building's former life as the A. France and Son funeral parlour where similar planking was put to use for coffins. But the decor, as invitingly old-fashioned as it is contemporary, conveys the idea of hoary-handed expertise, the atelier as emporium, and its spectacles as artisanal as craft gin or sourdough bread. Frame-making courses are another of the firm's offerings, and indicative of the yearning among consumers not just for products but also for experiences.

Recalling my own earliest encounters with opticians, where the examination parlours were grimly utilitarian and shared the ambience of dentists' consulting rooms, with almost the same wilted copies of *National Geographic* and the *Sunday Times* magazine laid out for visitors, it's a stark reminder of just how far we've come. On the one hand it exemplifies the gentrification – the expensification, arguably – of glasses; frame styles that were once available for nominal fees on the NHS are now for sale, if in slightly more refined and bespoke forms, as designer ranges. But equally it represents a delight in glasses for their sartorial sake and an overturning of centuries of anti-spectacle rhetoric, although eyewear, as hopefully we've seen, has always from its inception enjoyed moments of fashionability.

In a subsequent email exchange with John Dixon Salt, the curious figure of Horace Duke came up. Duke worked as a foreman at Marylebone Optical in Worthing and, according to Dixon Salt, was reputed to polish each pair of finished spectacles with a silk handkerchief. He was, nevertheless, better known as a local eccentric who spent his leisure hours cycling about the town in plus fours, a Harold Lloyd-style straw boating hat and a monocle, and waving at passing motorists when paused at roundabouts and major road junctions, a cigarette in a holder clamped tightly in his mouth. A mouth, it should be said, that often emitted obscenities. But in making a spectacle of himself, he looked the world in the eye through a lens. Something that all glasses wearers should do with pride, regardless of our prescriptions.

# THE HAPPY
# READER

With JARVIS COCKER (interviewed)
& urgent sci-fi classic WE (thoroughly investigated).

Bookish Magazine — Issue n° 10 — Winter 2017

Jarvis Cocker, cover star of *The Happy Reader* magazine.

# Acknowledgements

Thanks are first due to Sharmaine Lovegrove for introducing me to my editor Richard Beswick, who not only responded warmly to the idea of a book about glasses but also endured its somewhat protracted production and made invaluable suggestions on nipping the rather overlong draft into shape. I am extremely grateful to Daniel Balado for his diligent copy-edit, Rachel Cross for her proofreading, Nithya Rae for helping ease the manuscript into printed form and Linda Silverman for all her work on the pictures. Bo Diddley may well have sung 'You Can't Judge a Book by the Cover', but most people do. So I'd like to thank Michelle Thompson for the wonderful artwork that encases this volume and Charlotte Stroomer for overseeing the design process. Thanks to Grace Vincent for publicity and everyone else at Little, Brown for their efforts on behalf of the book.

This book would have been a far poorer thing without the assistance and immense knowledge of Neil Handley, curator of the British Optical Association Museum at the College of Optometrists and author of the definitive book on designer glasses, *Cult Eyewear*. During my visits to the museum and the college library, Handley was as essential a resource as the material held in the collection itself. He also generously replied to many additional queries by email and provided further material for me remotely, including most of the images in this book, after the library was closed to the public due to Covid-19 restrictions.

Thanks are due too to Daniel Hardiman-McCartney who

took the time out to speak to me in person at the College and also responded at length to my questions via email as well as supplying several articles that proved invaluable. No less giving of his time and wisdom in person and via email was John Dixon Salt, who invited me into his home, showed me his magnificent collection and supplied the photograph of his hand-crafted artificial eyes that appears in the book.

I am grateful to Ian Sanderson, the Office Manager of Savile Row Eyewear for giving me a guided tour of the Algha Works on Smeed Road. I'd also like to thank Virginia Ironside for providing me with a transcript of her interview with the legendary spectacle-maker Lawrence Jenkin. And thanks to Jack Bond and Andrew Wilson for answering my queries regarding Patricia Highsmith, Alfred Hitchcock and Miriam's spectacles in *Strangers on a Train,* and to Paul Kelly for scanning duties on various record sleeves.

As always, I am indebted to the staff at The British Library in St Pancras, The London Library in St James's, and Stoke Newington Library and Hackney Library services, who supplied so many of the records, books, journals, magazines and pamphlets pillaged to write this book.

I am immensely grateful to Peter Tomasevic for casting a professional eye over the manuscript. All errors that remain are, of course, entirely my own but his input was incredibly useful in clarifying a few points of detail.

I'd also like to thank Nick Rennison who again gave me some great feedback on the work in progress and also my brilliant and beautiful wife Emily Bick, for agreeing to do the same, especially after enduring the months of lockdown.

To friends, and family on both sides of the Atlantic, colleagues, collaborators, and previously kindly commissioning editors, festival bookers, event organisers and radio producers – thank you all for your support over these last couple of years. Be seeing you.

# Sources and select bibliography

This book could not have been written without the aid of numerous other books, journals, magazines, reports, pamphlets, newspapers, websites, novels, stories, memoirs, movies and songs. Back issues of *The Optician* and *The Newsletter of the Ophthalmic Antiques International Collectors Club* and the like were constant founts of information and inspiration, as were copies of trade promotional magazines such as *Wellsworth*, published by the American Optical Company in the opening decades of the twentieth century. The sources and select bibliography below should, I hope, give credit where credit is due and point those who want to know more in the right directions.

## Primary spectacle sources

Agarwal, Sunita, Pallikaris, Ioannis G., & Agarwal, Athiya, *Refractive Surgery* (London: Jaypee Brothers Medical Publisher Ltd, 2000).

Al-Khalili, J., 'In retrospect: Book of Optics', *Nature*, 518, 2015, pp. 164–165.

Azar, Dimitri T., Koch, Douglas, ed *LASIK (Laser in Situ Keratomileusis): Fundamentals, Surgical Techniques, and Complications* (Florida: CRC Press, 2002).

Bailey, Madeleine, 'Turning the Tide', *Acuity*, Spring 2019, pp. 18–23.

Barker, David, *How Glasses Caught a Killer: And Other*

*Stories of How Optics Changed the World* (feedaread.com publishing, 2015).

Barty-King, Hugh, *Eyes Right: The Story of Dolland & Aitchinson Opticians 1750–1985* (London: Quiller Press, 1986).

Bates, William Horatio, *The Bates Method for Better Eyesight Without Glasses* (New York: Henry Holt, 1943).

Bates, William Horatio, *The Cure of Imperfect Sight by Treatment without Glasses* (New York: Central Fixation Publishing Co, 1925).

The Beveridge Report Ad Hoc Committee, *The Place of the Optical Profession in the Health Services of the Nation* (London: Beveridge Report Ad Hoc Committee, Optical Profession (England), 1944).

Bilton, Nick, 'Disruptions: Why Google Glass Broke', *The New York Times*, 4 February 2015.

Bowden, Timothy J., *Contact Lenses: The Story* (Kent: Bower House Publication, 2009).

Brown, Vanessa, *Cool Shades: The History and Meaning of Sunglasses* (London: Bloomsbury 2015).

Browning, John, *How to Use our Eyes, and How to Preserve Them by the Aid of Spectacles* (London: Chatto & Windus, 1883 and 1892 edition).

Brueneni, Joseph, *More than Meets the Eye: The Stories Behind the Development of Plastic Lenses* (Pittsburgh: PPG Industries, 1997).

Cahan, David, *Helmholtz: A Life in Science* (Chicago: The University of Chicago Press, 2018).

Chance, James Frederick, *A History of the Firm of Chance Brothers & Co. Glass and Alkali Manufacturers* (London: printed for private circulation, 1919).

Collins, Edward Treacher, *The History & Traditions of Moorfields Eye Hospital. One Hundred Years of Ophthalmic Discovery and Development, etc* (London: H. K. Lewis & Co, 1929).

Corson, Richard, *Fashions in Eyeglasses* (London: Peter Owen, 1967).

Crestin-Billet, Frédérique (translated from the French by

Jonathan Sly), *Collectable Eyeglasses* (Paris: Flammarion; London: Thames and Hudson, 2004).

Darrigol, Olivier, *A History of Optics: From Greek Antiquity to the Nineteenth Century* (Oxford: OUP, 2012).

Davidson, Derek & MacGregor, Ronald, *Spectacles, Lorgnettes, and Monocles* (Princes Risborough: Shire, 2002).

Egerton, Samuel Y., *The Mirror, the Window, and the Telescope: How Renaissance Linear Perspective Changed Our Vision of the Universe* (Ithaca: Cornell University Press, 2009).

Fassell, Preston, 'Hindsight is 20/20: Aviator Eyeglasses', *20/20*, December 2013.

Fassell, Preston, 'Hindsight is 20/20: The Browline', *20/20*, January 2013.

Fontana, Michela, *Matteo Ricci: A Jesuit in the Ming Court* (London: Rowan and Littlefield, 2011 & 2015 editions).

Frank, Alex, *Oliver Peoples: California As We See It* (New York: Assouline, 2019).

Goes, Frank Joseph, *The Eye in History* (London: Jaypee Brothers Medical Publisher Ltd, 2013).

Gooding, Joanne, 'Rather unspectacular: design choices in National Health Service glasses', *Sound and Vision*, Spring 2017, http://dx.doi.org/10.15180/170703.

Gorin, George, *History of Ophthalmology* (Wilmington, Delaware: Publish or perish, 1982).

Gottschalk, Mary, 'Imagine Changing Glasses', *Seattle Times*, 13 March 1991.

Gross, Kim Johnson, Solomon, Michael, Stone, Jeff, *Chic Simple Components: Spectacles* (London: Thames and Hudson, 1994).

Handley, Neil, *Cult Eyewear: The World's Enduring Classics* (London: Merrill, 2011).

Heaf, Jonathan, ed, Gill A. A., introduction, *Forty Years of Vision and Style 1969–2009* (London: Cutler and Gross, 2009).

Herron, Estelle, 'Reflections: Fitting the Famous', *Optometric Management*, August 2011, https://www.optometricmanagement.com/issues/2011/august-2011/reflections.

Horner, Professor, *On Spectacles: their history and uses* (London: Baillière, Tidal & Cox, 1887).

Horsfall, Nicholas, 'Rome without Spectacles', *Greece & Rome*, 42 (1), April 1995, pp. 49–56, https://www.jstor.org/stable/643072.

Huxley, Aldous, *The Art of Seeing* (London: Chatto & Windus, 1943).

Ilardi, Vincent, 'Eyeglasses and Concave Lenses in Fifteenth-Century Florence and Milan: New Documents', *Renaissance Quarterly*, 29 (3), Autumn 1976, pp. 341–360, https://www.jstor.org/stable/2860275.

Ilardi, Vincent, *Renaissance Vision from Spectacles to Telescopes* (Philadelphia: American Philosophical Society, 2007).

Ings, Simon, *The Eye: a natural history* (London: Bloomsbury, 2007).

Ironside, Virginia, 'How I Live: Lawrence Jenkin, spectacle-maker', *The Idler*, 69, November/December 2019.

Johansen, T. K., *Aristotle on the Sense Organs* (Cambridge: CUP, 2008).

Kennedy, Maev, 'Spectacles provide clue to the secret of Turner's visual style', *Guardian*, 18 November 2003.

Kennedy, Pagan, 'Who Made That Eye Chart?', *The New York Times Magazine*, 24 May 2013.

Kennedy, Pagan, 'Who Made Those Aviator Sunglasses?', *The New York Times Magazine*, 3 August 2012.

Keynes, Milo, 'Why Pepys Stopped Writing his Diary: his dimming eyes and ill-health', *Journal of Medical Biography*, 5(1), February 1997.

King, Henry C., *The History of the Telescope* (London: Charles Griffin & Co Ltd, 1955, New York: Dover 2003).

Knight, Sam, 'The Long Read: The spectacular power of Big Lens', *Guardian*, 10 May 2018.

Law, Frank W., *The Worshipful Company of Spectacle Makers: a history* (London: The Company, 1979).

Leaver, Peter K., *The History of Moorfields Eye Hospital* (London: Royal Society of Medicine, 2004).

Leffler, Christopher T., Schwartz, Stephen G., Wainsztein, Ricardo D., Pflugrath, Adam & Peterson, Eric, 'Ophthalmology in North America: Early Stories (1491–1801)', *Ophthalmology and Eye Diseases*, 9, 2017, 1–51.

Levene, John R., *Clinical Refraction and Visual Science* (London: Butterworths, 1977).

Levy, Steven, 'Google Glass 2.0 Is a Startling Second Act', *Wired*, 10 July 2017, https://www.wired.com/story/google-glass-2-is-here/.

Lingberg, David C. C., *Theories of Vision from Al-kindi to Kepler* (Chicago: University of Chicago Press, 1996).

Lipow, Moss, *Eyewear: A Visual History 1491–Today* (London: Taschen, 2001).

Maldonado, Tomás, 'Taking Eyeglasses Seriously', *Design Issues*, 17 (4), 2001, pp. 32–43, https://www.jstor.org/stable/1511918.

Mann, I. & Pirie, A., *The Science of Seeing* (London: Penguin, 1946).

Margolin, Jane-Claude & Paul Bierent (English translation Tulett, Barry), *Pierre Marly: Spectacles and Spyglasses* (Paris: Editions Hoebeke, 1988).

Marmor, Michael F. & Albert, Daniel M., ed, *Foundations of Ophthalmology: Great Insights that Established the Discipline* (Cham: Springer International Publishing, 2017).

Martin, Benjamin, *An Essay on Visual Glasses, Vulgarly Called Spectacles etc.* (London: printed for the author, 1756).

Mazza, Samuel, *Spectacles*, (San Francisco: Chronicle Books, 1995).

Milburn, John R., *Benjamin Martin: author, instrument-maker and 'Country showman'* (Leiden: Noordhoff, 1976).

Mitchell, Margaret, *History of the British Optical Association 1895–1978* (London: The British Optical Association, 1982).

Murray, Simon & Albrechtsen, Nicky, *Fashion Spectacles, Spectacular Fashion* (London: Thames & Hudson, 2012).

*The Newsletter of the Ophthalmic Antiques International Collectors Club*, various issues from 1982 to 2019, https://oaicc.com/quarterly-journal/.

*The Optician*, London, various issues from 1891 to 2019.

*New Yorker* uncredited, 'Spectacles, Talk of the Town', *New Yorker*, 20 February 1960.

Orr, Hugh, *Illustrated History of Early Antique Spectacles* (Beckenham: Hugh Orr, 1985).

Pearl, Joanna, 'Which? reveals best and worst laser eye surgery companies', *Which*, 7 November 2019, https://www.which.co.uk/news/2019/11/which-reveals-best-and-worst-laser-eye-surgery-companies.

Pedersen, Nate, 'The Mysterious Disappearance – and Strange Reappearance – of Dr. William Horatio Bates', *Mental Floss*, 8 March 2018, http://mentalfloss.com/article/516460/mysterious-disappearance-and-strange-reappearance-dr-william-horatio-bates.

Poulet, W., (translated by Professor C. Blodi), *Atlas on the History of Spectacles* (Bonn: Wayborgh, 1978).

Power, D'arcy, 'Medical History of Mr and Mrs Samuel Pepys', *The Lancet*, 1 June 1895.

Rasmussen, Otto, *Chinese Eyesight and Spectacles* (Tonbridge: Tonbridge Free Press, 1946).

Rosen, Edward, 'The Invention of Eyeglasses', *Journal of the History of Medicine*, 1, 1956, https://www.jstor.org/stable/24619648.

Rosenthal, J. William, *Spectacles and Other Vision Aids: A History and Guide to Collecting* (San Francisco: Norman Publishing, 1996).

Sambrook, Stephen, *The Optical Munitions Industry in Great Britain, 1888–1923* (Abingdon: Routledge, 2015).

Segrave, Kerry, *Vision Aids in America: A Social History of Eyewear and Sight Correction* (Jefferson, North Carolina: McFarland & Co Inc, 2011).

Shilling, Donovan A., *A Photographic History of Bausch & Lomb* (Victor, NY: Pancoast Publishing, 2011).

Smith, Mark, A., *From Sight to Light: The Passage from Ancient to Modern Optics* (Chicago: University of Chicago Press, 2015).

Strauss, D. Pieter, 'Why Did Goethe Hate Glasses? Two

Puzzling Passages in the "Wahlverw and tschaften" and the "Wanderjahre"', *The Journal of English and Germanic Philology* 80 (2), April 1981, pp. 176–187.

Temple, Robert, *The Crystal Sun: Rediscovering a Lost Technology of the Ancient World* (London: Century, 2000).

Trevor-Roper, P. D., *The World Through Blunted Sight: An Inquiry into the Influence of Defective Vision on Art and Character* (London: Allen Lane, 1988).

*Vogue* uncredited, 'Beauty Bulletin: How Not to Miss a Thing ... The Techniques for Doing it Dashingly', *Vogue*, New York, 146 (1), 1 July 1965.

Wade, Nicholas, *A Natural History of Vision* (Cambridge, Mass: MIT Press,1998).

Wells, John Seolberg, *On long, short, and weak Sight and their treatment by the Scientific Use of Spectacles* (London, 1862).

*Wellsworth*, The American Optical Journal, Southbridge Mass, various issues from May 1916 to December 1934.

Willach, Rolf, *The Long Route to the Invention of the Telescope* (Philadelphia: American Philosophical Society, 2008).

Wilson, Graham A., Field, Amanda P., Fullerton, Susannah, 'The Big Brown Eyes of Samuel Pepys', *Archives of Ophthalmology*, 120, July 2002.

Wilson, Graham A., Ravin, James, 'Blinking Sam: The Ocular Afflictions of Dr Samuel Johnson', *Archives of Ophthalmology*, 22, September 2004.

Wilson, Ryan, 'Vision Care, Fashion Frames: Movie stars look great in glasses so why shouldn't you?', *Cincinnati Magazine*, 30 (3), December 1996.

Winkler, Wolk, ed, *A Spectacle of Spectacles: Exhibition Catalogue* (National Museum of Scotland, Edinburgh/Leipzig: Edition Leipzig, 1988).

Wodehouse, P. G., 'In Defense of Astigmatism: A Brief in Favor of Specs, Pince-nez and Goggles', *Vanity Fair*, January 1916, https://archive.vanityfair.com/article/1916/1/in-defense-of-astigmatism.

## Secondary reading

Abel, Richard, ed, *Encyclopedia of Early Cinema* (Abingdon: Routledge, 2004).

Amann, Elizabeth, *Dandyism in the Age of Revolution: The Art of the Cut* (Chicago: The University of Chicago Press, 2015).

Ashley, Benedict M., *The Dominicans* (Eugene, Oregon: Wipf and Stock Publishers, 1990).

Bentley, James, *Restless Bones: The Story of Relics* (London: Constable, 1985).

Bosworth, Patricia, *Jane Fonda: The Private Life of a Public Woman* (Boston: Houghton Mifflin Harcourt, 2011).

Bradley, Simon, *The Railways: Nation, Network and People* (London: Profile Books, 2015).

Braun, Michael, *Love Me Do: The Beatles' Progress* (London: Penguin, 1977).

Bray, Christopher, *Michael Caine: A Class Act* (London: Faber & Faber, 2005).

Brock, William H, *William Crookes (1832–1919) and the Commercialization of Science* (Abingdon: Routledge, 2008).

Bryne Curtis, Emily, *Glass Exchange between Europe and China: 1550–1800* (Farnham: Ashgate, 2009).

Caine, Michael, *What's It All About?* (London: Arrow, 2010).

Carlin, Martha, *Medieval Southwark*, (London: Hambledon Press, 1996).

Carr, Roy, Case, Brian, Dellar, Fred, *The Hip: Hipsters, Jazz and the Beat Generation* (London: Faber & Faber, 1986).

Carreri, Patrizia Maria, Serraino, Diego, 'Longevity of popes and artists between the 13th and the 19th century', *International Journal of Epidemiology*, 34, 2005, pp. 1435–1444.

Chamberlain, E. R., *The Bad Popes* (Stroud: The History Press, 2003).

Clair, Colin, *A History of European Printing* (London: Academic Press, 1976).

Cohen, Jean-Louis (introduction) and Benton, Tim (chapter introductions), *Le Corbusier le Grand* (London: Phaidon, 2014).

Cohodas, Nadine, *Spinning Blues Into Gold: The Chess Brothers and the Legendary Chess Records* (London: Aurum, 2000).

Connolly, Ray, *Being John Lennon* (London: Weidenfeld & Nicolson, 2018).

Coomes, David, *Dorothy L. Sayers: A Careless Rage for Life* (Oxford: Lion, 1992).

Cordle, Celia, *Out of the Hay and into the Hops: Hop Cultivation in Wealden Kent and Hop Marketing in Southwark, 1744–2000* (Hatfield: University of Hertfordshire Press, 2011).

D'Agostino, Annette M., *The Harold Lloyd Encyclopedia* (London: McFarland, 2004).

Dardis, Tom, *Harold Lloyd: The Man on the Clock* (London: Penguin, 1983).

Deighton, Len, *Action Cook Book: Len Deighton's Guide to Eating* (London: Harper Perennial, 2009 edition)

Didier Aaron Inc, catalogue, *Horace Vernet 1789–1863: Incroyables et merveilleuses: 25 Watercolours from the Collection of the Duchesse de Berry* (London: Hazlitt, Gooden & Fox, 1991).

Dringoli, Angelo, *Merger and Acquisition Strategies: How to Create Value* (Cheltenham: Edward Elgar Publishing Ltd, 2016).

Dringoli, Angelo, *Corporate Strategy and Firm Growth: Creating Value for Shareholders* (Cheltenham: Edward Elgar Publishing Ltd, 2011).

Dubois, J. Harry, *Plastics History U.S.A.* (Boston: Cahners Books,1972).

Dundaway, David, *Aldous Huxley Recollected: An Oral History* (New York: Carroll & Graf, 1995).

Eisenstein, Elizabeth L., *The Printing Revolution in Early Modern Europe* (Cambridge: CUP, 2012).

Ellis, Markman, *The Coffee House: A Cultural History* (London: Weidenfeld & Nicolson, 2011).

Epstein, Daniel Mark, *The Ballard of Bob Dylan: A Portrait* (New York: Harper Perennial, 2011).

Flint, Anthony, *Modern Man: The Life of Le Corbusier, Architect of Tomorrow* (Seattle: New Harvest, Amazon Publishing, 2014).

Flowers, Benjamin, *Skyscraper: The Politics and Power of Building*

*New York City in the Twentieth Century* (Philadelphia: University of Pennsylvania Press, 2009).

Freeman, Charles, *Holy Bones, Holy Dust: How Relics Shaped the History of Medieval Europe* (New Haven, Connecticut: Yale University Press, 2011).

Fullerton, John & Söderbergh Widding, Astrid, *Moving Images from Edison to the Webcam* (Sydney: John Libbey and Company Publishers, 2000).

Giles, George Henry, *The Ophthalmic Services under the National Health Service Acts, 1946–1952* (London: Hammond, Hammond & Co, 1953).

Godard, Simon, *Mozipedia: The Encyclopedia of Morrissey and the Smiths* (London: Ebury, 2012).

Goodwin, George, *Benjamin Franklin in London: the British life of America's Founding Father* (London: Weidenfeld & Nicolson, 2016).

Gordon, Ian, *The Persistence of an American Icon: Superman* (New Brunswick: Rutgers University Press 2017).

Gordon, Michael R., *Murder Files from Scotland Yard and the Black Museum* (Jefferson, North Carolina: Exposit/McFarland & Co Inc, 2018).

Green, Matthew Dr, 'The surprising history of London's fascinating (but forgotten) coffeehouses', *Daily Telegraph*, 6 March 2017.

Gregorin, Christina, Heyl, Norbert, Scarabello, Giovanni, *Venice Master Artisans* (Ponzano/Treviso: Grafiche Vianello, 2005).

Guiles, Fred Lawrence, *Norma Jean: The Life of Marilyn Monroe* (London: W. H. Allen, 1969).

Hart, Anne, *Agatha Christie's Miss Marple: The Life and Times of Miss Jane Marple* (London: HarperCollins, 2014 edition).

Hayes, R. M., *3-D Movies: A History and Filmography of Stereoscopic Cinema* (Jefferson, North Carolina: McFarland & Co Inc, 1999 edition).

Hiney, Tom, *Raymond Chandler: A Biography* (London: Vintage 1998).

Hutchinson, Robert, *The Last Days of Henry VIII: Conspiracy,*

*Treason and Heresy at the Court of the Dying Tyrant* (London: Orion, 2005).

John, Elton, *Me: Elton John* (London: Pan Macmillan, 2019).

Kercher, Stephen E., *Revel with a Cause: Liberal Satire in Post-War America* (Chicago: University of Chicago Press, 2006).

Larman, Alexander, *Blazing Star: The Life and Times of John Wilmot, Earl of Rochester* (London: Head of Zeus, 2014).

Leaming, Barbara, *Marilyn Monroe: A Biography* (New York: Crown Publishing, 2000).

Le Corbusier (introduction by Cohen, Jean-Louis; translated by Goodman, John), *Towards an Architecture* (London: Frances Lincoln, 2008).

Lehmer, Larry, *The Day the Music Died: The Last Tour of Buddy Holly, the Big Bopper and Ritchie Valens* (London: Prentice Hall International, 1997).

Leland, John, *Hip, the history* (New York: Ecco, 2004).

Lewis, Roger, *The Life and Death of Peter Sellers* (London: Arrow, 1995).

Lindroth, Linda & Tornello, Deborah Newell, *Virtual Vintage: The Insider's Guide to Buying and Selling Fashion Online* (New York: Random House, 2002).

Lloyd, Harold, 'written in collaboration with', Stout, Wesley W., *An American Comedy* (London: Constable, 1971).

MacAdams, Lewis, *Birth of the Cool: Beat, Bebop, and the American avant-garde* (London: Free Press, 2001).

Man, John, *The Gutenberg Revolution: The Story of a Genius and an Invention that Changed the World* (London: Review, 2002).

Marcello, Patricia Cronin, *Gloria Steinem: A Biography* (Westport, Connecticut: Greenwood Press, 2004).

Mathieson, Kenny, *Giant Steps: Bebop and the Creators of Modern Jazz 1945–65* (Edinburgh: Payback Press, 1999).

McCray, W. Patrick, *Glassmaking in Renaissance Venice: The Fragile Craft* (Farnham: Ashgate, 1999).

Meade, Marion, *Dorothy Parker: What Fresh Hell is This?* (London: Heinemann, 1988).

Miles, Barry, ed, *John Lennon in His Own Words* (London: Omnibus Press, 1980).

Monroe, Marilyn with Hecht, Ben, *My Story* (Lanham, Maryland: First Taylor Trade Publishing, 2007).

Mouskouri Nana, with Duroy, Lionel; translated by Leggatt, Jeremy, *Memoirs* (London: Weidenfeld & Nicolson, 2007).

Murray, Nicholas, *Aldous Huxley: An English Intellectual* (London: Little, Brown, 2002).

Nachman, Gerald, *Seriously Funny: The Rebel Comedians of the 1950s and 1960s* (New York: Pantheon Books, 2003).

Newton, Francis (Hobsbawm, Eric), *The Jazz Scene* (London: Penguin, 1961).

Nicholson, Virginia, *Singled Out: How Two Million Women Survived Without Men After the First World War* (London: Viking, 2007).

Norman, Philip, *Buddy: The Definitive Biography of Buddy Holly* (London: Pan Books, 2009).

Norman, Philip, *John Lennon: The Life* (London: HarperCollins, 2008).

Paglia, Camille, *Sexual Personae: Art and Decadence from Nefertiti to Emily Dickinson* (New Haven, Connecticut: Yale University Press, 1990).

Pepys, Samuel, ed Latham, Robert & Matthews, William, *The Diary of Samuel Pepys Vol 1–9* (London: HarperCollins, 1995).

Perry, David M., *Sacred Plunder: Venice and the Aftermath of the Fourth Crusade* (University Park, Pennsylvania: Pennsylvania State University Press, 2015).

Pine, B. Joseph II, & Gilmore, James H., *The Experience Economy: Competing for Customer Time, Attention and Money* (Boston: Harvard Business Review Press, 2019).

Piper, Leonard, *Murder by Gaslight* (London: Michael O'Mara, 1991).

Rees, Fran, *Gutenberg: Inventor of the Printing Press* (Minneapolis: Compass Point Books, 2006).

Robinson, James, *Finer Than Gold: Saints and Relics in the Middle Ages* (London: British Museum Press, 2011).

Sanders, Dennis & Lovallo, Len, *The Agatha Christie Companion: The Complete Guide to Agatha Christie's Life and Work* (London: W. H. Allen, 1985).

Siegel, Jerry, Johns, Geoff, Shuster, Joe and various, *Superman: A Celebration of 75 Years* (Burbank: DC Comics, 2013).

Smiles, Sam, 'Turner's Last Works and his critics' in Amigoni, David & McMullan, Gordon, ed, *Creativity in Later Life: Beyond Late Style* (Abingdon: Routledge, 2018).

Starkey, David, ed, *The Inventory of King Henry VIII* (London: Harvey Miller for the Society of Antiquaries of London, 1998).

Steinberg, Avi, 'Checking Out,' *Paris Review*, 26 December 2012, https://www.theparisreview.org/blog/2012/12/26/checking-out/.

Steinem, Gloria, *Revolution from Within: A Book of Self-Esteem* (New York: Little, Brown, 1992).

Strathern, Paul, *The Medici: Godfathers of the Renaissance* (London: Jonathan Cape, 2003).

Stross, Randall E., *The Wizard of Menlo Park: How Thomas Alva Edison Invented the Modern World* (New York: Three Rivers Press/Crown Publishing, 2007).

Thomson, David, *Bette Davis* (London: Penguin, 2009).

Thomson, David, *Television: A Biography* (London: Thames & Hudson, 2016).

Vaughan, Herbert M., *The Medici Popes: Leo X and Clement VII* (London: Methuen, 1908).

Vogel, Michelle, *Marilyn Monroe: Her Films, Her Life* (Jefferson, North Carolina: McFarland & Co Inc, 2014).

Walker, Michael, *Hitchcock's Motifs* (Amsterdam: Amsterdam University Press, 2005).

Walsh Larry, ed, *Keith Haring: Haring-ism* (Princeton: Princeton University Press, 2020).

White, George R, *Living Legend: Bo Diddley* (Chessington: Castle Communications, 1995).

Williams, Tom, *A Mysterious Something in the Light: The Life of Raymond Chandler* (London: Aurum, 2012).

Wesley Wishart, Alfred, *A Short History of Monks and Monasteries* (Trenton: Albert Brandt Publisher, 1900).

Wilson, Andrew, *Beautiful Shadow: A Life of Patricia Highsmith* (London: Bloomsbury, 2003).

## Novels, stories, memoirs and verse

Bloch, Robert, 'The Cheaters', *Pleasant Dreams: Nightmares* (London: Ronald Whiting & Wheaton, 1967).

Calvino, Italo, 'The Adventure of a Near-Sighted Man', *Difficult Loves: Smog – A Plunge into Real Estate* (London: Vintage, 1999).

Chandler, Raymond, *The Little Sister* (London: Penguin, 1949).

Chandler, Raymond, *The Raymond Chandler Omnibus: Four Famous Classics (The Big Sleep, Farewell, My Lovely, The High Window, The Lady in the Lake)* (New York: Alfred A. Knopf, 1964).

Christie, Agatha, *An Autobiography* (London: Fontana, 1978).

Christie, Agatha, *A Caribbean Mystery* (London: Collins, 1964).

Christie, Agatha, *At Bertram's Hotel* (London: Collins, 1965).

Christie, Agatha, *Murder at the Vicarage* (London: W. Collins and Son, 1930).

Christie, Agatha, *Miss Marple and Mystery: The Complete Short Stories* (London: HarperCollins, 2011).

Christie, Agatha, *The Mirror Crack'd From Side to Side* (London: Collins, 1962).

Deighton, Len, *The Ipcress File* (London: Hodder & Stoughton, 1962).

Doyle, Arthur Conan, 'The Adventure of the Golden Pince-Nez', *The Return of Sherlock Holmes*, (London: Penguin, 2011 edition).

Eco, Umberto, *The Name of the Rose* (translated from the Italian by William Weaver) (London: Secker & Warburg, 1980).

Ellis, Bret Easton, *American Psycho* (London: Picador 40th Anniversary Edition 2012, 1991)

Fitzgerald, F. Scott, *This Side of Paradise* (London: Penguin, 1974 edition).

Fitzhugh, Louise, *Harriet the spy*, (New York: Harper & Row, 1966, c1964).

Hegley, John, *Glad to Wear Glasses* (London: Deutsch, 1990).

Highsmith, Patricia, *Strangers on a Train* (London: Vintage, 1999 edition)

Holtby, Winifred, *Poor Caroline* (London: Virago, 1985 edition).

Huxley, Aldous, *Antic Hay* (London: Flamingo, 1994 edition).

Knausgaard Ove, Karl, *The End: My Struggle Book Six* (London: Harvill Secker, 2018).

Lessing, Doris, *The Memoirs of a Survivor* (London: Picador, 1981 edition).

Mayor, Flora Macdonald, *The Rector's Daughter* (London: Virago, 1987 edition).

Parker, Dorothy, *The Collected Dorothy Parker* (London: Penguin, 2001 edition).

Prouty, Higgins Olive, *Now, Voyager* (London: Hodder & Stoughton, 1942).

Sayers, Dorothy L. (introduction by Walter, Harriet Dame), *Gaudy Night* (London: Hodder, 2009 edition).

Sayers, Dorothy L., *Unnatural Death* (London: Ernest Benn, 1927).

Sayers, Dorothy L, *Whose Body?* (London: T. Fisher Unwin, 1923).

Shakespeare, William, *As You Like It* (Oxford: OUP, 2008 edition).

Viorst, Judith, 'New York Visit 1969', *New York* magazine (7 April 1969).

Warner, Sylvia Townsend, *Lolly Willowes: or The Loving Huntsman* (London: Virago, 2012 edition).

Warner, Sylvia Townsend, *Scenes of Childhood* (London: Faber & Faber, 2011).

Warner, Sylvia Townsend, 'The Foregone Conclusion', *Selected Stories* (London: Virago, 2011).

# Picture Credits

## Prelims

Welby Fine Frames Ltd of Tunbridge Wells, trade advertisement 1970. Archives of British Optical Association Museum at the College of Optometrists.

## Introduction

NHS glasses range, NHS leaflet April 1985. Archives of British Optical Association Museum at the College of Optometrists.

## Chapter 1

Woodcut illustration from Sebastian Brant's *Das Narrenschiff* (The Ship of Fools) Basel: Johann Bergmann de Olpe, 11 Feb. (Fastnacht) 1494. Library of Congress LC-USZ62-110317.

Conspicilla Inuenta conspicilla sunt, quæ luminum, obscuriores detegunt caligines, engraving, Phis Galle ca 1600. Library of Congress LC-DIG-ppmsca-38361.

## Chapter 2

Portrait of Fernando Niño de Guevara, El Greco 1600. The Metropolitan Museum of Art, New York.

## Chapter 4

Edward Scarlett trade card, circa 1728–30. Archives of British Optical Association Museum at the College of Optometrists.

Benjamin Martin's Visual Glasses, 1756–8. Archives of British Optical Association Museum at the College of Optometrists.

Quizzing glass. Archives of British Optical Association Museum at the College of Optometrists.

## Chapter 5

Railway glasses, illustration by Robert H. F. Rippon, from Browning, John, *How to Use our Eyes, and How to Preserve Them by the Aid of Spectacles* (London: Chatto & Windus, 1883 and 1892 editions). Author's collection.

Pince-nez, illustration by Robert H. F. Rippon from Browning, John, *How to Use our Eyes, and How to Preserve Them by the Aid of Spectacles* (London: Chatto & Windus, 1883 and 1892 editions). Author's collection.

## Chapter 6

Bateman's Opticians, East Street, Brighton. Archives of British Optical Association Museum at the College of Optometrists.

Ophthalmoscope in action, illustration from Gritti, Rocco, *Dell'ottalmoscopa e delle malattie end-oculari per esso riconoscibili.* Patronation, Milan 1862. Archives of British Optical Association Museum at the College of Optometrists.

## Chapter 7

Harold Lloyd, movie magazine clipping 1920. Author's collection.

Fits U Windsor illustration, cover of *Wellsworth* magazine, November 1919. Archives of British Optical Association Museum at the College of Optometrists.

## Chapter 8

Portrait of Sylvia Townsend Warner by Harold Coster, half-plate film negative, 1934. © National Portrait Gallery, London.

Cat's eye style of glasses, Stanley Unger for Unger & Adcock, early 1950s, 'the 48/K with additional ear motif "Chinese Flame"'. Archives of British Optical Association Museum at the College of Optometrists.

## Chapter 9

Dizzy Gillespie portrait by Carl Van Vechten. Library of Congress, LC-USZ62-92016.

Buddy Holly, That 'Tex-Mex Sound', artist uncredited, Coral Mono FEP 2006/Vogue Records Ltd, UK 1964. Author's collection.

## Chapter 10

*The Ipcress File*, Panther Crimeband edition, 1966, cover art uncredited. Author's collection.

## Chapter 11

John Lennon and Yoko Ono. Blank Archives/Getty Images.

## Chapter 12

Gloria Steinem at news conference, Women's Action Alliance, photographer unknown. Library of Congress, LC-DIG-ppmsc-03684.

Couture Eyewear US advert, 1977. Archives of British Optical Association Museum at the College of Optometrists.

Getty Artist Keith Haring is photographed for the *Soho News* in May 1981, in New York. Photo by © Robin Holland/CORBIS OUTLINE/Corbis via Getty Images.

Far Too Stylish to Take Off, optician's board on Stoke Newington Church Street, 2020. Author's collection.

## Chapter 13

Handmade artificial eyes. Photograph courtesy of John Dixon Salt, with thanks for granting permission for its use here.

Cazals window display, opticians Kingsland Road, Dalston, 2020. Author's collection.

Jarvis Cocker, cover star of *The Happy Reader* magazine. © *The Happy Reader* with thanks to Seb Emina and Ralitsa Chorbadzhiyska for granting permission for its use here.

# Index

Page numbers in *italic* refer to images.